CLINICS IN DEVELOPMENTAL MEDICINE NO. 95/96

SEQUELAE OF LOW BIRTHWEIGHT: THE VANCOUVER STUDY

Clinics in Developmental Medicine NO. 95/96

SEQUELAE OF LOW BIRTHWEIGHT: THE VANCOUVER STUDY

Edited by:
HENRY G. DUNN

1986
Mac Keith Press
OXFORD: Blackwell Scientific Publications Ltd.
PHILADELPHIA: J. B. Lippincott Co.

First published 1986

British Library Cataloguing in Publication Data

Dunn, Henry
Sequelae of low birthweight: the Vancouver study.
1. Birth weight, Low — Complications and sequelae
I. Title
612.6 RJ281

ISBN (UK) 0-632-01468-7
(USA) 0-397-48002-4

Printed in Great Britain at The Lavenham Press Ltd., Lavenham, Suffolk

The Mac Keith Press is supported by **The Spastics Society,** London, England

Contents

FOREWORD — page ix
Pamela A. Davies

1. NEUROLOGICAL, PSYCHOLOGICAL AND OPHTHALMOLOGICAL SEQUELAE OF LOW BIRTHWEIGHT — 1
Henry G. Dunn

2. DESCRIPTION OF PRESENT STUDY — 23
Henry G. Dunn and Ann-Marie Robertson

3. PHYSICAL GROWTH — 35
Henry G. Dunn, Cara-Joy Hughes and Michael Schulzer

4. EVOLUTION OF DEVELOPMENTAL AND PSYCHOLOGICAL TEST SCORES — 54
Annetta K. McBurney and Linda C. Eaves

5. CLINICAL OUTCOME: NEUROLOGICAL SEQUELAE AND THEIR EVOLUTION — 68
Henry G. Dunn, Ann-Marie Robertson and John U. Crichton

6. MINIMAL BRAIN DYSFUNCTIONS — 97
Henry G. Dunn, Helena H. Ho and Michael Schulzer

7. STATISTICAL ANALYSIS OF MILD BRAIN DYSFUNCTIONS — 114
Martin L. Puterman and Henry G. Dunn

8. OPHTHALMIC DISORDERS — 127
Andrew Q. McCormick, Enid M. Tredger, Henry G. Dunn and Ruth V. E. Grunau

9. HEARING IMPAIRMENT AND ASSOCIATED FACTORS — 147
Bryan R. Clarke, Robert F. Conry and Henry G. Dunn

ADDENDUM: VESTIBULAR FUNCTION — 163
R. Patrick Gannon

10. COMMUNICATION SKILLS — 168
Dorothy M. Washington, Annetta K. McBurney and Ruth V. E. Grunau

11. EDUCATIONAL ACHIEVEMENT 179
Ruth V. E. Grunau

12. ENVIRONMENTAL FACTORS AND NEUROLOGICAL AND INTELLECTUAL FUNCTIONING IN RELATION TO SOCIAL GROWTH 205
Annetta K. McBurney and Ruth V. E. Grunau

13. PROSPECTIVE STUDY OF ELECTROENCEPHALOGRAMS 219
Henry G. Dunn, Norman L. Auckland and Morton D. Low

14. NEUROLOGICAL CORRELATIONS AND PREDICTIONS 238
Henry G. Dunn, Ann-Marie Robertson and Michael Schulzer

15. EVOLUTION OF MINIMAL BRAIN DYSFUNCTIONS TO THE AGE OF 12 TO 15 YEARS 249
Henry G. Dunn, Helena H. Ho, John U. Crichton, Ann-Marie Robertson, Annetta K. McBurney, Ruth V. E. Grunau and P. Susan Penfold

REFERENCES 273

INDEX 300

The following abbreviations and definitions are used throughout this book:

ADD	Attention deficit disorder
AGA	Appropriate weight for gestational age
EEG	Electroencephalogram
FBW	Full birthweight
GQ	General quotient (Griffiths)
LGA	Large for gestational age
LBW	Low birthweight (≤2500g)
MBD	Minimal brain dysfunction
Preterm	Less than 37 completed weeks gestation
Post-term	42 weeks or more gestation
RDS	Respiratory distress syndrome
ROP	Retinopathy of prematurity
SFD	'Small for dates' (but preferred term is SGA — see below)
SGA	Small (*i.e.* light) for gestational age
Term	From 37 to less than 42 completed weeks gestation
VLBW	Very low birthweight (≤1500g)

Contributors

NORMAN L. AUCKLAND	Formerly Director, EEG Laboratory, Vancouver General Hospital; Clinical Assistant Professor, Division of Neurology, Department of Medicine, University of British Columbia.
BRYAN R. CLARKE	Professor and Head, Department of Educational Psychology and Special Education, University of British Columbia.
ROBERT F. CONRY	Associate Professor, Department of Educational Psychology and Special Education, University of British Columbia.
JOHN U. CRICHTON	Professor and Head, Division of Neurology, Department of Paediatrics, University of British Columbia.
HENRY G. DUNN	Professor Emeritus and former Head, Division of Neurology, Department of Paediatrics, University of British Columbia.
LINDA C. EAVES	Psychologist, British Columbia's Children's Hospital, Vancouver; Research Associate and Psychologist, Division of Neurology, Department of Paediatrics, University of British Columbia.
R. PATRICK GANNON	Formerly Director, Audiology–Vestibular Unit, Vancouver General Hospital; Associate Professor, Division of Otolaryngology, Department of Surgery, University of British Columbia.
RUTH V. E. GRUNAU	Psychologist, British Columbia's Children's Hospital, Vancouver; Clinical Instructor, Department of Psychology, University of British Columbia.

HELENA H. HO	Clinical Assistant Professor, Department of Paediatrics, University of British Columbia.
CARA-JOY HUGHES	Formerly Lecturer, Department of Computer Science, University of British Columbia.
MORTON D. LOW	Director, Department of Diagnostic Neurophysiology, Vancouver General Hospital; Professor, Division of Neurology, Department of Medicine, University of British Columbia.
ANNETTA K. McBURNEY	Formerly Assistant Professor, Department of Psychology; Assistant Professor, Division of Neurology, Department of Paediatrics, University of British Columbia.
ANDREW Q. McCORMICK	Associate Professor, Department of Ophthalmology, University of British Columbia.
P. SUSAN PENFOLD	Associate Professor, Division of Child Psychiatry, Department of Psychiatry, University of British Columbia.
MARTIN L. PUTERMAN	Associate Professor, Faculty of Commerce and Business Administration, University of British Columbia.
ANN-MARIE ROBERTSON	Research Associate, Division of Neurology, Department of Paediatrics, University of British Columbia.
MICHAEL SCHULZER	Associate Professor, Departments of Statistics and Medicine, University of British Columbia.
ENID M. TREDGER	Research Associate, Department of Paediatrics, University of British Columbia.
DOROTHY M. WASHINGTON	Assistant Professor Emerita, Faculty of Education, University of British Columbia.

Foreword

Low birthweight represents one of the most important topics of research for those concerned with the fetus and newborn infant. Impaired fetal growth, the prevention or postponement of preterm birth, and the increased morbidity and mortality of those born too soon and too small are all among the early problems faced. But the challenge does not stop there. The later progress of the survivors has always been of continuing concern, as well as of considerable importance to individual children, to their families, and ultimately to society.

There have been innumerable accounts of various aspects of this later outcome from different parts of the world, but these studies have had two problems. They study populations where varying and complex neonatal intervention occurred, and secondly most studies have been concerned with the very young. Professor Dunn and his colleagues in Vancouver are among the very few to have overcome these limitations. The children they followed were born shortly before neonatal intensive care started, and the children have been followed through to school age. While this cannot be considered a total population study, and the authors were unable to follow one-fifth of their original low-birthweight group and nearly one-third of the controls, they have accomplished a most valuable and classic prospective survey. Neurological examination has been very detailed. The scope of the children's attainments considered, and the range of tests administered, are unusually wide. Ophthalmic disorders, hearing and vestibular impairment have rarely been sought so thoroughly. All the results have been analysed with meticulous care. A large literature has been carefully reviewed. Minimal brain dysfunction was the most common sequel at 6½ years; and the discussion of this 'diffuse and heterogeneous syndrome', and of the attention deficit disorder, are particularly helpful. A sub-sample of affected children and an equal number of controls were re-examined at 12 to 15 years, and the importance of socio-economic status, parental concern and the quality of the remedial management were among the variables most important for progress.

There has been a steady increase in survival of low-birthweight infants, especially at the lowest gestations, since the birth of the Vancouver cohort. The use of brain-imaging techniques in the early weeks of life is allowing fresh insight into the pathogenesis of intracranial lesions. It is the fervent hope of obstetricians and neonatologists that uniform application of knowledge gained in the last two decades or so may lead eventually to an irreducible minimum of adverse sequelae among survivors. But this study emphasises that much more will be needed for a successful outcome than excellent perinatal care. Just as important, and needing far more effort, is surveillance for neurodevelopmental delay and school learning difficulties, adequate and early help for any remediable defects detected, and above all an improvement in the environment in which the children grow up. If these are not forthcoming, the improved survival will be a hollow victory. The data set out here in such detail will allow future research workers in this field to determine how far these goals are being achieved.

PAMELA A. DAVIES
London, 1986

ACKNOWLEDGEMENTS

This follow-up study of children of low birthweight extended over more than 20 years and was aided by many friends and staff members. It was initiated by Dr. J. F. McCreary, when he was Head of the Department of Paediatrics, University of British Columbia, and supported by his successors Dr. Bruce D. Graham, Dr. Sydney Israels and Dr. Robert H. Hill. Funding was supplied by National Health Grants 609-7-115 and 610-1030-29 from Health and Welfare Canada, and by grants from the Vancouver Foundation and from Mr. and Mrs. P. A. Woodward's Foundation. We are grateful for the advice given by Dr. Ruth Griffiths in England and by staff of the Collaborative Perinatal Project in the United States, particularly the late Dr. Richmond S. Paine, Dr. John A. Churchill, Dr. Joseph S. Drage and Dr. Karin B. Nelson. At the University of British Columbia we are particularly indebted to Mr. Alvin G. Fowler and Mr. J. H. Bjerring at the Computer Centre, and to the Department of Biomedical Illustration for assistance with the Figures in this monograph. In the Division of Vital Statistics of the Provincial Government we were assisted by Mr. G. H. D. Renwick and Mr. J. Rowe. At the Vancouver School Board we received particular help from Dr. Norman Ellis. The Research Associates, computer analysts, nurse co-ordinators, secretaries and students who worked in the Study are too numerous to be named individually, but special mention should be made of Dr. Margaret R. Cox, who helped greatly as Research Associate to get the whole project launched in its early years. Finally, our thanks are due to Dr. Pamela Davies and to the staff of the Mac Keith Press in London, particularly Dr. Martin Bax and Mr. Bernard Hayes, for their valuable assistance in editing this Clinic.

1
Neurological, Psychological and Ophthalmological Sequelae of Low Birthweight

Henry G. Dunn

> *Prematurity is the most frequently recurring factor now involved in infant death and morbidity. As such it has become the largest single problem in contemporary pediatrics and obstetrics, as well as one of the major public-health problems of the present time. . .*
> *. . .Methods for studying the interaction of multiple events in the incidence of disease are still rudimentary. The problem of prematurity, therefore, is also presented as a model for the study of interacting multiple variables as they affect the occurrence of a disease state.* (Abramowicz and Kass 1966)

In the so-called developed countries about 4 to 8 per cent of all children are born weighing 2500g or less, and according to the definition established by the World Health Assembly in 1948 these infants were termed immature. It was further stated that a liveborn infant with a period of gestation less than 37 weeks, or specified as 'premature', may be considered as the equivalent of an immature infant (World Health Organization 1948-49). Many studies have endeavoured to assess the effects of 'prematurity' on mortality and morbidity among the affected children. The mortality rate has diminished with modern management. However, in the province of British Columbia, Canada, between 1958 and 1966 the first-year mortality was still about 18 per cent for infants with birthweights of 2500g or less, and about 40 per cent for those weighing 2000g or less (see Chapter 2, Tables 2-I and II). Morbidity also remained high, largely because of the immaturity of many physiological functions and poor resistance to infection.

With improved understanding of neonatal physiology, it has become possible to compensate for some of the effects of immaturity by careful monitoring and correction of defects in respiration, caloric intake, fluid and electrolyte balance, temperature control and other aspects. It has also been demonstrated that such careful correction would improve survival and prevent some brain damage.

However, in addition to immaturity, infants of low birthweight have other handicaps. First, there is frequently a background of low socio-economic status and 'single parents', an undue proportion of very young or elderly mothers, a tendency to be firstborn, to be the younger children in big families or to be one of multiple births. These factors lead to an increased risk of poor genetic endowment, non-stimulating environment, faulty diet and inadequate medical care. Second, such babies have an increased incidence of congenital malformations (Hess *et al.*

1934, Yerushalmy *et al.* 1965). Third, they are liable to be born following complications of pregnancy and labour which may lead to brain damage by anoxia or haemorrhage. And fourth, they have special risks of a disturbed mother-child relationship because of the prolonged early separation and lack of 'bonding' (Klaus *et al.* 1972, Leifer *et al.* 1972), lack of breast-feeding and the tendency for the mother to be inexperienced and to have anxious or ambivalent feelings about her tiny, unattractive offspring, who may succumb or survive in a damaged condition (Lynch 1975).

Follow-up studies

Long-term follow-up investigations of the effects of low birthweight were first organized by such pioneers as Ylppö (1919) in Europe, and Capper (1928) and Hess and co-workers (1934) in the United States. Benton (1940) reviewed these early studies of the physical and mental development of 'prematures' and concluded that most investigations indicated a higher incidence of serious intellectual impairment and of behavioural disturbance among children who had been born prematurely. However, the detailed findings varied considerably, and Benton pointed out four reasons why they did so: the use of 'clinical impression' instead of standardized tests, the lack of attention to socio-economic factors, the use of inadequate numbers and unsatisfactory control children, and biased selection of samples.

Since then, follow-up studies have become more sophisticated, and it is now realized that certain rules should be observed, namely:

(1) The children should be examined and documented by a standardized technique. Diagnostic labels should be as accurate as possible. It is realized that the patients may have multiple disabilities (*e.g.* spastic diplegia and retinopathy of prematurity), but these should be analyzed individually.

(2) The infants should be unselected, preferably from a specified area or hospital. Socio-economic factors and other variables, which are often interdependent, must be taken into consideration. For instance, in a British study of the height of children at seven years it was noted that sex, social class, parity, mother's height, birthweight, length of gestation, maternal smoking during pregnancy and maternal age each had a partial effect (Goldstein 1971). Ethnic origin may be an added factor.

(3) The numbers of children to be followed must be large enough for meaningful statistical analysis. If one wishes to compare the fate of the larger children of low birthweight with that of smaller ones, one has to make sure of having an adequate number of the latter.

(4) It is useful to study a control group of mature children concurrently. This has not always been considered necessary, *e.g.* in investigations concerning children of very low birthweight (McDonald 1962, Rossier 1962, Lubchenco *et al.* 1963*b*), but it becomes important when minor deviations from normal are analyzed. If siblings are used as controls, the genetic and social factors usually are comparable (within limits), but often the early development of older siblings is poorly documented, and maternal age and parity will differ. Random samples of children born in the same

hospital serving as controls tend to have a higher social status and a lower incidence of twins.

(5) Prospective investigations are considered better than retrospective ones, since the latter tend to begin with a selected sample, *e.g.* a clinic population, and often are hampered by poor documentation of the child's birth and early development. However, prospective studies often have a high 'attrition rate', since present Western populations are highly mobile and it may be hard to retain the parents' co-operation for a period of years. This introduces a possible bias, since the children with co-operative, intelligent parents or with disabilities requiring treatment are more likely to be retained in the study.

(6) Ideally, the persons evaluating the children's progress should not know the birth data and previous development, but such 'blind' techniques of assessment can be hard to arrange.

(7) To study major neurological and ophthalmological sequelae, children should be followed to the age of at least four years. When subsequent intelligence and 'minimal brain dysfunctions' (including learning disabilities) are to be explored and 'global' intelligence tests (Stanford-Binet, Wechsler) are to be applied, follow-up should extend to at least six to seven years.

Details of the desirable design and reporting of such studies have been discussed by Kiely and Paneth (1981) and Davies (1984), and suitable assessment techniques by Parmelee *et al.* (1976). A number of careful surveys of this type have been made in the last 25 years, particularly by Knobloch and Pasamanick and their associates (1956, 1960), Douglas (1956, 1960), Drillien (1961*a*, 1964), McDonald (1962, 1967) and Lubchenco and colleagues (1963*b*, 1972*a*). The results were reviewed by Wiener (1962, 1970), Drillien (1964), Harper and Wiener (1965), Abramowicz and Kass (1966) and Caputo and Mandell (1970). They need not be repeated in detail here, but some general conclusions should be noted:

(1) On the whole, the larger children of low birthweight do not show any marked impairment of mental ability compared with maturely born children from a similar environment. However, mild learning-problems are more frequent in the total 'premature' group. Thus, in British studies Douglas (1956, 1960) showed that at 11 years only 9.7 per cent of ex-premature children gained entry into grammar schools, compared to 22 per cent of controls; May (1958) noted that ex-premature boys at seven to eight years had significantly lower scores than controls in arithmetic tests; and Drillien (1969) found that even children with birthweights between 2001 and 2500g were at some disadvantage in normal school compared to those of full birthweight.

(2) Below the birthweight of about 2000g there is an increasing incidence of mental retardation and neurological defect as the birthweight decreases, and this cannot be accounted for solely by a poorer environment. Both birthweight and social status influence intellectual development (Knobloch and Pasamanick 1960, Drillien 1964).

(3) Knobloch and associates (1956, 1960) established the important concept of a 'continuum of reproductive casualty' among premature infants, which extends from death through severe neurological impairment (cerebral palsy, epilepsy, mental

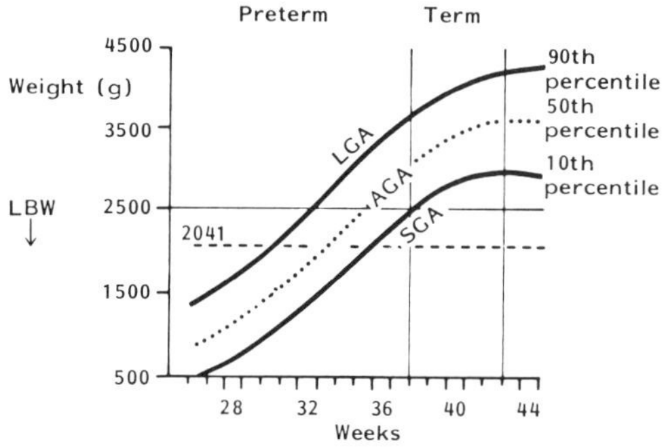

Fig. 1-1. Classification of newborn infants by birthweight and gestation (after Babson *et al.* 1970). Note that infants of low birthweight (LBW; ≤ 2500g) may be born preterm with appropriate gestational age (AGA) or at term and small for their gestational age (SGA). There is also an overlap group of SGA infants born preterm. In the LBW follow-up project in Vancouver, most of the study infants weighed ≤2041g (≤ 4½lbs). LGA = large for gestational age. Sex differences are omitted for the sake of clarity.

retardation) to behaviour disorders and reading disabilities. Other authors confirmed the frequent behaviour problems among these children, which were not explained by unfavourable social surroundings (Uddenberg 1955, Prechtl and Dijkstra 1960, Drillien 1964). Drillien (1964) postulated that 'minimal cerebral damage' might cause lowered resistance to environmental stress. She also noted that prematurely born children were more likely to be working below their intellectual capacity in school than maturely born children of similar intelligence and backgrounds.

(4) In the lower birthweight groups the incidence of serious sequelae used to be alarmingly high. McDonald (1962), in a large survey, found that 22.6 per cent of children with birthweights below 1800g had neurological or ophthalmological disorders at six to eight years. Knobloch and Pasamanick (1959) demonstrated that about half of all children with birthweights below 1500g had such sequelae, and Lubchenco and colleagues (1963*b*) found that two-thirds of children in this weight-group showed some visual or neurological defect at 10 years. Among 49 children with birthweights below 1360g, Drillien (1961*b*) found half to be ineducable in normal school because of physical or mental handicap, or both, and another quarter were dull children requiring remedial education within the normal school. Other studies had less discouraging results, even among children of very low birthweight (Dann *et al.* 1958, 1964; Rossier 1962), but in at least one of these studies this could be attributed partly to a high socio-economic level (Dann *et al.* 1964).

Categories of low-birthweight infants

Meanwhile it was evident that about one-third of infants in the developed countries with birthweights ≤2500g were actually born at term (at or after 37 completed weeks) when maternal health and medical care were good. The proportion was higher in an unfavourable socio-economic environment. Accordingly, in 1961 the Expert Committee on Maternal and Child Health, established by the World Health Organization, recommended that babies weighing ≤2500g should no longer all be referred to as 'premature' and that the concept of 'prematurity' in the definition should give way to that of 'low birthweight' (LBW). Lubchenco *et al.* (1963*a*) and others (Usher and McLean 1969, Babson *et al.* 1970) then devised intra-uterine growth curves from liveborn male and female birthweight data in relation to gestational age (after 24 weeks). 'Term' is now defined as from 37 completed weeks to less than 42 completed weeks of gestation (259 to 293 days), as measured from the first day of the last menstrual period (WHO 1977). Infants born before 37 completed weeks of gestation and whose weight lies between the 10th and 90th percentiles on such curves may be termed preterm 'appropriate for gestational age' (AGA). Infants whose weight is at or below the 10th percentile may be called 'small for gestational age' (SGA) (see Fig. 1-1), and have also been referred to as hypotrophic, dysmature or 'small for dates'.

In this way LBW children can be divided into two major categories—those who are born too early but from their weight are assumed to have grown appropriately (preterm AGA), and those born at the right time but who are assumed to be undergrown (term SGA). Infants in both categories may encounter difficulties, but the risks have been shown to be somewhat different (Table 1-I). It should be noted that SGA infants who are born preterm represent an overlapping group (preterm SGA) which is liable to have mixed handicaps.

The preterm AGA infant is exposed to all the well-known hazards of prematurity (Crosse and Hill 1975). The basic physiological functions, such as circulation, respiration, digestion, blood coagulation and temperature control are immature, poorly regulated and vulnerable, with consequent difficulty in adapting to extra-uterine life. Respiratory distress may develop because of immaturity of the lungs and lack of surfactant in the alveoli, and may lead to formation of hyaline membranes and risk of anoxia. The preterm infant is also subject to damage from excessive levels of oxygen in the bloodstream during treatment; this may result in retrolental fibroplasia (Ashton *et al.* 1953, Kinsey 1956, Patz 1957), which may be better termed retinopathy of prematurity (Heath 1950, McCormick 1977, Phelps 1981). It appears to occur particularly in the presence of contributory factors like low gestational age, apnoea and septicaemia (Gunn *et al.* 1980, Merritt *et al.* 1981, Rothberg *et al.* 1981).

The immature brain is soft and fragile. In anoxic-ischaemic encephalopathy, areas of periventricular leukomalacia may be formed, probably owing to failure of perfusion: this is liable to occur particularly in periventricular arterial end-zones, and secondary haemorrhage may ensue (Banker and Larroche 1962, De Reuck *et al.* 1972, Armstrong and Norman 1974). Such lesions probably represent the pathological substrate for cerebral palsy. In infants with birthweights ≤1500g and a gestational age of less than 32 weeks, a haemorrhage starting in the subependymal germinal layer over the head of the caudate nucleus is liable to rupture and to give rise to an intraventricular haemorrhage (IVH) (Larroche 1964, Fedrick and Butler 1970, Leech and Kohnen 1974, Hambleton and Wigglesworth 1976, Pape and Wigglesworth 1979). Infants who survive such IVH may develop post-haemorrhagic hydrocephalus (Larroche 1972, Lorber and Bhat 1974, Korobkin 1975). Bleeding may also occur elsewhere in the cerebral hemispheres, in cerebellum, in brainstem or into the subarachnoid or subdural spaces (Tsiantos *et al.* 1974, Volpe 1977, Norman 1978, Pape and Wigglesworth 1979). The liability to haemorrhage can be

TABLE 1-I
Hazards of low birthweight

	Preterm AGA	*SGA at term*
Congenital malformations	+	++
Transplacental infections	+	++
Intra-uterine hypoxia	+	++
Respiratory difficulties		
Hyaline membrane disease	++	0
Meconium aspiration	+	++
Pulmonary haemorrhage	+	++
Apnoeic attacks	++	+
Metabolic difficulties		
Hypoglycaemia	+	++
Metabolic acidosis	+	++
Hypocalcaemia	+	++
Jaundice, kernicterus	++	+
Alimentary difficulties		
Inability to suck or swallow	++	0
Functional intestinal obstruction, enterocolitis	++	+
Other hazards		
Polycythaemia	0	++
Anaemia	++	0
Cerebral haemorrhage	++	0
Cerebral oedema, neuronal necroses	+	++
Retinopathy of prematurity	++	+
Sensorineural deafness	++	+
Liability to infection	++	+
Difficulty in maintaining body temperature	++	+
Withdrawal syndrome (maternal drug abuse)	+	++
Renal function	Urine concentration reduced	Normal

0 = incidence as in normal term infant; + = more common than in normal term infant; ++ = found mainly in group designated.
Modifed from Robinson (1971).

increased by immaturity or defects of coagulation mechanisms (Gray *et al.* 1968, Chessells and Wigglesworth 1972, Barnard *et al.* 1979, Setzer *et al.* 1982); by hypothermia (Chadd and Gray 1972); by hypoxia, as in hyaline membrane disease (Harrison *et al.* 1968, Wigglesworth *et al.* 1976); and by associated hypotension and reduced cerebral blood-flow (Lou *et al.* 1977, Fujimura *et al.* 1979), with failure of autoregulation (Lou *et al.* 1979, Robinson 1979, Milligan 1980); and also by cerebral overperfusion and fluctuations in blood pressure, as with intravenous fluid overload and with pneumothorax (Hill *et al.* 1982).

Recently the diagnosis of such intracranial haemorrhages has been greatly facilitated by the advent of computerized tomography (CT) and ultrasound studies. At birthweights of ≤1500g the frequency of subependymal haemorrhages (SEH) and IVH has been found to be surprisingly high (Scott *et al.* 1974, Burstein *et al.* 1977). In one series of 46 consecutive VLBW infants, 20 had evidence of IVH and six developed ventricular enlargement on CT scans (Papile *et al.* 1978). In a larger series of 191 infants of less than 35 weeks gestation, 40 per cent were shown to have

SEH or IVH, or both, and among the survivors 22 per cent developed severe progressive hydrocephalus (Ahmann *et al.* 1980). Among VLBW infants requiring assisted ventilation, 21 of 30 (70 per cent) were shown to have intracranial haemorrhage on CT scan (Lee *et al.* 1979). There appears to be a poor correlation between CT-scan and clinical evidence of mild to moderate degrees of intracranial haemorrhage, and many infants make a surprisingly good recovery, even from IVH (Krishnamoorthy *et al.* 1979). The ultrasound technique appears to be at least as sensitive as CT scanning in experienced hands for diagnosing small haemorrhages, and is also useful in follow-up (Pape *et al.* 1979, 1981; London *et al.* 1980; Bejar *et al.* 1980).

Hyperbilirubinaemia also may occur in preterm AGA infants, even without any distinct primary cause such as sepsis or haemolytic disease, and may lead to kernicterus even when serum bilirubin levels are below 20mg per cent (Stern and Denton 1965), particularly in conjunction with anoxia. Kernicterus, in turn, may be the forerunner of choreo-athetoid cerebral palsy and sensorineural hearing-loss. A characteristic form of cerebral palsy—spastic diplegia or paraplegia—is often found among the neurological sequelae of prematurity, and is compatible with normal intelligence.

In contrast to the preterm AGA baby, the SGA infant born at term has more mature physiological processes, particularly as far as the nervous system and renal function are concerned. However, SGA infants may have suffered subacute or chronic anoxia, or malnutrition *in utero*, with consequent growth retardation (Gruenwald 1963). If there has been severe fetal deprivation, brain development may be impaired. These infants are also liable to develop neonatal hypoglycaemia, which may cause brain damage (Cornblath *et al.* 1959, Neligan *et al.* 1963, Haworth and McRae 1965, Cox and Dunn 1967). Further, among SGA infants of whatever gestational age there is a higher incidence of major and minor congenital defects than among the purely immature (Warkany *et al.* 1961, Yerushalmy *et al.* 1965, Scott and Usher 1966, Drillien 1968, Crichton *et al.* 1971). Whereas preterm infants frequently develop anaemia, SGA infants are liable to have increased haematocrit and polycythaemia, with the so-called hyperviscosity syndrome (Kontras 1972, Gross *et al.* 1973, Amit and Camfield 1980, Black *et al.* 1982), in which cerebral perfusion may be impaired and infarcts ensue. Among SGA infants there is a group with intra-uterine infection (*e.g.* rubella) and another in which the mother has taken excessive amounts of alcohol or drugs (medical and non-medical), which may have a lasting effect on the infant (Usher 1970, Miller and Hassanein 1973, Fedrick and Adelstein 1978). Some may be small for genetic reasons or because of 'maternal constraint' of intra-uterine growth (Dawkins 1965, Ounsted 1966, Ounsted and Ounsted 1968, Johnstone and Inglis 1974). It will be evident that SGA infants are a heterogeneous group who can be divided into many aetiological categories (Scott and Usher 1966, Drillien 1970, Usher 1970, Fedrick and Adelstein 1978, Bard 1978).

The brain of these infants is relatively heavy, and its development is consistent with length of gestation rather than birthweight. Autopsies commonly have demonstrated oedema and other changes associated with hypoxic-ischaemic encephalopathy (Volpe 1976), but not the haemorrhages in the germinal matrix encountered in preterm infants. Neuronal necrosis is found particularly in the motor cortex, hippocampus and pontine nuclei, rather than in the central grey-matter, where it may be found in the immature infant. Larroche and Haggai (1967) postulated that such necroses require a certain degree of cellular maturity and would be consistent with greater maturation of the brain of SGA infants. Lesions caused by hypoglycaemia and hypoxia are similar in morphology (Banker 1967, Chase 1973, Norman 1978).

Follow-up studies have shown an increased prevalence of mental retardation and seizures among these children (McDonald 1967, Drillien 1970), and a slight deficit in stature and head-circumference may persist (Sinclair and Coldiron 1969, Babson 1970, Fitzhardinge and Steven 1972*a*, Bjerre 1975*b*, Neligan *et al.* 1976). Girls normally have lower mean birthweights than boys, so it is not surprising that SGA girls are more frequent than SGA boys among LBW infants. In one study in New York City, 4.5 per cent of female and 2.9 per cent of male white infants were born at 37 or more weeks gestation weighing ≤2500g; the corresponding figures for black infants were 6.8 per cent of females and 4.7 per cent of males (Yerushalmy *et al.* 1965). The neonatal mortality rate for the girls of either race was only about half that for the boys, and one may speculate whether this was due, at least partly, to SGA infant girls being closer to their normal state than boys. LBW girls as a group also generally have a lower morbidity rate and fewer neurological sequelae than boys.

From all this it is evident that long-term studies of the physical and mental development of LBW children now have to differentiate between preterm AGA infants and SGA infants, who may be preterm or term and who have grown inadequately *in utero*. It is also clear that in any comparison between these categories the influence of socio-economic status, sex, multiple births and other variables has to be taken into consideration.

Our group of investigators was among the first to study the development of LBW children in that manner (Eaves *et al.* 1970). It was noted that, in general, SGA children, whether preterm or term, obtained higher scores (uncorrected for conceptional age) than preterm AGA children on the Griffiths Mental Development Scale up to the age of 12 months, but slightly lower scores on the Stanford-Binet test at 2½ and four years and on the Wechsler (WISC) Full-scale IQ at 6½ years. However, the latter differences were only significant in a few weight-groups. In either category the effect of birthweight on IQ became less marked at 2½ to four years, whereas the effect of socio-economic status only became definite at that age. Brandt and Schröder (1971) similarly found that the achievements of preterm AGA children on the Griffiths Scale exceeded those of preterm SGA children by the age of 18 months if no correction for gestational age was applied. If such a correction was made, the differences in Griffiths GQ in favour of the AGA children were even more marked.

In 1971 we reported in our follow-up study that a significantly lower proportion of all SGA than of preterm AGA LBW children were at the expected grade placement in school at eight years and had normal electroencephalograms (EEGS)

(Dunn *et al.* 1971). Drillien (1972) also noted that fewer of the SGA infants were normal when examined at the age of one to three years compared to preterm infants of appropriate weight. This made her suspect that the more frequent malformations among SGA children might share a cause with the subsequent handicaps, and this cause might be operative in early pregnancy and then not be influenced greatly by perinatal care. Fitzhardinge and Steven (1972*b*) pointed out that major neurological sequelae were uncommon in a group of SGA children born between 1960 and 1966, with an incidence of only 1 per cent for cerebral palsy and 6 per cent for convulsions. However, *minimal brain dysfunction*, characterized by hyperactivity, short attention-span, learning difficulties, poor fine co-ordination and hyperreflexia, was diagnosed in 25 per cent. Speech defects and poor school-performance were also common, and EEG abnormalities, predominantly mild and diffuse, were seen in about two-thirds.

Francis-Williams and Davies (1974) performed Wechsler, Bender Gestalt and reading tests on 105 children at four to 12 years who had weighed ≤1500g at birth between 1961 and 1968. There was a significant difference between the mean Full-scale IQ of 99.2 for 72 preterm AGA children and the mean of 92 for 33 SGA children. Learning difficulties were present in 20 per cent, often with normal intelligence.

A detailed follow-up study comparing the outcome for infants of short gestation (<255 days) with that for 'light-for-dates' children was reported by Neligan and colleagues in Newcastle, England, in 1976. It should be noted that both groups included children of normal birthweight. At five years 59 children of short gestation were compared with 67 who were 'rather light for dates' (birthweight between 5th and 10th precentiles), 74 who were 'very light for dates' (birthweight on or below fifth percentile) and 186 random control children. The study was repeated at six and seven years. Extensive psychological tests showed that both categories had impaired performance over a wide range of cognitive and sensorimotor functions, but the adverse effects of being born too small were more severe than the effects of being born too soon. There was a consistent gradient between the controls, the 'rather light-for-dates' and the 'very light-for-dates' groups. Social class and sex had important modifying effects. Behaviour and temperament were also more abnormal among the study children than the controls, and the 'very light-for-dates' children had more abnormal behaviour than those of short gestation. Abnormal neurological signs were significantly more common in the 'very light-for-dates' group than in the control group, while the short-gestation group differed less from the controls. These differences in the status of the different groups persisted when the effects of six biological, clinical and environmental associated factors had been allowed for (*e.g.* mother's height and her care of the child).

Recent improvements in the outlook for LBW infants

Mortality

Since the early 1950s there has been a steady improvement in the survival rate of LBW infants. While stillbirths and mortality during the first 28 days fell throughout

TABLE 1-II

Birthweights ≤2500g as percentage of livebirths*

1968	7.3	1973	6.7
1969	7.4	1974	6.4
1970	7.2	1975	6.2
1971	7.1	1976	5.9
1972	6.4	1977	5.8

*Livebirths for which weights were stated.
Source: British Columbia, Ministry of Health Division of Vital Statistics (1978).

this period, mortality on the first day of life did not begin to fall in England and Wales until the mid-1960s, and then it improved in all birthweight groups (Pharoah and Alberman 1981). Since about 1965 the annual neonatal mortality rate for VLBW infants (≤1500g) has fallen more steeply than before (McDonald 1981). This has coincided with the advent of intensive-care nurseries and the introduction of improved techniques of obstetric monitoring and paediatric care (Lubchenco *et al.* 1974, Teberg *et al.* 1977, Thompson and Reynolds 1977). It seems probable that the improved perinatal care is a major factor responsible for the declining mortality of LBW infants, not only in the United Kingdom (Pharoah and Alberman 1981) but also in North America (Lee *et al.* 1980). However, social, biological and demographic changes may also play a part (Knobloch *et al.* 1982). Indeed in some parts of the world there has been a reduced frequency of low birthweight generally, *e.g.* in Sweden (Hagberg *et al.* 1973), temporarily in the United Kingdom (Ashford *et al.* 1969), and also recently in the United States (Lee *et al.* 1976, 1980; Chase 1977; Kessel *et al.* 1984). The diminished frequency of low birthweight, expressed as the percentage of livebirths, in British Columbia over the decade from 1968 to 1977 is shown in Table 1-II.

It has been suggested that this reduction in the number of LBW infants in some areas is caused partly by the prevention of unwanted pregnancies, but this is doubtful (Morris *et al.* 1973). The easier availability of elective or therapeutic abortion, improved nutrition and antenatal care and other factors may play a part. Also, it should be noted that the *over-all* neonatal mortality rates in some North American, British and Scandinavian hospitals has been reduced from about 15 to 25 to about eight to 14 per 1000 livebirths (Thompson and Reynolds 1977). In British Columbia the mortality rate has diminished not only for LBW infants but also among babies >2500g, or full birthweight (FBW), and the total infant mortality in 1977 had fallen to 1.3 per cent (Table 1-III).

In the management of the preterm infant, the provision of adequate warmth and humidity has been supplemented by attention to metabolic requirements and early administration of intravenous fluids, with adequate caloric and nutrient content to prevent dehydration, starvation, hypoglycaemia and hyperbilirubinaemia. Early detection and prompt management of intra-uterine asphyxia, adequate resuscitation at birth, prevention of postnatal ventilatory failure and hypoxia by oxygen administration, and ventilatory support by intermittent positive

TABLE 1-III
Infant mortality in British Columbia by birthweight

	≤2000g	*2001-2500g*	*>2500g*	*Total*
1958				
Livebirths	802	1750	36,748	39,300
Total deaths first year	347	118	507	972
Infant mortality (%)	43.3	6.7	1.4	2.5
1966				
Livebirths	811	1506	30,512	32,829
Total deaths first year	324	90	335	749
Infant mortality (%)	40.0	6.0	1.1	2.3
1977				
Livebirths	732	1422	34,717	36,871
Total deaths first year	203	53	233	489
Infant mortality (%)	27.7	3.7	0.7	1.3

Data include weighed infants only.
Source: British Columbia, Ministry of Health Division of Vital Statistics (1980).

and continuous distending pressure are critical to improving the rates of mortality and handicap among LBW infants. In order to prevent cerebral anoxia, ischaemia and haemorrhage, circulatory, metabolic and acid-base disturbances must be minimized and corrected early. The effects of oxygen administration must be monitored closely by intermittent sampling of gas in arterial blood (umbilical or peripheral) and by continuous oxygen monitors (transcutaneous or intravascular) if the deleterious effects of hypoxaemia or hyperoxia are to be avoided. Potentially neurotoxic blood-levels of bilirubin must be prevented by phototherapy and, if necessary, exchange transfusion. Bacterial infection may be a contributory cause of jaundice, particularly in the preterm newborn, and must be diagnosed early and treated promptly to reduce the risk of neonatal meningitis, with its grave neurological sequelae. Cerebral blood-flow and intracranial pressure may be monitored and intracranal haemorrhages are investigated with ultrasound and CT scans. By these and other factors mortality in the various weight categories has been reduced considerably, *e.g.* to about 15 per cent in the birthweight category between 1001 and 1500g in major centres (*Lancet* 1980). Even infants with birthweights of 751 to 1000g are beginning to have a more than even chance of survival (Papageorgiou 1977, Bowes *et al.* 1979, Hack *et al.* 1979, Roberton 1979, Yu and Hollingsworth 1980).

Morbidity

Whether there has been a similar reduction in sequelae among LBW infants is a more difficult and controversial question. First, most recent studies have been concerned with the outcome for VLBW survivors in a particular hospital. There is a dearth of statistics for *all* LBW children (≤2500g), particularly on a regional basis. The results in intensive-care nurseries depend on the proportion of extramural ('outborn') infants *vs.* those born in the hospital itself, and also on the extent of the 'catchment area', the acceptance rate, the social and racial composition of the population and other variables. Second, there well may have been more reduction in the morbidity of preterm AGA babies with respect to anoxia and cerebral haemorrhage than in the morbidity of SGA infants with congenital defects or infections like rubella originating earlier in pregnancy (see Kumar *et al.* 1980). Third, the follow-up period frequently has been too short to determine the prevalence of neurological sequelae accurately (*e.g.* sensorineural hearing-loss). Fourth, there are difficulties in defining handicaps of LBW children: most authors refer to major and minor handicaps, but do not always agree on the definitions (*Lancet* 1980). In general, a major handicap would prevent a child from attending a normal school, and would include more than minimal cerebral palsy, an IQ below 70, epilepsy and severe deafness or visual loss. Minor handicap is more difficult to define, since it includes many problems which border on normality, such as learning disabilities and other 'minimal brain dysfunctions'. It has been suggested that it takes about three years of follow-up to detect all the major handicaps and up to a decade for minor handicaps (*Lancet* 1980; see also Chapter 5, Fig. 5-1). Fifth, it should be noted that, in terms of the community, the number of LBW children with neurological defects will increase if the mortality rate falls and the morbidity rate remains unchanged. To quote Paneth *et al.* (1981): '. . . in order to avoid an increase in the prevalence rates of impairment in the population, the morbidity rates among the low-birthweight [infants] must actually decline by 35 to 39 per cent'.

Since 1971 there have been many enthusiastic reports about the improved outlook for LBW and VLBW survivors (Rawlings *et al.* 1971, Calame and Prod'hom 1972, Stewart and Reynolds 1974, Davies and Stewart 1975, Mercer *et al.* 1978, Hack *et al.* 1979, Bosch and Kowalewski 1981). Rawlings and associates in London, England, and Calame and Prod'hom in Lausanne, Switzerland, were among the first to report remarkable reductions in the prevalence of disabilities among LBW survivors. The British group claimed that 86.7 per cent of 68 children with birthweights under 1501g were neurologically and developmentally normal at a mean conceptional age of 2 years 3 months. Stewart and Reynolds evaluated 95 children of similar very low birthweight born between 1966 and 1970 and claimed that 90.5 per cent had no handicaps at a mean age of 5 years 2 months. The Swiss authors claimed that 75 per cent of 66 surviving VLBW infants showed normal development between 15 months and 4½ years; 10.5 per cent were considered neurologically abnormal and 14 per cent were 'doubtful'. Mercer and colleagues also claimed that of 88 VLBW survivors only 11.4 per cent had neurological handicaps.

More extensive reviews have revealed more moderate results. Thus Jones and colleagues (1979) at the Hammersmith Hospital, London, found that of 357 VLBW (501 to 1500g) liveborn babies between 1961 and 1975, about 60 per cent died, and 5.3 per cent had a major and 5.6 per cent a minor handicap. There was no significant improvement in the proportion of handicapped children among the VLBW babies throughout the 15-year period. Stewart and colleagues (1981) at University College Hospital, London, surveyed the world literature and concluded that in developed countries the prevalence of major handicaps among VLBW survivors had been high until 1960 and since then had remained 'stable and relatively low at 6 to 8 per cent of VLBW *livebirths*' (not survivors). Silverman (1981) pointed out that the complexity of the relevant variables (*e.g.* changes in maternal age and parity, shift in social class and sampling distortions) made such calculations very unreliable. Horwood *et al.* (1982) made a retrospective study of the morbidity among all VLBW survivors in an urban southern-Ontario county for the periods July 1964 to December 1969 and January 1973 to December 1977. They sent questionnaires to parents and obtained reports of 'major damage' for 13 of 121 children (11 per cent) in the first period and for 18 of 134 (13 per cent) in the second period. They concluded that neonatal intensive care was associated with significant reduction of mortality (from 89.4 to 77.6 per cent) but no significant change in morbidity. On the other hand, Knobloch and colleagues (1982) found that in the birthweight group 1001 to 1500g the incidence of major neuropsychiatric disability for infants born between 1975 and 1980 was 17 per cent, compared to an incidence of 48 per cent in a similar group of infants examined by the same technique in 1952. It would seem that the proportion of handicapped VLBW children was highest before 1955, especially with respect to blindness from retrolental fibroplasia, and partly because of early starvation and other damaging regimes (McDonald 1981).

Cerebral palsy

The difficulty in assessing morbidity is well illustrated with respect to cerebral palsy. The incidence of spastic diplegia, which in the past has represented about one-third of cases of cerebral palsy in childhood, ranged from 10.3 to 32 per cent in three surveys of surviving infants with birthweights ≤1500g who were born before 1965 (Lubchenco *et al.* 1972*a*, Wright *et al.* 1972, Davies and Tizard 1975). Since then its incidence in children of similar birthweight in five hospitals is reported to have fallen to 5 per cent or less (Alden *et al.* 1972, Calame and Prod'hom 1972, Fitzhardinge and Ramsay 1973, Stewart and Reynolds 1974, Davies and Tizard 1975). In Sweden, Hagberg and colleagues (1975*a,b*) demonstrated an over-all fall in the rate of cerebral palsy during the years 1954 to 1970, and this was largely attributable to a reduction of nearly 50 per cent in spastic and ataxic diplegia among LBW infants. A significant decrease in the incidence of spastic diplegia among VLBW children was also reported in a British study (Davies and Tizard 1975). These studies provided circumstantial evidence for the predominantly perinatal origin of these forms of cerebral palsy. However, since 1970 there has been no further decrease in the incidence of cerebral palsy reported from Sweden, and there has even been a slight increase in mild spastic diplegia with normal intelligence, mainly among LBW infants with birthweights of 1001 to 1500g (Hagberg 1979; Hagberg *et al.* 1982, 1984).

In Western Australia, the falling neonatal mortality rate for LBW infants between 1966 and 1975 coincided with a slight *increase* of spastic cerebral palsy in these LBW children, despite a reduction in the incidence of spastic diplegia among bigger infants (Dale and Stanley 1980). Originally those authors also thought that the total incidence of cerebral palsy was falling (to 1.6 per 1000), but later Stanley (1982) had to withdraw this conclusion since further cases had been ascertained.

Although generally the diagnosis can be established by the age of one year, Stanley thought that the earliest age for definitive ascertainment and assessment of incidence would be five years. Kiely and colleagues (1981*a,b*) also advised against too early ascertainment. Paneth *et al.* (1981) estimated that in the 1970s about 6 to 9 per cent (mean 8.1 per cent) of VLBW survivors had cerebral palsy, and this is not greatly different from the 9 per cent found by Ellenberg and Nelson (1979) in the National Collaborative Perinatal Project in the United States. Although the incidence of cerebral palsy has fallen to about 1.5 per 1000 livebirths in Sweden, the VLBW preterm children still represent quantitatively the largest risk-group for the condition. There is some evidence that the type of cerebral palsy may be changing, as VLBW infants develop more spastic quadriplegia than diplegia (Teberg *et al.* 1982), but this is still controversial.

Other sequelae

The incidence of retinopathy of prematurity has fallen, largely because blood-oxygen levels are monitored more carefully (Stewart and Reynolds 1974, Davies and Tizard 1975). However, despite monitoring, it is still fairly common among VLBW infants who require oxygen therapy, particularly in the lowest birthweight categories below 1001g, though it tends to be milder than in the past (Mushin 1974, McCormick 1977, Pape *et al.* 1978, Rothberg *et al.* 1981). It has been claimed that sensorineural deafness has diminished to less than 2 per cent for infants with birthweights below 1500g (Stewart and Reynolds 1974, Davies and Tizard 1975, Mercer *et al.* 1978), but a recent careful study again showed sensorineural hearing-loss in 9 per cent of VLBW children at a mean age of 6.5 years (Abramovich *et al.* 1979).

With respect to mental development, McDonald (1967) found that the mean IQ of 1066 children with birthweights $<$1800g was 96.4, and Drillien (1964) reported a mean IQ of only 82.5 when the birthweight was 1360g or less. By 1974, Francis-Williams and Davies calculated a mean WISC Full-scale IQ of 97 for 105 children between the ages of four and 12 years with birthweights $\leq$ 1500g born between 1961 and 1968. Stewart and Reynolds even claimed that 65 children of the same very low birthweight, born between 1966 and 1970, obtained IQ scores on various psychological measures at a mean age of 3½ years with a distribution of values 'no different from that of their parents'.

In neonatal centres receiving LBW infants from other hospitals the results tend to be less satisfactory than in units caring for 'inborn' babies (Fitzhardinge *et al.* 1976, Pape *et al.* 1978). Concomitant intra-uterine growth retardation may also be an additional risk-factor for preterm VLBW infants (Commey and Fitzhardinge 1979, Hack *et al.* 1979). Babies with marked birth asphyxia, subsequent severe respiratory failure, neonatal seizures or abnormal neurological status and marked intraventricular haemorrhage are particularly liable to have serious residual handicaps (Fitzhardinge and Ramsay 1973, Roberton and Tizard 1975, Calame *et al.* 1976). Among the survivors of intraventricular haemorrhage, hydrocephalus may develop insidiously and has a serious prognosis (Larroche 1972, Lorber and Bhat 1974, Korobkin 1975, Papile *et al.* 1978, Chaplin *et al.* 1980). In addition to the problems resulting from asphyxia, extreme immaturity and severe intra-uterine growth retardation, neonatal meningitis also remains an occasional complication, with grave consequences for future brain function.

On the whole, since 1960 there does seem to have been some improvement in the outlook for LBW children. Before 1965, 20 to 50 per cent of VLBW survivors had a major neurological handicap, whereas now the rate is about 10 to 20 per cent (Mercer *et al.* 1978, Jones *et al.* 1979, Kitchen *et al.* 1979) and is reported to be even lower in a few centres (Stewart and Reynolds 1974, Hommers and Kendall 1976). For babies with birthweights below 1001g, the prevalence of major handicaps is usually 20 to 35 per cent (Alden *et al.* 1972, Stewart *et al.* 1977, Black *et al.* 1977, Pape *et al.* 1978, Ruiz *et al.* 1981, Knobloch *et al.* 1982, Kitchen *et al.* 1984). Frequently they also have a significantly small stature (Bethenod *et al.* 1979). Since 1965, many more VLBW infants have been salvaged, and it seems premature to draw any firm conclusions concerning the proportional rate of major sequelae in *all* LBW children in the population.

In our own follow-up study, which had its intake of LBW neonates from 1959 to 1966, we had only one survivor with birthweight below 1001g and we cannot shed much light on the problem of changes in morbidity, but we endeavoured to make a detailed study of the natural history of the neurological and ophthalmological disorders and we hope that our data will form a suitable basis for analysis and comparison in demonstrating recent progress (Dunn *et al.* 1980).

Minimal brain dysfunctions

We have already referred to earlier follow-up studies which showed that even LBW children with relatively high birthweights (2001 to 2500g) were liable to have learning problems in school (Douglas 1956, 1960; Knobloch *et al.* 1956; May 1958; Kawi and Pasamanick 1959; Drillien 1964; Wiener *et al.* 1965; Corrigan *et al.* 1967; Bjerre and Hansen 1976). We also noted the concept of a 'continuum of reproductive casualty' in LBW children, which extends from death and severe neurological impairment to behaviour disorders and reading disabilities (Knobloch *et al.* 1956, Knobloch and Pasamanick 1959). Drillien (1964) showed that 'prematurely born' children, particularly boys, were liable to be unsettled or maladjusted at school at 6½ to 7½ years, as rated by class-teachers. Conversely, Kawi and Pasamanick (1959) found significantly more LBW births among poor readers than among controls, and the differences were not accounted for by socio-economic status, maternal age or number of previous pregnancies. Meier (1971) reported a LBW rate of 20 per cent in a population of children with learning disabilities, compared to 5 per cent of controls. Balow and colleagues (1975/76) have reviewed the evidence for a significant relationship between perinatal events and subsequent reading disability.

In the past, such children with learning and behaviour problems often were considered 'brain damaged', even if they had normal intelligence. Their disabilities ranged widely in the motor, sensory, cognitive and emotional spheres. They were considered liable to exhibit an 'organic behaviour syndrome' (Kahn and Cohen 1934; Bradley 1937, 1957; Strauss and Lehtinen 1947; Rosenfeld and Bradley 1948;

Strauss and Kephart 1955; Bender 1956; Eisenberg 1957). This syndrome consists of hyperkinesis, distractability and short attention-span, mood swings, irritability, temper tantrums, unpredictability, impulsiveness and perseveration, and is often associated with anxiety and antisocial behaviour. The World Health Organization prefers the term 'hyperkinetic syndrome' (Rutter *et al.* 1969), but it is doubtful whether hyperkinesis is an essential component, particularly for older children. Neurological examination of these children may reveal 'soft signs' such as apraxias, agnosias, asymmetries of muscle tone or tendon reflexes, and poor co-ordination of fine movements. Psychological assessment may also point to particular difficulties, for example in drawing, concept formation, rote memory or copying designs in the Bender Gestalt test. EEGs frequently are abnormal and even liable to show epileptiform discharges.

This wide concept of brain-damage syndromes has been criticized, particularly from a psychiatric viewpoint (Pond 1961, Schulman *et al.* 1965, Rutter 1977, Shaffer 1978, Rutter *et al.* 1980). It was also noted that there was a genetic component, with predominance in males, and frequently there was no history of any damaging event. Accordingly, at a conference in 1962 an interdisciplinary study-group attempted to reach common ground and substituted the term 'minimal cerebral dysfunction' (Mac Keith 1963), which emphasized functional and developmental aspects. Later, in the United States, a committee under the direction of Clements (1966) defined the 'minimal brain dysfunction syndrome' as referring to '. . . children of near average, average, or above average general intelligence with certain learning or behavioural disabilities ranging from mild to severe, which are associated with deviations of function of the central nervous system. These deviations may manifest themselves by various combinations of impairment in perception, conceptualization, language, memory, and control of attention, impulse or motor function'.

Several books have described various aspects of this syndrome (Wender 1971, de la Cruz *et al.* 1973, Walzer and Wolff 1973, Gross and Wilson 1974, Anderson and Halcomb 1976, Denhoff and Stern 1979, Rie and Rie 1980, Nichols and Chen 1981), and in our view it remains a useful clinical unitary concept. Its weakness is its diffuseness and the absence of any single pathognomonic sign or of exact diagnostic criteria. Rutter and colleagues (1970) have stated that 'to put all the different syndromes into the same ragbag is to lose valuable information'. Gomez (1967) also called for more specific neurological diagnoses. On the other hand, Pond (1961) stated that 'the poverty of our methods of localizing brain damage makes it impossible to implicate any particular area of the brain' when children have difficulty in learning. Paine *et al.* (1968) concluded that the pattern of abnormalities in individual children with minimal brain dysfunction (MBD) 'reflects a complex matrix of underlying dimensions, some innate, some traumatic and some psychosocial'. It seemed desirable that the syndrome should be subdivided (Birch 1964, Rodin *et al.* 1964, Rutter *et al.* 1970), and statistical techniques have been used to analyze the condition (Lucas *et al.* 1965, Werry 1968, Paine *et al.* 1968, Conners 1973). However, Paine and colleagues (1968) found a disappointing lack of correlation between data collected under different headings, and Werry (1968) concluded that factor analysis of multidisciplinary measures did not tap a single unitary dimension of MBD, but rather a series of developmental dimensions which might be impaired singly or in combination. The use of cluster analysis by Conners (1973) did not appear to lead to clinically meaningful subgroups.

Even in the more restricted field of reading disabilities, Denckla (1977) defined five subsyndromes but also found marked overlap of neurological findings and presumptive aetiology in the different types. The utility of proceeding within the concept of MBD proved to be that it freed the investigator from the pursuit of elusive 'pure' syndromes. The usefulness of including many heterogeneous subsyndromes under the label of MBD certainly may be questioned, but as Accardo (1980) points out, in the absence of a generally accepted system of such classification there are two alternatives: (1) to avoid any diagnostic label and simply describe the strengths and weaknesses of each particular child from as many viewpoints as is practicable; or (2) to use a global term like MBD or specific learning disability, recognize its limitations and supplement it with the same description as in (1).

Among LBW children, behavioural abnormalities akin to the 'organic behaviour syndrome' have long been recognized (Shirley 1939, Drillien 1964). Fitzhardinge and Steven (1972*b*) diagnosed 25 per cent of 96 term SGA infants later as having 'minimal cerebral dysfunction, characterized by hyperactivity, short attention-span, learning difficulties, poor fine co-ordination and hyperreflexia'. Those authors also found an excess of diffuse, mild EEG abnormalities and delayed development of expressive and receptive language. Bjerre (1975*b*) diagnosed MBD in 13 (9.4 per cent) of 139 LBW children at five years on the basis of detailed neurological examination. Denhoff and colleagues (1972) developed a Birth Stress Index and a First Year Stress Index and related these to outcome in their sample of children in the Collaborative Study in the United States. No significant relationships were established between the Birth Stress Index ratings and the seven-year outcome as measured by the WISC, Wide Range Achievement Test (WRAT) and a screening test (MSSST) for learning disability, but the First Year Stress Index did show a significant correlation with both WRAT and MSSST, demonstrating the association between early abnormal neurological findings and later inefficient learning skills and poor school performance. Similarly, Drillien (1972) and colleagues (1980) suggested that transient dystonia and other abnormal neurological signs in the first year of life, exhibited by over 40 per cent of infants with birthweights ≤2000g, might lead on to MBD and were predictive of schooling difficulties. In another follow-up study, Calame *et al.* (1976) expressed concern that transient neurological abnormalities in high-risk newborns might herald speech delay, behavioural problems, perceptual-motor and other disturbances in the preschool period, and subsequent learning disabilities in school. This fits with the concept of MBD and also shows that the total number of later neurological sequelae may prove to be greater than was thought during infancy.

The findings in our own study are similar and, as will be discussed later, MBD proved to be the most common neurological sequel of low birthweight at 6½ years. It was found in 61 (18 per cent) of 335 LBW children followed to school-age, compared to only nine (6.5 per cent) of 139 control children of full birthweight. Further analysis showed considerable overlap between the various features of the 'organic behaviour syndrome' (including short attention-span and hyperactivity), clumsiness, learning disabilities and manifestations of associated emotional disorders. We followed the practice of Paine *et al.* (1968) that the diagnosis of *minimal* brain dysfunction should be confined to children with a 'global' IQ of at least 80, and we insisted that it should not be based on abnormal behavioural and psychological findings alone, but that there also should be some abnormality of neurological status and/or EEG.

Forty of the 61 LBW children with MBD in our study were re-examined at the ages of 12 to 15 years, along with LBW control children who had been considered neurologically normal at 6½ years, and with FBW control children. We were able to confirm the finding of previous authors that the manifestations of MBD change with age (Wender 1971, Denhoff 1973), since hyperkinesis tended to subside in the teen years, whereas brief attention-span, distractability, irritability and low frustration threshold, singly or in combination, more often continued to be major problems, along with learning disabilities and poor social adaptation (Laufer *et al.* 1957, Menkes *et al.* 1967, Weiss *et al.* 1971, Cohen *et al.* 1972).

It has been proposed that children with mild brain-damage are abnormally vulnerable to emotional stress (*e.g.* Drillien 1964, Rutter *et al.* 1970). Pincus and Glaser (1966) reviewed the MBD syndrome in children and concluded that the basic aetiology of behavioural symptoms associated with brain damage was not known, but was probably related to a combination of environmental and organic factors. Boydstun *et al.* (1968) studied physiological and motor conditioning and generalization of 26 children with MBD, compared to controls, and concluded from the differences that motivational as well as cognitive defects might be organically based. Hanvik *et al.* (1961) found evidence of cerebral dysfunction in 59 per cent of 148 children aged seven to 14 years who were referred to a child-guidance clinic. Rutter (1977) confirms that brain damage is accompanied by a greatly increased rate of psychiatric disorder, but like Pond (1961) questions the concept of a 'brain damage syndrome'. He also maintains that the association between brain damage and low birthweight or neonatal difficulties is weak. More recently, his team of researchers examined 60 boys aged between five and 11 years who had been referred to a child-psychiatric clinic and measured their hyperactivity on the Conners Teacher and Parent Questionnaires and by systematic time-sampled observations of behaviour during psychological testing (Sandberg *et al.* 1978). There were low and statistically insignificant correlations between these different measures of hyperkinesis, whereas overactivity correlated highly with conduct disturbance. After comprehensive examination it was concluded that there was no evidence for the validity of a broad concept of a hyperkinetic syndrome. Nevertheless, seven children were overactive in all situations studied, and these seemed to differ significantly from their peers with respect to neurological anomalies, erratic responses on the Matching Familiar Figures Test, and early onset of hyperkinesis.

It is perhaps unfortunate that so much emphasis has been placed on hyperkinesis in MBD, since overactivity has been notoriously difficult to measure, even with actometers (Schulman and Reisman 1959) and other technical aids, and may have many different causes (Mac Keith 1974, Rie 1975, Stephenson 1975, Rapoport and Ferguson 1981, Ross and Ross 1982). It is also highly dependent on the child's mood, environment, age and other factors. Shaffer *et al.* (1974) made objective measurements for four groups of boys with and without conduct disorder and with and without associated brain injury, using an actometer and a Werry and Sprague Activity Rating Scale. They concluded that overactivity is a function of psychiatric disturbance, rather than of an abnormality of the central nervous system. This work requires further confirmation (see Barkley 1981, Ross and Ross 1982), and it might be advisable to try to distinguish 'situational' from 'true' hyperactive children, since the latter are liable to show more abnormal conduct (Schleifer *et al.* 1975, Campbell *et al.* 1977). Even then, the measurement of other aspects of the 'organic behaviour syndrome' may be more rewarding, such as the deficit in attention (Luria 1959, Stevens *et al.* 1967, Crichton and Mackoff 1969, Dykman *et al.* 1971). It is noteworthy that the American Psychiatric Association (1978) adopted the term 'attention deficit disorder' (ADD) to describe this kind of behaviour.

In the context of the present discussion, it is evident that prospective follow-up studies of LBW infants should concern themselves not only with the gross neurological defects which can be detected in the first few years, but also with school performance (Alm 1953; Douglas 1956, 1960; Kawi and Pasamanick 1958, 1959; May 1958; Drillien 1964, 1969; De Hirsch *et al.* 1966; Corrigan *et al.* 1967; Wiener *et al.* 1968; Horn *et al.* 1969; Balow *et al.* 1975/76; Bjerre and Hansen 1976) and with this wide MBD syndrome. Estimates of the prevalence of MBD will depend, of course, on the diagnostic criteria used. Thompson and Reynolds (1977) have emphasized that additional follow-up studies are needed to define these disabilities of LBW children more clearly, and so understand the extent of brain damage among survivors of intensive care. We hope that our own study will supply some baseline data for future research along these lines.

Prediction and the LBW infant 'at risk'

Nancy Bayley (1958), one of the originators of developmental assessments, stated that such tests were of great value in judging and diagnosing a child's current status, but of very little use in predicting what the child's IQ would be. However, Knobloch *et al.* (1956) showed that the correlation of Gesell DQ scores at 40 weeks and three years for 300 LBW children was 0.5 for the total group, and 0.75 if there was neurological or intellectual impairment. Similarly, Illingworth and Birch (1959) demonstrated that developmental and physical assessment was of particular predictive value for retarded children; in the first two years mental retardation was forecast correctly for 83 of 100 children, as shown by an IQ (mostly Terman-Merrill) of 75 or less at the age of five to 10 years. Thus prediction clearly is better for children with impaired brain function or at the lower end of the near-Gaussian distribution of intelligence than for shades of difference within the normal population.

It is also established that the risk for neurological and intellectual sequelae in LBW children is inversely related to both birthweight and socio-economic status (Knobloch *et al.* 1956; Drillien 1959, 1961*a*, 1964; Robinson and Robinson 1965; Wiener *et al.* 1968; Eaves *et al.* 1970; Gröpl and Derbacher 1971). In addition, the length of gestation has to be considered; preterm children ultimately tend to have slightly better intelligence and school performance than SGA children (Horn *et al.* 1969; Eaves *et al.* 1970; Parmelee *et al.* 1970; Neligan *et al.* 1976). Sex also is an important factor, since language development and early educational achievement, particularly reading, are generally better for girls than for boys in most Western countries, and in both categories of LBW children (AGA and SGA) boys appear to be consistently more vulnerable than girls with respect to physical growth, cognitive function, behaviour and neurological signs (Drillien 1959, 1964; Davie *et al.* 1972; Neligan *et al.* 1976). Obviously many other factors in the family and maternal history, pregnancy, delivery and postnatal course are liable to influence the prognosis in individual cases. The question is how to calculate the prognosis most accurately in this multifactorial situation.

Donovan *et al.* (1962) studied 192 newborn infants and found high correlations between two independent examiners in their impressions of neurological normality or abnormality. However, 80 per cent of the suspected abnormal infants were normal at one year, so no significant relationship could be established. Mundo-Vallarta and Robb (1964) selected 57 newborn (including 40 'premature') infants with perinatal complications and found a significant correlation between neurological findings in the neonatal period and the subsequent status at one year. However, nearly half of those initially considered abnormal were normal by one year. For fullterm infants, Prechtl (1967) developed a standardized quantitative neurological examination technique, and when this was refined by correlation with 42 obstetric risk-items for 150 neonates with abnormal neurological signs, 73 per cent still showed abnormal findings two to four years later. Parmelee *et al.* (1970) analyzed the results of expert neonatal neurological and EEG examinations of 'prematures' in Paris and correlated them with the findings later in childhood (mostly at two to six years). Of the children considered abnormal on neonatal examination, only 26 per cent remained 'pathological'; 32 per cent became normal and 42 per cent were considered doubtful. All these investigators found that babies initially considered normal on neurological examination had a low frequency (2.5 to 14 per cent) of abnormal findings on follow-up. On the other hand, a higher proportion (27 to 80 per cent) of those initially considered abnormal seemed to improve spontaneously.

Meanwhile, Graham *et al.* (1962) had studied the psychological findings at three years for 355 children who had had perinatal anoxia or other potentially damaging experiences as newborns. Preterm children showed significant impairment on cognitive and perceptual-motor measures, but differed from fullterm children in that there was no difference between those who had had anoxia and those who had not. This was interpreted as supporting the hypothesis that the immature organism is more resistant to anoxia than the more mature. With respect to the whole cohort, however, the children who did not suffer a major handicap as a result of anoxia apparently were not untouched, and the findings supported the concept of minimal brain-damage.

Later data from the US Collaborative Study showed that deviant performance on the Bayley test at eight months and on neurological examination at one year could be predicted more reliably by combining two perinatal factors, such as abruptio placentae plus Apgar score of 6 or less (Niswander *et al.* 1966), or low birthweight plus low Apgar score at five minutes (Drage and Berendes 1966). The Minnesota sample of the study showed that the Bayley Mental Scale at eight months for 536 fullterm children was correlated meaningfully with the four-year Binet IQ, though the highest relationship of the latter was with socio-economic status (Ireton *et al.* 1970).

Werner *et al.* (1968), in their extensive studies on the island of Kauai, Hawaii, like some of the other investigators, found that prediction of intelligence and achievement at 10 years was improved by combining several factors, such as the Cattell DQ at 20 months (which was the best single predictor), paediatrician's rating, social quotient, perinatal stress score, and parental socio-economic status. For children with Cattell DQs below 80, a combination of infant test-scores and paediatrician's ratings yielded a multiple R of 0.80 with 10-year IQ. Smith *et al.* (1972) extended this technique by using more factors and sequential prediction stages. The relevance of such studies to the establishment of criteria for infants 'at risk' was discussed by Parmelee and Haber (1973).

Drorbaugh and colleagues (1975) isolated a high-risk group of LBW newborns by combining four factors: gestational age of 33 weeks or less, premature rupture of membranes, low Apgar score at five minutes and respiratory distress. However, this high-risk subgroup had only a greater than 50:50 chance of falling into an adverse category at seven years. In another study of 137 LBW children and 96 full-sized controls, Goldstein *et al.* (1976) related 35 maternal and infant variables to Cattell DQ at one year. When DQ was corrected for gestational age, three factors remained significantly related to outcome: the strongest was 'delivery and related variables', followed by 'complications' and 'prematurity'. Other investigators found that major neurological sequelae among VLBW infants were most strongly associated with a neonatal history of seizures and intracranial haemorrhage (Fitzhardinge *et al.* 1976, Nelson and Broman 1977).

Computerized tomography has demonstrated a correlation between the amount of intraventricular haemorrhage and the severity of neurological impairment (Krishnamoorthy *et al.* 1979, Ahmann *et al.* 1980). Further, initial apnoea of five minutes or more, recurrent apnoea and severe respiratory distress in infants with birthweights ≤1250g have a significant association with subsequent limited mental development and other neurological sequelae (Bacola *et al.* 1966, Fitzhardinge and Ramsay 1973, Ziegler *et al.* 1976). For VLBW infants, hypothermia and severe neonatal acidaemia, with blood pH below 7.2, have also been reported to correlate significantly with developmental delay (Pape *et al.* 1978, Mercer *et al.* 1978). With respect to Apgar scores, Nelson and Ellenberg (1979) found that a score of three or less at five minutes, and particularly at 10 minutes, indicated a significant risk of subsequent cerebral palsy.

The neonatal examination of LBW infants has been refined by the techniques and scoring systems devised by Howard *et al.* (1976), Saint-Anne Dargassies (1977) and Dubowitz and co-workers (1980). Newer technical aids such as the CT scan and sonogram to demonstrate intracranial haematomas and infarcts will aid prognostic accuracy. Meanwhile, we hope to contribute the results from discriminant analysis of our own cruder data.

Summary

The handicaps affecting LBW infants have been analyzed with increasing sophistication in long-term follow-up studies during the past 60 years. It has been shown that there is an increasing incidence of mental retardation and neurological deficit as birthweight decreases, and this cannot be accounted for solely by lower socio-economic status. By 1960 the important concept of a 'continuum of reproductive casualty' in LBW children had been established, which extends from death through severe neurological impairment (cerebral palsy, mental retardation, epilepsy) to behaviour disorders, reading disabilities and what are now widely called 'minimal brain dysfunctions'.

The incidence of serious sequelae used to be alarmingly high in the lower-birthweight groups. In the respective birthweight ranges, sequelae appear to have become less frequent since about 1965 under the impact of neonatal intensive-care units, improved obstetrics and some social changes, but with increased survival of VLBW infants the total prevalence of sequelae in the population may not have been reduced.

In analyzing outcome for LBW infants, those who are born before 37 completed weeks of gestation with a weight appropriate for their gestational age should be distinguished from those whose birthweight is at or below the 10th centile, so that they are unduly light, or SGA. The latter category may be subdivided into those who are born after at least 37 weeks gestation and others who are born preterm.

In determining the incidence of mild sequelae among LBW children, one difficulty lies in the lack of clearly defined diagnostic criteria for 'minimal brain dysfunction' and its diffuse features, with interdependent neurological, intellectual and behavioural components. Since this diffuse syndrome is not uncommon in the general population, the contribution of LBW to its causation requires clarification. The nature and pathogenesis of the hyperkinetic or 'organic' behaviour syndrome which is said to be a characteristic component of minimal brain dysfunction, also needs further study.

Recently attention has been devoted to the identification of the LBW infant 'at risk' and the prediction of future disabilities from findings in infancy, which are of major interest in public health. Since the neurological, intellectual and behavioural sequelae are of multifactorial origin, attempts are being made to use factor and discriminant analyses to predict by establishing cumulative risk-scores.

It is hoped that the results of this prospective study, which had its intake of LBW newborns between 1959 and 1966, will contribute to the clarification of some of these problems.

2
Description of Present Study

Henry G. Dunn and Ann-Marie Robertson

The present investigation was planned in 1957-58. Its main purpose was to study the evolution of neurological and ophthalmological defects in LBW children prospectively from the newborn nursery to school and to correlate the early findings with later status. In order to obtain a cohort of children with a high frequency of disabilities, it was decided to concentrate on 500 infants with birthweights ≤2041g (4½lbs). It was hoped that this investigation not only would be of academic interest but also would yield useful data concerning the early diagnosis and the prognosis of neurological and ophthalmological defects in such children, and would even benefit the children in the study group to some extent by leading to the early detection of defects, some of which might be remediable. The question of a control group was discussed, but the majority of members of the Steering Committee* felt that the cohort might be divided into subgroups (according to birthweight, length of gestation, social class and other factors) which could be compared with each other, and that full-birthweight (FBW) control children were not required. FBW infants were not included in the British survey of LBW infants (≤1800g) by Dr. Alison McDonald with the Society of Medical Officers of Health, the results of which were published between 1962 and 1967.

Pre-coded forms were devised on the basis of our initial experience and were modelled on those used by the US National Institutes of Health for the Collaborative Perinatal Project, which had just begun. In October 1958 we started to take infants into the study from the Premature Nursery (later renamed the Intensive Care Nursery) of the Vancouver General Hospital. The original intention was to examine all infants in the nursery with a birthweight ≤2041g, but some died before they could be examined by the research assistants, and in a few cases consent was not given by the parents or attending physician. The children in the study were examined at regular intervals, as will be described below, and by 1964 it had become evident that *minor* deviations from normal were common, particularly minimal brain dysfunction (Crichton *et al.* 1971), minor congenital defects (Crichton *et al.* 1972*b*) and slight impairment of physical growth and intellectual development (Eaves *et al.* 1970). The Steering Committee then reversed its decision about a control group and decided to study at least 200 FBW infants

*The Steering Committee initially was under the chairmanship of Dr. J. F. McCreary, then Professor and Head, Department of Paediatrics, University of British Columbia. It included Dr. F. E. Bryans, Head, Department of Obstetrics and Dr. S. Segal, Head, Division of Neonatology, Department of Paediatrics (University of British Columbia); Dr. A. F. Hardyment, who was in charge of the Newborn Nurseries at Vancouver General Hospital; and Dr. H. G. Dunn and D. C. Kendall, Ph.D., Head, Department of Special Education (University of British Columbia). In 1959 Dr. H. G. Dunn became Project Director.

TABLE 2-I
Births and infant deaths by weight groups*, British Columbia 1958

	Birthweights (g)			
	≤2000	*2001-2500*	*≥2501*	*Total*
Livebirths	802	1750	36,748	39,300
Deaths: < 7 days	301	77	150	528
7-27 days	29	15	65	109
28 days-1 year	17	26	292	335
Deaths in first year: total	347	118	507	972
%	43.3	6.7	1.4	2.5

*Weighed infants only.
Source: British Columbia Ministry of Health Division of Vital Statistics (1980).

TABLE 2-II
Births and infant deaths by weight groups*, British Columbia 1966

	Birthweights (g)			
	≤2000	*2001-2500*	*≥2501*	*Total*
Livebirths	811	1506	30,512	32,829
Deaths: < 7 days	296	43	91	430
7-27 days	18	7	30	55
28 days-1 year	10	40	214	264
Deaths in first year: total	324	90	335	749
%	40.0	6.0	1.1	2.3

*Weighed infants only.
Source: British Columbia Ministry of Health Division of Vital Statistics (1980).

prospectively. All were of similar socio-economic status to the LBW cohort, all were born in the same hospital, and the same methods were used as with the LBW infants. However, while the intake of 501 children with birthweights ≤2041g occurred from the end of 1958 to the early months of 1965, the FBW controls were taken into the study from the end of 1964 to the spring of 1966. This flaw in the design restricts the usefulness of the control data, but fortunately there was relatively little change in the nursery management of the newborn during those years, as will be discussed later.

Background statistics

In 1958 Canada stood 12th among other countries of comparable social development in her infant mortality rate of 30 per 1000 livebirths, and 8th in her neonatal mortality rate* of 19 per 1000. Of all the infants who died, 64 per cent in 1956-58 and 65 per cent in 1959 (*i.e.* nearly two-thirds) did so in the first four weeks, and 31.3 per cent in 1956-58 and 32.5 per cent in 1959 (*i.e.* nearly one-third) did so on the first day. The causes of neonatal mortality in Canada were tabulated

*Neonatal mortality refers to deaths below the age of four weeks.

as the following percentages: immaturity* 24.9, asphyxia and atelectasis 16.1, congenital malformations 15.6, birth injuries 15.5, respiratory infections 6.1, erythroblastosis fetalis and haemorrhagic disorders 5.1, and other and unknown causes 16.7. It was noted further that immaturity was also associated with deaths from other causes in an approximately equal number of cases (Dominion Bureau of Statistics 1960). Thus the prime importance of 'immaturity' as a cause of infant mortality is evident.

In British Columbia the mortality figures were only slightly lower than for Canada as a whole (Statistics Canada 1972). In 1958 the infant mortality rate was 27 per 1000 livebirths and the neonatal mortality rate was 17 per 1000. Mortality was consistently higher among male than female infants, and there was little change in death rates on the first day during the years 1958 to 1966, whereas the total infant and neonatal mortality rate continued to decline (Department of Health Services and Hospital Insurance 1964, 1968). These were the years when newborn infants were taken into our study. Tables 2-I and II show the infant mortality figures for 1958 and 1966, analyzed by weight-group.

It can be seen that approximately 40 per cent of infants with birthweights ≤2000g and 6 per cent with birthweights 2001 to 2500g in British Columbia died during the first year of life, even at the end of this period.

The birth and death figures for Vancouver General Hospital during the years 1958 to 1965 are shown in Table 2-III, together with those for British Columbia.

Since the completion of the intake of newborn infants into the study in 1966 there has been a further reduction in infant mortality in British Columbia, but it remains greater for male than for female infants (under six months). After 1966 the first-day mortality rate also began to decline, probably at least partly because of the establishment of intensive-care nurseries (see Pharoah and Alberman 1981).

Infant mortality in the weight groups <2500g has also declined. In 1977 the rate was 27.7 per cent for infants with birthweights <2000g and 3.7 per cent for those weighing 2001 to 2500g (see Chapter 1, Table 1-III). Total infant mortality in 1977 was only 1.3 per cent and the rate among FBW infants (>2500g) had fallen to 0.7 per cent. This suggests that the reduced infant mortality was also partly due to other factors, such as improved obstetric care and maternal health, and perhaps also to removal of unwanted infants by abortion.

Description of cohort

The cohort of LBW infants enlisted for prospective study in the newborn nursery during the years 1959 to 1964 comprised 388 of the 578 born in the hospital who weighed <2000g. Additional infants admitted to the study at the end of 1958 and at the beginning of 1965 raised the number to 412. Many who died during the first day were not examined by the research assistants and were not included in the study. Otherwise no selection procedure was used, and whenever the parents and physicians gave permission the LBW infants in the appropriate weight-range were

*In 1969 procedures were intensified for confirming the specific cause of death among infants. Figures for 'immaturity' then declined, and pulmonary complications, including hyaline membrane disease, are now registered as cause of death more commonly than 'immaturity'.

TABLE 2-III

Births and deaths of LBW infants in British Columbia (BC) and Vancouver General Hospital (VGH), 1958-1965

		Infants weighing ≤2000g					*Infants weighing 2001-2500g*		
		BC births	*VGH births*				*BC births*	*VGH births*	
		N	*N*	*Deaths in 1st year*	*Follow-up study Intake*	*Follow-up study Deaths*	*N*	*N*	*Deaths in 1st year*
1958	M	394	43	23	9	5	796	100	10
	F	408	56	28	11	1	954	124	9
1959	M	406	49	32	24	7	761	89	8
(approx)	F	403	55	18	21	1	888	105	7
1960	M	383	42	23	27	8	785	84	9
	F	395	44	16	34	5	881	103	6
1961	M	382	43	21	25	4	750	93	9
	F	425	44	14	32	2	863	93	5
1962	M	405	51	27	34	10	777	83	5
	F	409	57	18	44	5	885	109	4
1963	M	422	46	19	36	10	716	71	3
	F	395	55	21	44	11	829	103	3
1964	M	439	54	22	38	7	727	94	4
	F	371	38	10	29	1	809	90	2
1965	M	396	52	19	1	—	670	73	2
	F	398	51	17	3	—	800	81	2
Total	M	3227	380	186	194	51	5982	687	50
%				48.9		26.3			7.3
	F	3204	400	142	218	26	6909	808	38
%				35.5		11.9			4.7

included. Since the initial plan was to study infants with birthweights <2041g, a group weighing between 2001 and 2041g was also admitted, and occasionally a baby weighing between 2042 and 2500g was added for a special reason (*e.g.* as the twin of a study infant). 72 babies in the range 2001 to 2500g were accepted. Another 17 LBW infants born elsewhere and transferred to Vancouver General Hospital as neonates were included for prospective correlations, but in some respects are analyzed separately. This brings the total number of LBW children in the study to 501.

The 203 FBW control infants were intentionally selected largely from public wards so as to reduce their mean social status to that of the LBW group. Otherwise they were taken at random whenever permission was given, and no attempt was made to match the controls closely with the study infants.

Twins were included in both groups, but were the expected higher proportion among the LBW infants. There were 100 twins (52 male, 48 female), including 39 twin pairs. There were also four triplets and one set of quadruplets among the 501 LBW infants, and only two twin pairs among the 203 FBW controls.

Infants of unmarried mothers were not excluded, and were followed with the assistance of the child-welfare authorities.

TABLE 2-IV

Details of all singletons admitted to study

Birthweight (g)			*LGA*		*AGA preterm*		*SGA preterm and term*		*<27 wks, or unknown gest.*	*Total*
	M	*F*	*M*	*F*	*M*	*F*	*M*	*F*		
LBW infants										
≤1000	8	8	—	—	2	3	2	2	7	16
1001-1250	20	19	—	—	9	12	7	6	5	39
1251-1500	29	34	—	—	19	20	7	12	5	63
1501-1750	43	54	—	—	22	25	18	28	4	97
1751-2000	71	64	—	1	34	33	34	26	7	135
2001-2250†	19	23	1	—	7	7	10	16	1	42
2251-2500†	1	—	—	—	1	—	—	—	—	1
Total	191	202	1	1	94	100	78	90	29	393
			LGA		*AGA*		*SGA*		*Unknown gest.*	
Control infants										
2501-2750	5	6	—	—	—	1	5	4	1	11
2751-3000	7	15	—	—	6	7	—	6	3	22
3001-3250	21	22	—	—	17	20	—	—	6	43
3251-3500	25	26	—	—	23	24	—	—	4	51
3501-3750	16	17	—	—	15	17	1	—	—	33
3751-4000	18	6	—	1	17	5	—	—	1	24
4001-4250	6	3	3	3	3	—	—	—	—	9
≥4251	3	3	3	2	—	1	—	—	—	6
Total	101	98	6	6	81	75	6	10	15	199

†See text for explanation of small numbers in these two birthweight groups.

On the basis of gestational age (calculated from the mothers' dates) and birthweight, the children were classified according to the fetal-growth curves devised by Babson *et al.* (1970) in Portland, Oregon, where the climate and altitude are similar to those of Vancouver. Thus preterm infants with birthweights appropriate for gestational age (AGA) are those born before 37 completed weeks gestation (World Health Organization 1977), calculated from the first day of the last menstrual period, and whose birthweights lie between the 11th and 89th percentiles. Infants with birthweights at or below the 10th percentile are SGA (small for gestational age), and may be preterm or term (37 to less than 42 completed weeks gestation). Those with birthweights above the 90th percentile are large for gestational age (LGA) and may also be preterm or term. Similarly, the FBW controls may be classified into three groups, those between the 11th and 89th percentiles being of appropriate weight for gestational age (AGA). Table 2-IV shows the total number of singletons admitted to the study, listed according to birthweight, sex and relationship of birthweight to gestational age.

No SGA infants had a gestation of less than 30 weeks. About 6 per cent of the FBW control infants were in the LGA and 8 per cent in the SGA categories. In contrast, 168 singletons and 22 twins, or more than one-third (38 per cent) of the LBW children were SGA. As shown in Table 2-V, the SGA group could be further subdivided into 98 preterm and 70 fullterm infants. Similarly, the twins were analyzed according to sex, birthweight and gestational age (Table 2-VI). In this

Table 2-V

Total SGA LBW singletons admitted to study

Birthweight (g)	*Preterm*		*Fullterm*		*Total*		*Total*
	M	*F*	*M*	*F*	*M*	*F*	
≤1000	2	2	—	—	2	2	4
1001-1250	7	6	—	—	7	6	13
1251-1500	3	10	4	2	7	12	19
1501-1750	13	16	5	12	18	28	46
1751-2000	14	13	20	13	34	26	60
2001-2250	5	7	5	9	10	16	26
2251-2500	—	—	—	—	—	—	—
Total	44	54	34	36	78	90	168

Table 2-VI

Details of all twins admitted to study

Birthweight (g)			*LGA*		*AGA preterm*		*SGA preterm and term*		*< 27 wks, or unknown gest.*	*Total*
	M	*F*	*M*	*F*	*M*	*F*	*M*	*F*		
LBW infants										
≤1000	1	2	—	—	—	2	1	—	—	3
1001-1250	4	3	—	—	3	1	1	2	—	7
1251-1500	8	7	—	—	5	6	2	1	1(M)	15
1501-1750	11	9	—	—	7	6	4	3	—	20
1751-2000	10	20	—	—	9	14	1	5	1(F)	30
2001-2250	17	7	1	2	15	4	1	1	—	24
2251-2500	1	—	—	—	1	—	—	—	—	1
Total	52	48	1	2	40	33	10	12	2	100
			LGA		*AGA*		*SGA*		*Unknown gest.*	*Total*
Control infants										
2501-2750	—	1	—	—	—	1	—	—	—	1
2751-3000	—	—	—	—	—	—	—	—	—	—
3001-3250	1	1	—	—	1	1	—	—	—	2
3251-3500	1	—	—	—	1	—	—	—	—	1
≥3501	—	—	—	—	—	—	—	—	—	—
Total	2	2	—	—	2	2	—	—	—	4

case the intra-uterine growth curves of Naeye *et al.* (1966) were used as the basis for classification. There were 64 LBW twins (38 female, 26 male) in pairs of like sex, and 14 LBW and four control twins in pairs of unlike sex. Another 22 LBW twins were admitted to the study without their co-twin. Among the 100 LBW twins there were 11 with birthweights more than 25 per cent below their bigger co-twin, so they may be defined as 'runt' twins (Babson *et al.* 1964).

Racial origin

Most of the children in the study were caucasian. Among the 335 children followed to the age of 6½ years there were 15 native Indians, 17 Orientals and three of East Indian origin. For mixed-race marriages the mother's race was used for classification. The 203 FBW controls included 15 non-caucasians. The non-caucasian children are excluded from some analyses of physical and mental development in view of their different norms.

Significant findings within cohort

A detailed analysis was made of the historical, social and physical data of the mothers in the study cohort and of their infants. It is only possible to give here the significant conclusions of this analysis, but full details are available from the author.

The mothers of the LBW infants differed significantly from those of the FBW controls in the following respects:

(1) a higher proportion had had at least one abortion;
(2) a higher proportion had had a previous LBW infant, and also more than one LBW infant;
(3) a more frequent history of hypertension (BP >140/90);
(4) a more frequent history of neurological or psychiatric disorder;
(5) a more frequent history of other diseases (*e.g.* allergies);
(6) more familial congenital anomalies;
(7) mothers of LBW singletons had a lower mean weight before pregnancy than mothers of FBW singletons.

The mothers of preterm AGA LBW infants differed significantly from those of SGA LBW infants in the following respects:

(1) a lower proportion had had a previous LBW infant, and also fewer had more than one LBW infant;
(2) they had a greater mean height than mothers of SGA infants, and also than mothers of twins born at term;
(3) they had a greater mean weight than mothers of SGA infants born at term.

During pregnancy the mothers of LBW children differed significantly from the mothers of the FBW controls in the following respects:

(1) a greater proportion were suspected of dietary inadequacy;
(2) toxaemia was more frequent;
(3) vaginal bleeding was more frequent (placenta praevia and abruptio, or 'other');
(4) weight gain in excess of 9kg was less common;
(5) they more commonly smoked more than 10 cigarettes a day.

During pregnancy the mothers of preterm LBW infants differed significantly from those of SGA infants in the following respects:

(1) a smaller proportion were suspected of dietary inadequacy;
(2) hyperemesis was more frequent;
(3) toxaemia was less frequent;
(4) vaginal bleeding was more frequent;
(5) anaemia (haemoglobin level <10g per cent) was more frequent;
(6) they less commonly smoked more than 10 cigarettes a day.

During delivery the LBW infants differed significantly from the FBW controls in the following respects:

(1) in a greater proportion the membranes had ruptured more than 12 hours before delivery;

(2) breech presentation and delivery, and abnormal presentation in general, were more frequent;
(3) forceps were used less often;
(4) they had a lower number of high (≥7) Apgar scores;
(5) they were cyanosed more frequently;
(6) resuscitation was required more frequently.

During delivery the preterm AGA LBW infants differed from the SGA LBW infants in the following respects:
(1) in a greater proportion the membranes had ruptured more than 12 hours before birth;
(2) fetal distress occurred less often;
(3) resuscitation was required more often.

They were also cyanosed more frequently, but the difference just failed to reach significance ($p = 0.07$).

During the neonatal period the LBW infants differed significantly from the FBW controls in the following respects:
(1) respiratory difficulties were more frequent;
(2) oxygen therapy was given more often;
(3) hypothermia (<35.5°C) was noted more often on admission to the nursery, and rectal temperature more often remained below 35.5°C;
(4) on average, feedings were commenced later, and more often by gavage;
(5) exchange and other blood transfusions, intravenous and oxygen therapy and antibiotics were required more often;
(6) twitching occurred more frequently.

They also had convulsions more frequently, but the difference just failed to reach significance ($p = 0.07$).

During the neonatal period the preterm AGA LBW infants differed significantly from the SGA LBW infants in the following respects:
(1) respiratory difficulties were more frequent;
(2) oxygen therapy was given more often;
(3) hypothermia (<35.5°C) was more likely to persist after admission to the nursery;
(4) on average, feedings were commenced later, and more often by gavage;
(5) exchange and other blood transfusions, intravenous and oxygen therapy, and antibiotics were required more often;
(6) they had fewer minor congenital defects (Crichton *et al.* 1972*b*).

In general, preterm SGA infants were intermediate between preterm AGA and term SGA infants in the frequency of abnormalities.

Method of follow-up

The following protocol was drawn up for the prospective follow-up study of the children in the project.

Nursery assessment

Summary forms were completed with details of the course of pregnancy and delivery, previous maternal health, family and social history: these were completed by research assistants from hospital records and interviews with the mothers. The research assistants also performed repeated physical examinations of the infants, with emphasis on neurological status. If any abnormality was suspected the infant was referred to a neuropaediatric consultant. A staff ophthalmologist performed an ophthalmoscopic examination and retinoscopy. An EEG was recorded after incubator care had ended (omitted for the control infants).

Follow-up home visits
These were carried out by research assistants when the children were three, six, 12 and 18 months old, and again at 2½, four and 6½ years of age. Complete physical examinations were carried out, again with emphasis on neurological status. Developmental testing was performed using the Griffiths (1954) technique for children under two years and the Crawford Small Parts Dexterity Test and a further check on socio-economic status at 6½ years.

Home visits were found to be most suitable early in the study because mothers often found it inconvenient to bring the children back to hospital for examination and so were liable to default. Home visits also gave the physician and psychologist an opportunity to study the social situation, maternal efficiency and the mother-child relationship in the home setting. When the children had to be brought back to hospital for consultation, EEG or other special examinations, car transportation was provided.

Other assessments
A repeat EEG was recorded at about the age of one year. Home visits were made by the psychologist and the children were tested with the Stanford-Binet (Form L-M) and the Vineland Social Maturity Scale at 2½ years; with the Stanford-Binet and Vineland tests, Graham-Ernhart Block Sort Test, Porteus Maze and Goodenough-Harris Drawing Test at four years; and with the Wechsler Intelligence Scale for Children (WISC), Bender Visual-Motor (Gestalt) Test, Knox Cubes, Vocal Encoding (from Illinois Test of Psycholinguistic Ability), Goodenough-Harris Drawing Test and Benton Sentence repetition at 6½ years.

The children's eyes were examined by a staff ophthalmologist* at four and 6½ years. This included ophthalmoscopy, refraction, and evaluation of visual acuity, muscle balance and stereopsis.

Speech and hearing were evaluated by a speech pathologist** at four years, and this included the Hejna test of articulation. Audiometry was performed at 6½ years†, and EEG was repeated at about 6¾ years.

Educational achievement was also assessed from several sources. Copies of school reports and record cards were examined, and when the study children were in Grade 1 their teachers completed a Haggerty-Olson-Wickman behavioural guide: in the case of the LBW children this was also completed for two control children in the same class, of the same sex and with normal birthweight. The

*Mostly by Dr. A. Q. McCormick (see Chapter 8).
**Miss D. M. Washington, M.A.; †B. Clarke, Ph.D. (see Chapter 10).

teachers also completed a special check-list concerning the child's behaviour and ability in various subjects (also for classroom controls). Stanford Achievement Tests were used in Grades 1 and 3, and again for two classroom controls.

Neuropaediatric consultations* were arranged for all infants considered to be abnormal by the research assistants. Referrals to other specialists were also made in some cases, *e.g.* otologist, psychiatrist, speech and hearing clinic, cerebral palsy clinic.

All data were entered on the precoded examination forms and then transferred onto special code-sheets which were sent to the Division of Vital Statistics of the Department of Health Service in the provincial government. There the information was punched onto two sets of IBM cards, and one set was sent to the computer centre at the University of British Columbia for recording onto tapes and for analysis.

The nurse co-ordinator and the secretary made intensive efforts to maintain contact with the study children through public-health and social-welfare authorities, as well as through private physicians. When study families moved without leaving their new address, contact was re-established by sending prepaid reply postcards (with the help of the Family Allowances Division of the Department of National Health and Welfare). Private physicians and public-health staff also were informed of the findings.

Social class

This was determined on the basis of the Hollingshead Two-factor Index (1957) by interview with the mother. The index is based on the father's professional status and educational attainments. Social class was recorded on a detailed form before the infant's discharge from the nursery and was brought up to date when the children were seen again at 6½ years, when a new form was completed. Social class was not analyzed for infants who died during the first few weeks.

Early social-class (SC) analysis was available for 342 LBW children. For 333 of these it was updated at 6½ years, when 32 had a lower SC and 29 a higher SC, so the net change was negligible. Similarly, early SC analysis was available for 164 FBW children. For 139 of these it was updated at 6½ years, when 13 children were in a lower class and 16 in a higher one, so again the net change was insignificant. The analysis for the various categories of children in the seventh year of the study is shown in Table 2-VII.

It will be seen that the social status of the FBW control children who were selected largely from public wards appears even slightly lower than that of the LBW families. However, when classes I to III are combined and compared with classes IV and V, the social-class distribution is not significantly different in the two categories ($\chi^2 = 4.15$, NS).

When the social-class distribution of the preterm AGA LBW children in our study is compared to that of the SGA LBW children born at term, there is no significant difference. In this repect our data differ from those of Bjerre and

*Dr. H. G. Dunn or Dr. J. U. Crichton.

TABLE 2-VII
Social-class analysis of children in 7th year of study

Birthweight group	*N*	*Social class* I	*II*	*III*	*IV*	*V*
LBW (≤2041g):						
Preterm AGA	182	8.8	4.4	15.9	36.3	34.6
Preterm SGA	69	5.8	7.2	8.7	37.7	40.6
Term SGA	60	6.7	8.3	8.3	35.0	41.7
All LBW	333*	8.1	5.4	12.3	35.1	39.0
FBW controls (>2500g)	139	5.8	5.0	7.9	43.9	37.4

*Inluding 22 children with uncertain gestational age or LGA, *i.e.* not definitely SGA or preterm. Two children were excluded whose social class was uncertain.

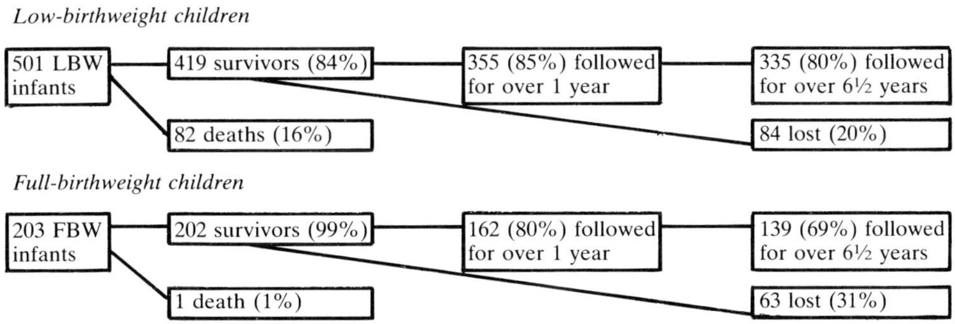

Fig. 2-1. Flow chart of children in study.

Värendh (1975) and of Neligan *et al.* (1976), who found that the social status of the families was lower for preterm AGA than for SGA children.

Completeness of follow-up

Complete follow-up to the age of 6¾ years proved possible for 335 of the 501 LBW children (about 80 per cent of survivors) and for 139 of the 203 FBW infants (about 69 per cent) (Fig. 2-1). The data for these complete cases filled 43 IBM cards for each child.

A total of 82 LBW children died, mostly during the first few months of life. 41 of these were preterm AGA and 30 were SGA. These represent mortality rates of 15 and 16 per cent, respectively. Among the controls, only one died during the first year, and another died of leukaemia at four years. A further 84 LBW children and 63 controls survived but were lost to follow-up, despite our best efforts: this was usually because the family had moved away, and only occasionally because consent for follow-up was withdrawn.

Our original purpose of studying 500 children with birthweights ≤2041g prospectively to the age of 6½ years has been carried out reasonably successfully. It seems satisfactory to have 80 per cent of the survivors available for analysis, considering our highly mobile North American population.

Discussion

Because of the change to the metric system since this study began, infants who weighed 2000 to 2041g at birth are now less easily classified in the analysis. We also have a few others who need to be kept somewhat separate, *viz.* the 35 non-caucasians, the 17 'outborn' children admitted to Vancouver General Hospital as neonates, and a few infants with birthweights 2041 to 2500g who were followed for special reasons, such as being twins of study children. However, this leaves a reasonable cohort of about 250 LBW children for analysis of long-term development. In retrospect, one might wish for a matched group of simultaneously born mature controls, but Drillien (1958) has pointed out the futility of most attempts at close matching. Wright *et al.* (1972) did attempt very close matching of controls and 'blind' evaluation, but this was largely retrospective and failed to distinguish subgroups of LBW children who now require separate analysis. Also, the important socio-economic status was not well controlled and, not surprisingly, 'a nearly significant difference in paternal income favouring the control subjects was detected'.

It is generally agreed that socio-economic status is one of the most important factors influencing the neurological and mental development of LBW children (Dann *et al.* 1964, Robinson and Robinson 1965, Eaves *et al.* 1970, Neligan *et al.* 1976, Dunn 1984), and that low birthweight is correlated with low socio-economic status (Drillien 1957, Baird 1964, Butler and Alberman 1969, Birch and Gussow 1970, Bjerre and Värendh 1975, Dowding 1981). Hence when random control children of full birthweight are selected for comparison they are likely to be of higher socio-economic status than the LBW children. Since we were interested in studying the effect of early birth and also of intra-uterine growth retardation on the development of the nervous system, we wished to compare the LBW children with FBW controls of similar social-class. Therefore we deliberately included babies of mothers in public rather than private wards. As shown in Table 2-VII, we almost exceeded our aim, but not to a significant extent. From the educational point of view, we safeguarded ourselves by comparing our alumni further with classroom control children of the same sex and of full birthweight, in addition to our own FBW controls.

In a long-term study of this kind it is inevitable that there will be changes in the pattern of care during the course of the project. However, the changes that did occur had the effect of causing distinct improvements in the weight-related prognosis for LBW infants. Although present-day methods in the care of these infants have become much more complex than those used during the study period, and the prognosis for survival is now greatly improved, we hope that the analysis of our long-term results will still be of value in elucidating the natural history of brain dysfunction in children of low birthweight, and in serving as a baseline for comparison in the future.

3 Physical Growth

Henry G. Dunn, Cara-Joy Hughes and Michael Schulzer

In 1919, Ylppö was one of the first to notice that the physical growth of LBW babies is considerably impaired during the first three to five years. Mohr and Bartelme (1934) found that among the 'prematurely born': (1) boys tend to weigh more than girls (mean 1877g for 93 boys *vs.* 1787g for 134 girls); (2) children with lower birthweights (≤1500g) tend not to reach the mean weights attained by the larger (>2000g) 'prematures' and are liable to remain permanently below normal; (3) twinning exerts an unfavourable effect on the weight curve; and (4) these infants' head circumference may become large in the early weeks, but usually this does not persist.

The preterm and term AGA and SGA classification referred to previously is recent, so the findings of earlier studies cannot be compared in detail. However, Douglas and Mogford (1953), among others, realised that a proportion of 'premature' infants were really LBW babies born at term, and that maternal height and weight bore a relationship to the ultimate height and weight of the children. Drillien (1958) agreed that genetic factors were important and found them to be interrelated with environmental ones, such as diet and maternal efficiency. She also noted that environmental factors appeared to exert a more marked influence on the growth of the 'prematurely born' than of mature controls, and that 'premature' singletons reared in the most favourable conditions had very nearly caught up with mature controls in height and weight by two years.

In 1964, Babson *et al.* showed that among twin pairs of dissimilar size at birth, the smaller or 'runt' twin tended to remain significantly lower in stature, weight and head circumference than the other. Later, Babson (1970) demonstrated that preterm AGA infants generally 'catch up' in height and weight and approach the measurements of FBW infants by one year, whereas SGA infants tend to grow at a slower level. The growth curves of these categories were nearly parallel if plotted against gestational rather than chronological age. Head circumference of the preterm AGA children increased at an accelerated rate one to two months after birth, so as to approach (or even temporarily surpass) the expected mean curve for normal fetal growth, and then remained normal. By contrast, the curve for the head circumference of undersized SGA infants was less likely to attain normal measurements by one year.

Several other workers have also noted that SGA children have reduced growth and a slight deficit in ultimate stature and head circumference (Sinclair and Coldiron 1969, Fitzhardinge and Steven 1972*a*, Bjerre 1975*a*, Neligan *et al.* 1976, Chamberlain and Simpson 1977, Mau 1977, Brandt 1978). Fitzhardinge and Steven (1972*a*) reported that 'catch-up' growth in a group of SGA infants brought the average weight from well below the third percentile at birth to a point between the

10th and 25th percentiles at six months, but 35 per cent of these children were still at or below the third percentile for height at six years of age. On the other hand, in occasional SGA children growth velocity in the first year far exceeded that of FBW infants, so that they attained normal measurements. After the age of six months the growth velocity of SGA children did not differ significantly from that of FBW controls. Cruise (1973) confirmed that SGA infants grew at a slower rate than AGA preterm infants in the first year and had smaller mean measurements at one to three years. She found that the greatest 'velocity growth' occurred during the first 13 weeks, and that head circumference showed the greatest increment at that time. Martell and co-workers (1978) also calculated that preterm and SGA infants had faster rates of growth than FBW controls during the first six months. They further reported that preterm infants generally caught up with term infants by the age of three years, whereas SGA children did not.

As mentioned in Chapter 1, the SGA children are a heterogeneous group, and one may anticipate that they are liable to grow particularly poorly if they: *(a)* have genetic defects or antenatal infections like rubella; *(b)* have a family history of small stature (Ounsted 1966, Falkner 1973); or *(c)* are born with reduced length and head circumference in relation to their gestational age, suggestive of 'chronic fetal distress' (Gruenwald 1963), *i.e.* prolonged intra-uterine growth retardation (Warkany *et al.* 1961, Lubchenco 1976, Davies *et al.* 1979). In recent years it has become possible to document intra-uterine growth by serial ultrasonic cephalometry, and it has been shown that those SGA children whose skull growth had begun to slow *in utero* before 34 weeks menstrual age* were more likely to have a length and weight below the 10th percentile at birth and subsequent slow growth. When the onset of growth failure had occurred before 26 weeks menstrual age there was also a lower DQ at follow-up to about four years (Fancourt *et al.* 1976), and neurological examination at six years revealed a greater frequency of minor brain dysfunctions (Harvey and Wallis 1979). Brandt (1978) drew the following conclusions from her extensive studies: (1) If nutrition and care are adequate, the growth pattern of AGA preterm infants depends largely on postmenstrual (so-called 'conceptional') age, irrespective of postnatal (chronological) age. (2) Head growth is least affected after a short period of under-nutrition and with adequate nutrition is the first to regain the original growth pattern. Initial retardation of weight is compensated for earlier than retardation of length. (3) In preterm infants the difference between corrected and uncorrected age becomes non-significant for weight after two years, for supine length/height after 3½ years, and for head circumference after 1½ years. (4) Catch-up growth of head circumference of SGA infants seems to occur only in the first six to eight postnatal months. Infants who exhibit this have a significantly more favourable prognosis for intellectual development than those who do not. In accordance with Brandt's conclusions, our results will be presented largely with respect to conceptional age in infancy and chronological age later.

*Calculated from first day of mother's last menstrual period and synonymous with the less accurate term 'gestational age'.

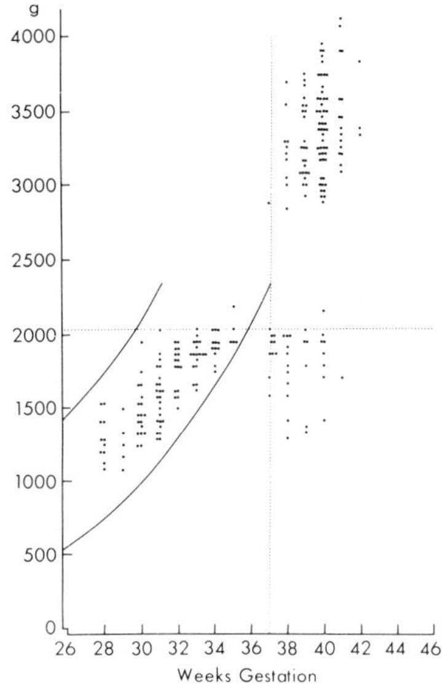

Fig. 3-1. Scattergram of cases used in most analyses.

Material and method

Chapter 2 gives a complete description of the organization of the study. 335 of the 501 LBW children and 139 of the 203 FBW controls were followed prospectively to the age of more than 6½ years. The children were examined in the newborn nursery and at three, six, 12 and 18 months, as well as at 2½, four and 6½ years of age. Caucasian singletons of low and full birthweight who had at least three complete individual examinations were used in the construction of growth curves. The numbers varied at different ages, and the range of numbers in each category is indicated in the legends to the curves (Figs. 3-2 to 3-10).

Children with chromosome defects and those with uncertain gestational age were excluded from the samples. Two children were eliminated from the analysis of growth because they were either grossly overweight or extremely tall at the time they were last measured, and thus would skew the growth curves. The preterm SGA infants were excluded from most graphs and calculations in order to show the contrast between the growth of preterm AGA and term SGA infants more clearly. The LBW sample of singletons then consisted of 111 preterm infants who had an appropriate birthweight (11th-89th percentiles for gestational age) and 39 term infants who were small for gestational age. There were 112 FBW children. These groups are shown in Figure 3-1.

In the nursery, infants were weighed on baby scales, or on spring scales if in the incubator, recording accurately to the nearest ounce. These weights were converted to grams for entry into the charts and computer files. Afterwards the children were weighed to the nearest pound on a spring-balance scale at home visits, mostly dressed in light indoor clothing, without shoes. The weight percentiles for gestational age were determined according to the norms by Babson *et al.* (1970)

for singletons, but using the WHO definition of 'preterm', and by Naeye *et al.* (1966) for twins. At subsequent age-levels, percentiles were derived from the Studies of Child Health and Development, Harvard School of Public Health (Nelson *et al.* 1969).

The norms for neonatal length and head circumference in relation to gestational age were taken from the data of Lubchenco *et al.* (1966). Crown-heel length measurements were made with the baby recumbent and both legs extended on a portable measuring board with a movable foot-piece. The head circumference was measured with a tape and reported as the largest occipito-frontal measurement. Both length and head circumference were recorded to the nearest centimeter in the computer. From the age of three months estimations of percentiles of length/height and head circumference were again derived from the Harvard norms (Nelson *et al.* 1969). However, to determine velocity of growth from increments, we avoided jumping from one set of norms to another. We used the Lubchenco norms to 42 weeks in relation to earlier measurements and the Harvard norms at birth (term, *i.e.* 40 weeks postmenstrual age) in relation to later data, if necessary with extrapolations for intermediate weeks. From the age of 1½ years standing height was measured in centimeters. After the age of three years the norms of Nellhaus (1968) were used for head circumference. A proportion of children were not seen at exactly the intended age-levels because of illness, absence on holidays, and various other reasons. In such cases the measurements were included in the formation of the growth curves, the actual time of measurement being used.

The data for the growth curves for weight, length/height and head circumference were modelled by third-order polynomial-splines. One serious disadvantage of a polynomial approximation is that the nature of the polynomial over an entire range is determined by its behaviour in a relatively small portion of the region. A higher-order polynomial merely provides more oscillatory character. However, polynomial splines can greatly reduce this problem by using pieces determined by polynomials to model the data. Each polynomial approximates the data in its own time-segment, relatively independently of the other areas. Dependence is imposed by restrictions of continuity at the segment boundaries where two polynomials meet (de Boer and Rice 1968*a,b;* Merchant 1974).

The boundary points for the polynomial segments are known as 'knots'. The growth curves were modelled using two interior knots and three polynomial segments. In general the curves were relatively insensitive to the position of the knots, and spline-smoothed curves of approximately the same continuous contour were derived for several different knot positions. For chronological data the knots usually were located at 40 and 150 weeks, allowing the initial growth-pattern some degree of independence fom the one-year to the three-year plateau. Where tail distributions at the 6½-year measurement period were a problem, the second knot was put further out on the time axis to minimize the tail effect on the central growth-portion. Any isolated tail measurement (*e.g.* one over 400 weeks) was deleted from the data set if it forced a sharp rise or fall in the tail segment of the curve. Knots for the gestational-age data were handled in a similar manner.

It is appreciated that such polynomial curves are not highly exact, *e.g.* with

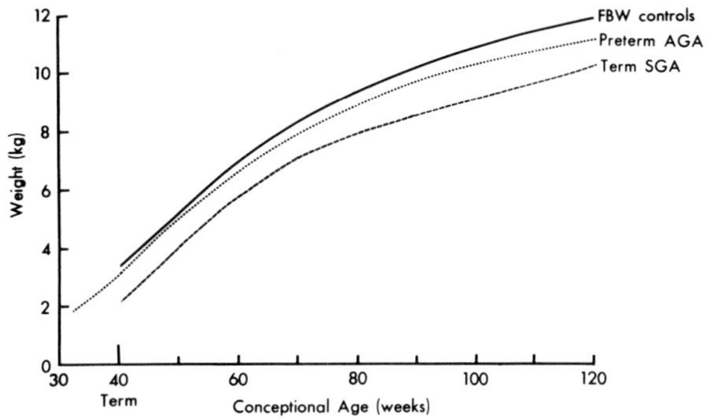

Fig. 3-2. Weight *vs.* conceptional age for singletons (infancy). Range of N: FBW controls 74-112, preterm AGA 73-111, term SGA 26-36.

respect to the time-points when the growth lines for different categories cross. Accordingly we have pooled the data for singletons of both sexes in the Figures in this chapter to show the general trends of growth. More detailed analysis for each sex was performed by statistical comparison with North American standards. For this purpose we compared the three groups (FBW, term SGA, preterm AGA) statistically with respect to height, weight and head circumference at different ages along their development. Since the age-groupings (birth, three months, six months, *etc.*) were rather wide, each child's measurements were standardized by subtracting the corresponding 'expected' value (50th percentile) obtained from the standard reference (population) curves for the same sex, taken at the same gestational (or chronological) age as specified above. Analysis of variance was then performed at each age-level, comparing the adjusted measurements of the three groups of children separately for each sex. Duncan's multiple contrast method was employed to sort out differences when they were significant.

Similar analyses were performed to compare growth *velocity* in the three groups of children over successive intervals between observations. To this end, again, measurements were adjusted by sex and gestational (or chronological) age, as before. Each child's increment (or decrement) in the adjusted measurements (relative to the corresponding standard values) was calculated and divided by the corresponding time-lapse, yielding a relative rate of growth. These quantities were analyzed in the same manner as indicated above, over each pair of successive time-points. Analyses were performed both on raw rates and on logged rates, and no important differences were observed between the two methods.

Results

Weight

When plotted against conceptional age, the mean weights of preterm AGA singletons appear to be close to those of FBW controls throughout the first 1½ years after birth (Fig. 3-2). This close relationship is not apparent when the mean weights of the preterm infants are plotted against chronological age, because their weight curve is shifted to the right, *i.e.* forward in time, so the preterm infants appear to be different from the FBW controls (Fig. 3-3). On the other hand, the SGA infants have

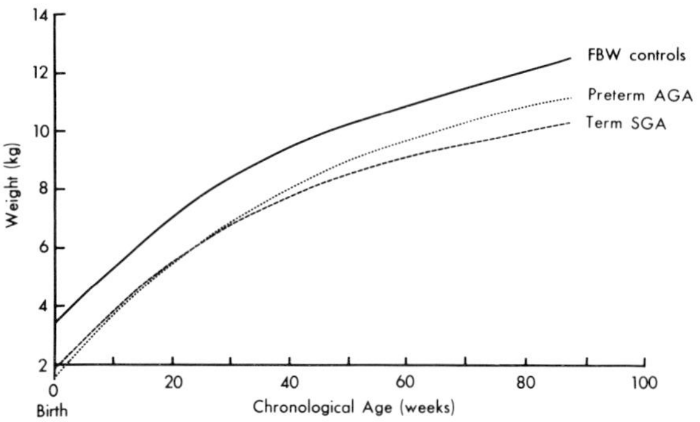

Fig. 3-3. Weight *vs.* chronological age for singletons (infancy). Range of N: FBW controls 74-112, preterm AGA 73-111, term SGA 26-36.

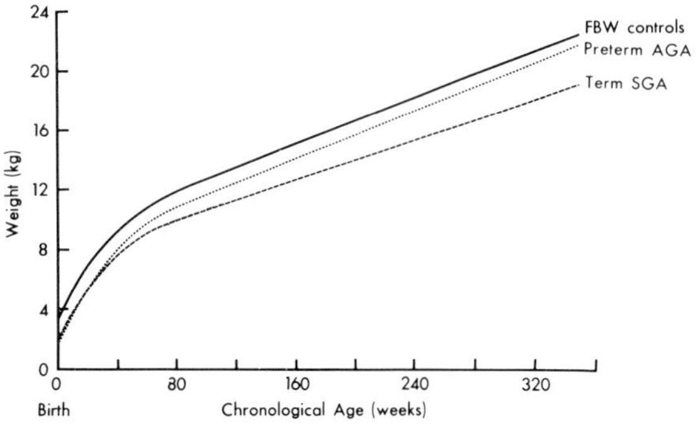

Fig. 3-4. Weight *vs.* chronological age for singletons (to 6½ years). Range of N: FBW controls 74-112, preterm AGA 67-96, term SGA 25-34.

mean weights which are distinctly lower throughout than those of the preterm AGA and FBW infants when plotted against conceptional age (Fig. 3-2). At 60 to 70 weeks conceptional age the two LBW growth-curves are somewhat closer together, and this suggests greater 'catch-up' by the SGA group in the first six months after term. When plotted against chronological age, the mean weights of the SGA infants start close to those of the preterm AGA group, but within about one year they fall below the mean weights of the preterm AGA infants (Fig. 3-3), and remain distinctly lower beyond the age of six years (Fig. 3-4). In contrast, the mean weights of the preterm AGA approach those of FBW control children in the first six years (Fig. 3-4).

Statistical analysis* shows that, as expected, the mean birthweight of SGA infants at term is significantly lower in relation to their gestational age than that of the other two categories when compared to normal intra-uterine growth data. The mean birthweight of AGA male babies is also significantly lower for their gestational age compared to FBW control children, but this difference is not significant for female newborns.

Comparisons were then carried out at 53, 66, 92 and 118 weeks conceptional age. In both sexes the term SGA children remained significantly lower in weight throughout than the FBW controls. The preterm AGA were intermediate. The

*The statistical tables are obtainable from the authors.

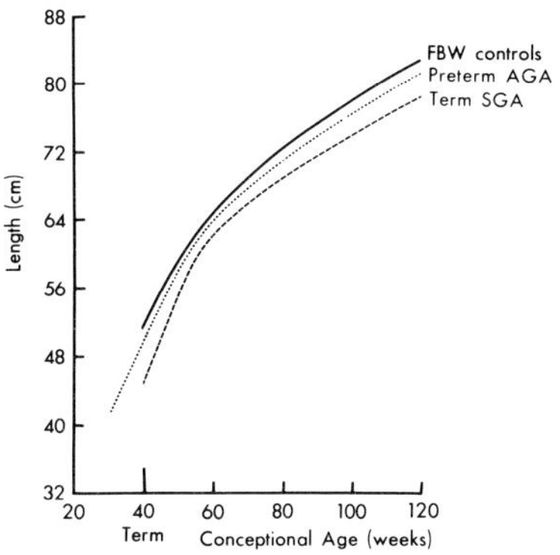

Fig. 3-5. Length *vs.* conceptional age for singletons (infancy). Range of N: FBW controls 77-111, preterm AGA 79-85, term SGA 21-31.

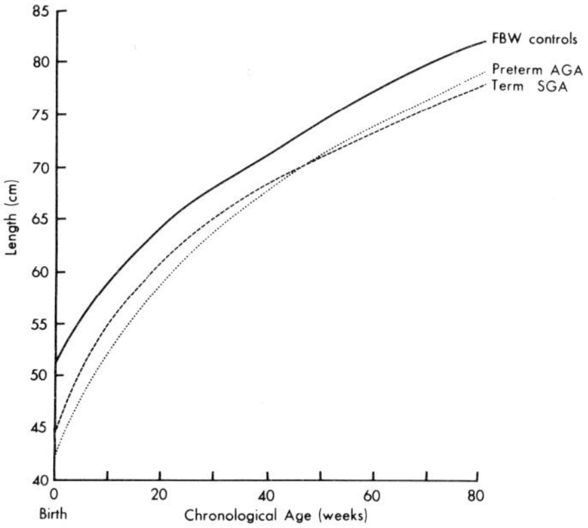

Fig. 3-6. Length *vs.* chronological age for singletons (infancy). Range of N: FBW controls 77-111, preterm AGA 79-85, term SGA 21-31.

females among them continued to be indistinguishable from FBW controls up to 66 weeks (six months after term), but one year later they were indistinguishable from term SGA infants and significantly lighter than the FBW controls. The same order persisted to the age of 6½ years, but the differences became less significant. The term SGA males remained significantly lighter than the preterm AGA, who in turn remained significantly lighter than the FBW controls right up to the age of 6½ years, except that the difference from the FBW children was not significant at 53 and 66 weeks. While the above differences for males were highly significant ($p = 0.000$) throughout, the level of significance of the difference for females was more variable, ranging from 0.001 to 0.02, and at 6½ years it was only 0.066.

Analysis of the velocity of weight gain in comparison with standard norms showed that the female SGA babies gained significantly more than the preterm AGA baby girls during the interval from birth to 13 weeks after term ($p = 0.01$). Afterwards no significant differences in the rate of weight gain between the three categories can be demonstrated. For boys, no significant differences in rates of gain can be demonstrated at any time.

Length/height

When conceptional age is used on the time axis (Fig. 3-5), the FBW controls and AGA preterm infants have mean length measurements close to each other at term and largely parallel growth curves during the subsequent 1½ years. Initially the mean length measurements for the SGA infants appeared to be well below those for preterm babies, but by six months after term the two means were closer to each other, suggesting relatively greater growth velocity in length by the SGA children. Figure 3-6 illustrates the growth curve in length, using the chronological age. As with weight, the SGA infants appear to have mean length measurements above those of preterm AGA infants initially, but subsequently fall behind within a year.

TABLE 3-I

Mean differences from head-circumference norms for different birthweight categories according to conceptional age

		FEMALES					MALES				
				Analysis of variance					Analysis of variance		
Age	*Category*	*N*	*Mean difference from HC norm (cm)*	*SD within groups*	*F prob. between groups*	*Duncan 0.05 level*	*N*	*Mean difference from HC norm (cm)*	*SD within groups*	*F prob. between groups*	*Duncan 0.05 level*
Birth	Preterm AGA (prem.)	44	−0.523				51	0.239			
	Term SGA	15	−2.127	1.232	0.000	SGA <prem.<FBW	16	−1.519	1.449	0.000	SGA <prem.<FBW
	FBW controls	51	0.351				52	0.842			
53 wks	Preterm AGA (prem.)	34	0.785				37	0.887			
	Term SGA	12	−0.783	1.294	0.000	SGA≈FBW <prem.	12	−1.983	1.460	0.000	SGA <FBW<prem.
	FBW controls	39	−0.215				34	0.094			
66 wks	Preterm AGA (prem.)	39	0.603				42	0.214			
	Term SGA	13	−0.562	1.387	0.004	SGA≈FBW <prem.	13	−1.415	1.429	0.002	SGA <FBW≈prem.
	FBW controls	48	−0.300				52	−0.364			
92 wks	Preterm AGA (prem.)	41	0.249				46	−0.296			
	Term SGA	10	−1.190	1.406	0.018	SGA <FBW≈prem.	15	−1.900	1.485	0.0015	SGA <FBW<prem.
	FBW controls	44	0.005				45	−0.940			
118 wks	Preterm AGA (prem.)	42	0.036				49	−0.606			
	Term SGA	9	−0.933	1.451	0.187	NS	18	−1.811	1.547	0.004	SGA <prem.≈FBW
	FBW controls	49	−0.043				46	−0.361			

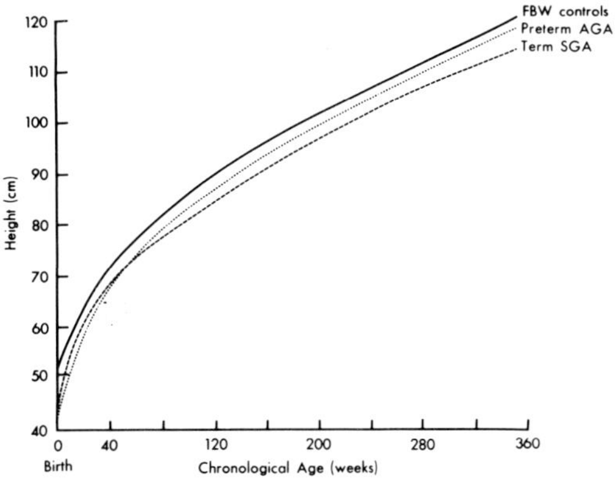

Fig. 3-7. Length/height *vs.* chronological age for singletons (to 6½ years). Range of N: FBW controls 77-111, preterm AGA 79-85, term SGA 21-31.

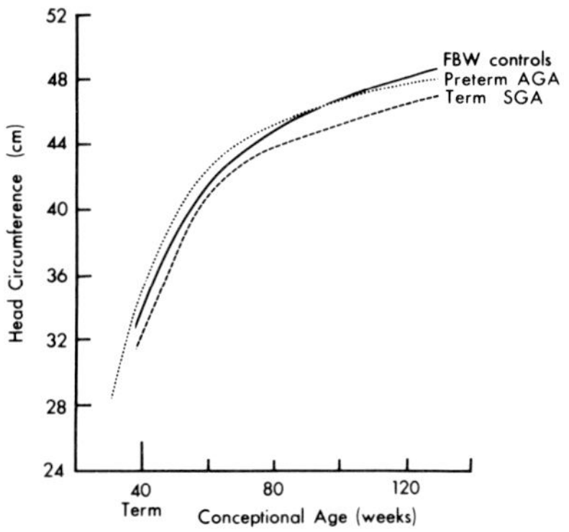

Fig. 3-8. Head circumference *vs.* conceptional age for singletons (infancy). Range of N: FBW controls 74-111, preterm AGA 67-96, term SGA 25-34.

The term SGA children continue to be shorter than preterm AGA children in the first six years (Fig. 3-7).

Statistical analysis shows that from birth to 6½ years the male SGA term infants are significantly smaller than the male AGA preterm, as well as the FBW control children. At birth the male preterm AGA babies also have a significantly shorter mean length than the FBW controls, but at fixed conceptional ages during infancy their weights are not significantly different from those of FBW controls. From the age of 2½ to 6½ years the AGA preterm children again have a significantly intermediate position ($p = 0.000$). For girls the trend is similar, except that the preterm AGA become indistinguishable from FBW in length only at 92 weeks conceptional age (one year after term), and after 2½ years the level of significance changes from $p = 0.000$ to $p = 0.035$ at 6½.*

The velocity of longitudinal growth in the different categories of children was also analyzed. As with weight, the SGA females appear to grow faster between birth and 53 postmenstrual weeks (13 weeks after term) than either of the other categories ($p = 0.007$). For males the difference failed to reach significance.

In general, Figures 3-5 to 7 confirm the findings in the literature that attempts at catch-up growth by SGA infants occur chiefly in the first three to six months after term and are unsuccessful.

Head circumference

Table 3-I shows that in comparison to the norms for the respective gestational age by Lubchenco *et al.* (1966) the mean head-circumference at birth was significantly bigger in our FBW control than in the preterm AGA infants, and again significantly bigger in the latter than in term SGA babies. However, Figure 3-8 suggests that

*It may be noted that at 6½ years a different (slightly taller) Harvard standard population is used, and the height of all our categories is slightly reduced in comparison.

TABLE 3-II

Mean differences from head-circumference norms for different birthweight categories according to chronological age

		FEMALES					MALES				
				Analysis of variance					*Analysis of variance*		
Age (yrs)	*Category*	*N*	*Mean difference from HC norm (cm)*	*SD within groups*	*F prob. between groups*	*Duncan 0.05 level*	*N*	*Mean difference from HC norm (cm)*	*SD within groups*	*F prob. between groups*	*Duncan 0.05 level*
2½	Preterm AGA (prem.)	44	−0.196				48	−0.840			
	Term SGA	10	−1.790	1.501	0.007	SGA <prem.≈FBW	18	−2.517	1.398	0.000	SGA <prem.<FBW
	FBW controls	46	−0.141				42	−0.100			
4	Preterm AGA (prem.)	50	−0.184				51	−0.351			
	Term SGA	14	−1.207	1.492	0.050	SGA <prem.≈FBW	19	−1.605	1.309	0.000	SGA <prem.≈FBW
	FBW controls	49	−0.125				41	0.100			
6½	Preterm AGA (prem.)	51	−0.167				54	−0.182			
	Term SGA	14	−1.007	1.447	0.044	SGA≈prem. prem.≈FBW SGA<FBW	20	−1.925	1.289	0.000	SGA <prem.<FBW
	FBW controls	49	0.121				44	0.468			

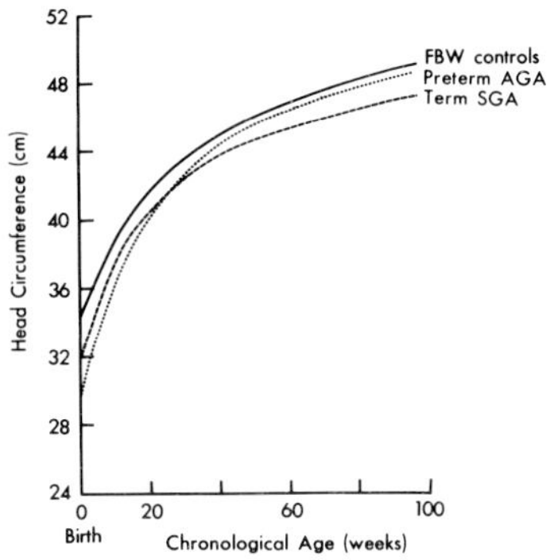

Fig. 3-9. Head circumference *vs.* chronological age for singletons (infancy). Range of N: FBW controls 74-111, preterm AGA 67-96, term SGA 25-34.

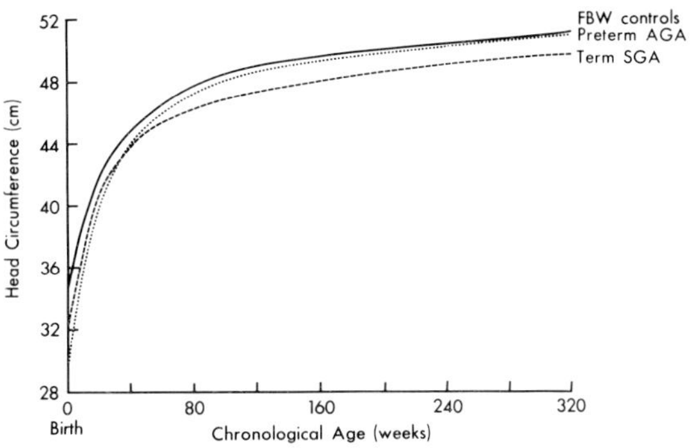

Fig. 3-10. Head circumference *vs.* chronological age for singletons (to 6 years). Range of N: FBW controls 74-111, preterm AGA 67-96, term SGA 25-34.

when term is reached the AGA preterm infants' head circumference exceeds that of the FBW control children. If this were to be considered a dubious 'tail' phenomenon in the polynomial curve, it is certainly supported by the figures for head circumference in Table 3-I, which show the heads of the preterm AGA to be significantly bigger than those of the FBW infants in comparison to normal standards by the age of 53 postmenstrual weeks, *i.e.* three months after term.

Figure 3-8 also suggests that the head circumference of the SGA group approaches that of the FBW controls at about 55 to 65 weeks conceptional age. This is confirmed in Table 3-I with respect to SGA girls, who at 53 and 66 weeks have a mean head-size which is not significantly smaller than that of the FBW group, though it always remains further below the normal standards. However, the growth velocity of the head, in contrast to that of weight and length, is never significantly greater in term SGA than in preterm AGA infants. The attempt at catch-up head growth by SGA infants appears to cease at about 92 weeks, *i.e.* around the end of the first year after term. The slight (but often significant) superiority in head circumference of the AGA preterm infants, compared to that of the FBW controls, also appears to subside at about 100 weeks, so that there is no significant difference between these categories at 118 postmenstrual weeks, *i.e.* 1½ years after term. Subsequently the FBW controls take the lead, though their mean head-circumference usually is not significantly bigger than that of the ex-preterm, and both are very close to the Nellhaus (1968) norms. However, the mean head-size of the SGA children remains distinctly smaller (Table 3-II). When head growth is plotted according to chronological age (Figs 3-9 and 10), the mean head-circumference of the FBW control children exceeds that of the AGA preterm group throughout, but by the age of four years the difference is non-significant in girls.

Relationship of head size to neurological and psychological outcome

The close relationship between head circumference and brain development in the

TABLE 3-III

Correlation of head-circumference in infancy with intellectual and neurological outcome

	N	*Mean WISC Full-scale IQ at 6½ yrs*	*p*		*Neurological outcome at 6½ years* *Normal*	*Abnormal*	*p*
SGA children with head circumference <10th percentile at birth	42	91.0	t = 2.0829 p<0.05		18	24	$\chi^2 = 6.767$ p<0.05
SGA children with head circumference >10th percentile at birth	24	100.8			19	5	
LBW infants with head circumference <3rd percentile at 1 yr	38	85.0	t = − 3.37 p = 0.001	N 42	15	27	$\chi^2 = 6.735$ p<0.01
LBW infants with head circumference >3rd percentile at 1 yr	187	95.5		198	117	81	
All SGA children with head circumference <10th percentile at birth and at 6½ yrs	11	73.4	t = − 3.86 p<0.001		2	9	$\chi^2 = 2.466$ NS
All SGA children with head circumference <10th percentile at birth and >10th percentile at 6½ yrs	31	97.3			16	15	
Term SGA children with head circumference <10th percentile at birth and 6½ yrs	9	72.3	t = −4.10 p<0.001		1	8	$\chi^2 = 3.715$ 0.05<p<0.10
Term SGA children with head circumference <10th percentile at birth and >10th percentile at 6½ yrs	19	101.4			11	8	

TABLE 3-IV

Comparison of intellectual and neurological outcome for SGA infants with small head-circumference at birth and different body lengths

	N	*Mean WISC Full-scale IQ at 6½ yrs*	*p*	*Neurological outcome at 6½ years* Normal	Abnormal	*p*
SGA children with head circumference <10th percentile at birth and with length >10th percentile	39	92.6	t = 0.32	19	20	$\chi^{2*} = 0.1956$
SGA children with head circumference and length <10th percentile at birth	32	91.0	NS	13	19	NS

*Corrected.

first year has been established by many authors (Ylppö 1919, Bray *et al.* 1969, Winick and Rosso 1969, Dobbing 1970, Babson and Henderson 1974, Cooke *et al.* 1977). Accordingly it has been suggested that the head circumference at birth and the catch-up head growth by one year may have prognostic significance for intellectual development (Nelson and Deutschberger 1970; Avery *et al.* 1972; Brandt 1973, 1978; Babson and Henderson 1974; Gross *et al.* 1978; Stave and Ruvalo 1980, Gross and Eckerman 1983). It has also been suggested that the prognosis may vary according to the degree of growth retardation associated with reduction of head circumference, yielding various patterns of retarded fetal growth (O'Connell *et al.* 1965, Woods *et al.* 1979). Therefore we decided to correlate these measurements for our LBW children, and particularly for SGA children, with intellectual and neurological outcome at 6½ years.

In Table 3-III the mean WISC Full-scale IQ scores and neurological outcome at 6½ years for different groups of LBW children are analyzed according to head circumference in infancy. The first comparison is between SGA children with a head circumference less than the 10th percentile at birth and those above that level. This shows that both psychological and neurological outcome are just significantly better ($p<0.05$) for those with a bigger head. A similar analysis at one year shows that LBW infants with a head circumference above the third percentile have a significantly better intellectual and neurological outcome than those with a head size below that level, *i.e.* with significantly small heads.

We then compared SGA infants who exhibited catch-up growth of the head with those who did not do so to any marked extent. SGA infants with a head circumference less than the 10th percentile at birth and still at 6½ years had significantly lower mean WISC IQ scores at the latter age compared to those whose head circumference increased beyond the 10th percentile ($p<0.001$). However, the neurological outcome of these two groups was not significantly different, possibly because the numbers were too small. When the term SGA children alone were considered in an analogous fashion with respect to head circumference at birth and at 6½ years, the ultimate mean WISC Full-scale IQ at the latter age was again quite significantly better for those with bigger heads, and neurological outcome also appeared to be better, though the difference just failed to reach significance

(0.05<p<0.10).

The analysis in Table 3-IV was designed to answer the question whether IQ is related to stature, in addition to head circumference. It suggests that reduced stature is not associated with increased intellectual or neurological handicap over that of small head-circumference by itself.

The above results led to further investigation of the relationship between IQ (adjusted for social class) at 6½ years, as compared to the population mean, by regression analysis. The highly significant relationship between IQ and social class described in Chapter 4 was confirmed again, and controlling for this the difference between each infant's head-circumference and the population mean (according to Nellhaus 1968), corrected for conceptional age, was calculated ($\triangle$HC). Using multiple regression (orthogonal polynomials), the adjusted IQ was regressed on $\triangle$HC and on $(\triangle \text{HC})^2$. This technique examines both the linear (*i.e.* direct) and the quadratic relationship between head circumference and IQ. In the latter, IQ increases directly with head circumference up to a maximum; beyond this point, as the head gets very large the IQ begins to fall.

For 114 LBW *boys* the results of this analysis indicated significant linear ($p<0.0005$) and quadratic ($p<0.025$) relationships. Mean IQ rose as head circumference increased from 5.8cm below the population mean to 3.3cm above the mean. However, beyond this size, as head circumference increased further, IQ began to decrease.* For 106 LBW girls, only a significant linear relationship could be demonstrated ($0.0005<p<0.005$), extending from 5cm below the population mean to 3.9cm above the mean. There was no significant quadratic relationship with fall in IQ beyond that point. The reason for the difference in the relationship between IQ and head circumference for boys and girls at 6½ years is not clear. It could be partly the result of greater morbidity among boys with larger heads.

The following conclusions may be drawn:

(1) SGA infants with a head circumference below the 10th percentile at birth have a significantly lower mean WISC Full-scale IQ score and more abnormal neurological status at 6½ years than SGA neonates with normal head-size.

(2) LBW infants in general with a head circumference below the 3rd percentile at one year similarly have significantly lower mean IQ scores and worse neurological outcome at 6½ years.

(3) The mean WISC Full-scale IQ at 6½ years is significantly lower and the neurological outcome at that age almost significantly worse if *term* SGA children with a head circumference below the 10th percentile do not exhibit catch-up growth of the head beyond the 10th percentile by the age of 6½. In the total SGA group the importance of such catch-up growth can also be shown with respect to ultimate mean IQ, but is not significant for neurological outcome.

(4) Body length below the 10th percentile at birth does not appear to add significantly to the adverse prognosis for SGA newborns with head circumferences

*Relationship between IQ (adjusted for social class) and head circumference was approximated by the following formulae: *Boys:* IQ (adjusted) = 2.380 + 3.412 $\triangle$HC −0.785 $(\triangle \text{HC})^2$; *Girls:* IQ (adjusted) = 1.57 + 2.63 $\triangle$HC −0.327† $(\triangle \text{HC})^2$.

†Non-significant.

below the 10th percentile.
(5) Regression analysis of IQ (adjusted for social class) and head size demonstrates that among LBW children at 6½ years there is a linear relationship between head circumference and IQ. For boys this increase extends from 5.8cm below the population mean to 3.3cm above the mean, and as head circumference increases beyond this point IQ begins to fall in a quadratic relationship. For girls, IQ rises in a linear relationship alone from 5cm below the population mean to 3.9cm above the mean, and there is no significant quadratic relationship or reduction of IQ beyond that point.

Discussion

The term 'catch-up growth' was coined in an important paper by Prader and colleagues (1963), which dealt with compensatory growth after illness or starvation in children. It implies the concept of 'developmental canalization', *i.e.* each child has a genetically predestined normal channel of growth which is to be attained, maintained and, if necessary, regained.

Weight

Brandt (1978) found that the extra-uterine weight-curve of preterm AGA infants at 32 to 39 postmenstrual weeks tended to follow approximately the 10th percentile of so-called intra-uterine curves. If they remain healthy and obtain an adequate calorie intake they will then begin to 'catch up', but at term and one month later their weight may still be significantly lower than that of FBW controls. Two months after term they will usually no longer be significantly lighter than FBW infants, and after that there is no significant difference in weight growth, though the preterm infants tend to have non-significantly lower values (perhaps at least partly explained on genetic grounds). This is largely confirmed in our studies. The AGA preterm LBW infants of either sex who had survived to three months after term (53 weeks postmenstrual age) were not significantly lighter than the FBW controls, whereas on average they were significantly heavier than the SGA infants of the same conceptional age, in comparison with normal standards.

This order of FBW weights being highest, preterm AGA intermediate and term SGA lowest continued until the age of 6½ years. Our results differed slightly from Brandt's in that the ex-premature *boys* gained relatively less well than the girls and retained a significantly lower weight than FBW controls, perhaps partly because of greater morbidity. Our data also differed in one respect from those of Cruise (1973), since the velocity of weight gain in the first 13 weeks after term in our series was greatest among the SGA infants and significantly greater for SGA baby girls than for AGA preterm girls, the FBW controls being intermediate. This may indicate that SGA infants (at least the girls) have a brief but intensive period of neonatal catch-up gain, while the preterm infants are still ailing. However, it is evident that the catch-up weight gain by the AGA preterm infants is maintained better after the first three to six months, though the differences in growth velocity are not statistically significant (see Figs. 3-2 and 4). In any event, 'true prematures' generally find and follow their weight channel in the first year if the brain is intact and they are fed adequately, and will then be close to FBW controls in weight.*

The situation is much more complex for SGA infants. If the cause of their hypotrophic condition is a severe congenital defect (*e.g.* Down syndrome, Russell-Silver dwarfism, idiopathic microcephaly) or an antenatal infection (*e.g.* rubella), they are well-proportioned but have restricted growth-potential. On the other hand, if they are SGA because of maternal or placental disease resulting in malnutrition and/or hypoxia, their potential for growth may be better. These are the infants who may exhibit catch-up growth after reaching extra-uterine life and thus a better environment and food supply. However, if the intra-uterine malnutrition has progressed to such an extent that not only weight but also length and finally head circumference (*i.e.* brain development) have become affected, then the number of cells in the body and even in the brain may become restricted and the potential for catch-up gain and growth will become limited (Gruenwald 1963, Winick 1968, Winick and Rosso 1969, Dobbing 1974).

Our finding that SGA term infants have a greater mean rate of weight gain than the AGA preterm group between birth and the age of three months after term is in keeping with studies by Davies (1981), who found their rate of growth exceeding that of AGA preterm infants over the first six months. It is clear that the attempt at catch-up by SGA infants usually is inadequate to get them to the normal range. After the first six months their velocity of gain is no different from that of the other categories, so they are doomed to remain lighter. However, Kitchen *et al.* (1980) found that 19.6 per cent of their sample of VLBW infants were SGA at birth, whereas by eight years only 7.6 per cent remained below the 10th percentile for weight. According to Lubchenco (1976), complete catch-up by SGA infants is most likely to occur if they are low only in weight and not in height or head circumference, *i.e.* probably have had only a short period of intra-uterine malnutrition. Such wasted-looking infants tend to have a low 'ponderal index' ($g/cm^3 \times 100$) (Miller and Hassanein 1971), and Davies *et al.* (1979) documented more rapid catch-up during the first month by such babies than by non-wasted SGA infants.

Length/height

As with weight, our data show that the length of FBW control infants is fairly close to North American norms, and again the term SGA infants appear to grow faster than the controls in the first three months. There is also a suggestion of further catch-up growth among male infants at 66 to 92 postmenstrual weeks (*i.e.* six to 12 months) so that catch-up for length may continue somewhat later than for weight. However, as is shown in Figure 3-5, the growth curve settles below that for AGA prematures about a year after birth, and subsequently there is no difference in growth velocity, so that the mean height of SGA children at 6½ years is significantly lower than that of FBW controls, and also somewhat lower than that of AGA prematures (significantly so in males). Davies and Beverley (1979) found that SGA babies increased their weight relatively more than their length in the first postnatal

*One exception to this rule may be a proportion of VLBW AGA children (birthweight ≤1250g) who exhibit growth failure after a stormy neonatal course (Bethenod *et al.* 1979, Kumar *et al.* 1980).

year, so in spite of continuing to be lighter and shorter they become better proportioned (and the ponderal index rises). Fitzhardinge and Steven (1972) considered height a better indicator of growth than weight for SGA children and found that increases in head circumference paralleled increases in height.

Head circumference

Head circumference is of particular interest, as it reflects the growth of the brain. Again the mean measurements of our FBW control children are fairly close to North American norms. Interestingly, the AGA 'true prematures' take the lead over the FBW infants before the conceptional age of 53 weeks (Table 3-I), and Figure 3-8 suggests that this already happened at term. The head circumference of the AGA preterm group then remains significantly bigger than that of FBW controls for the first year after term. This phenomenon, sometimes known as 'pseudo-hydrocephalus of prematurity', has been noted by other authors. Babson (1970) found that this catch-up in head size coincided with the unridging of sutures and an extension of the area of reflected light on transillumination of the skull. He concluded that it might be due to 'late oedema of prematurity' and to the increased subarachnoid and subdural space in the preterm infant. The relatively large head-circumference also may be at least partly attributable to preterm infants being hypotonic and nursed on their side, so that the head is liable to become dolichocephalic from lateral postural flattening. The circumference of the more elongated ellipse would thus be increased from that of the normal more rounded head (Baum and Searls 1971).

Fujimara and Seryu (1977) noted that term AGA and SGA infants exhibited a steady slowing in growth rate of the head from birth, whereas preterm AGA infants of less than 36 weeks gestation showed an increasing velocity of head growth, with the maximum occurring 30 to 40 days after birth. The net effect was that at a given conceptional age their head circumference was greater than that of FBW term infants, at least within the first five postnatal months. Brandt (1978) found that the velocity of growth of AGA preterm infants' heads only exceeded that of fullterm controls significantly in the fourth month after term, and that from term to six years the head-circumference curves of the preterm AGA and fullterm infants were identical. In our cohort the FBW control group ended up with slightly bigger heads than the AGA preterm group, but the difference was only significant for boys in comparison with Nellhaus norms (Fig. 3-10 and Table 3-III).

For SGA infants, head circumference and its development are of particular importance. Davies (1980) found that SGA babies showed a marked increase in head circumference in the first three months after birth, with a more gradual continuation of this trend over the next three months. Brandt (1978) studied 43 such infants and found that they could be divided into two groups: (1) those with catch-up growth of head circumference and favourable mental development; and (2) those without catch-up growth of the head and with less favourable development. There were no cases for whom these associations did not hold.

Analysis of our SGA cases supports the view that head circumference below the 10th percentile calls for careful follow-up in view of the serious prognosis if no catch-up occurs. Gross and Eckerman (1983) have devised normative head-growth curves for sequential plotting of the circumference of VLBW infants. Brandt (1978) speculated on possible benefits of high-calorie feedings to improve brain growth during the critical postnatal period. It appears that on generous breast-milk feedings in the first month, SGA neonates may indeed at least equal the head-growth velocity of AGA infants, but complete catch-up of head size cannot be accomplished (Rosegger *et al.* 1980). Optimal milk formulae to increase brain development of LBW infants have been discussed by Davies and Davis (1970), Davies and Evans (1978), D'Souza and Black (1979) and Lucas *et al.* (1984).

Summary

Polynomial growth-curves with splines are presented for 111 preterm AGA, 39 term SGA and 112 FBW control singletons, demonstrating their mean weight, length/height and head circumference from birth to various age-levels in terms of both conceptional and chronological age. In addition, the three categories have been compared with North-American standards in statistical tabulations for each sex, and the velocity of growth in terms of weight and length/height has also been determined in relation to such norms.

For *weight*, term SGA infants tend to remain significantly below the other two categories from birth to the age of 6½ years, but for females the difference is not clear-cut at some age-levels. Term SGA infants make an attempt at catch-up between birth and the conceptional age of 53 weeks (three months after term), which fades out about three months later. AGA preterm infants are closer to FBW controls in mean weight from term onwards but remain lighter, though the difference at four and 6½ years is significant only for boys.

For *length/height*, the *male* SGA infants are significantly smaller than the male preterm AGA infants from birth to 6½ years, but again the difference is not so clear-cut for girls. Term SGA infants again appear to make an attempt at catch-up between birth and three months after term, but this fades out within a year. Preterm AGA infants of both sexes get very close to FBW controls in mean length about six months after term but do not catch-up completely; at 6½ years the difference remains significant only for boys.

Mean *head circumference* is significantly bigger among FBW controls than for preterm AGA infants at birth, but at term the latter begin to have a slightly bigger mean head-size than the controls, and this excess continues through the first year after term. Subsequently the FBW control children have the biggest mean head-size until the last measurement at 6½ years, but the difference from the mean head-size of preterm AGA children is not significant for girls, and the measurements in both sexes are close to the Nellhaus (1968) norms. Growth velocity of the heads of SGA infants (as distinct from growth rate in terms of weight or length) is never significantly greater than the velocity for AGA preterm children of either sex, even during the initial attempt at catch-up between birth and three months after term.

Our data also show that head circumference below the 10th percentile at birth indicates a more adverse outcome, as measured by WISC Full-scale IQ scores and neurological status at 6½ years, than head size between the 10th and 90th percentiles. The most serious situation arises when the head circumference is below the 3rd percentile at birth or at one year and there is no catch-up head-growth into the normal range. At 6½ years there is a linear relationship between WISC Full-scale IQ and head circumference for both sexes, but for males there is also a quadratic relationship, indicating that IQ begins to decrease beyond a certain maximum.

Acknowledgements: The authors are indebted to Drs. Debra M. Millar, Elizabeth Cosulich and Jennifer G. Bell for their assistance with these studies.

4

Evolution of Developmental and Psychological Test Scores

Annetta K. McBurney and Linda C. Eaves

Longitudinal studies of the relationship between low birthweight and subsequent psychological test scores were discussed in Chapter 1. Several large studies have followed 'premature' infants from infancy to school-age, with the general finding that *small* intellectual deficits and mild learning disabilities are associated with low birthweights. These problems increased with decreasing birthweight.

Compared to controls, 'premature' children did less well at eight and 11 years (Douglas 1956, 1960), and the lighter the infant the greater the deficit in developmental quotient at four years (Drillien 1961*a*, 1964). Differences of five IQ points were found at six to seven years, and of six points at ages eight to 10, in favour of the fullterm controls (Wiener *et al.* 1968). McDonald (1967) eliminated twins and those with cerebral palsy, blindness, deafness or an IQ below 50 from her analysis. The average IQ of the remaining sample with birthweights ≤1800g was 102.4, although those with birthweights ≤1350g were an average of five IQ points lower than those between 1350 and 1800g. Mild learning disabilities were more prevalent among LBW children, but the larger ones did not have marked impairment of cognitive functioning. However, as birthweight decreased below about 2000g there was an increasing frequency of mental retardation, not solely accounted for by poorer social environment.

Studies of LBW children which distinguished between (1) 'true prematures' ('born too soon'; Neligan *et al.* 1976) of appropriate weight for gestational age and (2) 'small-for-dates' (SFD) children, who were fullterm but light in weight ('born too small'; Neligan *et al.* 1976) have shown that 'true prematures' scored lower on tests of mental development up to 12 months uncorrected chronological age, but slightly higher at 2½, four and 6½ years (Eaves *et al.* 1970, Brandt and Schröder 1971). Neligan *et al.* (1976) found impaired performance in both groups, with those 'born too small' scoring the lowest, though not significantly below the short-gestation group up to six years of age. Francis-Williams and Davies (1974) found the IQ of the SGA VLBW sample to be significantly lower than that of the preterm AGA at four to 12 years.

That the effects of high social-class ameliorate the effects of low birthweight has been shown in several studies (Dann *et al.* 1958, 1964; Werner *et al.* 1968; Eaves *et al.* 1970; Davie *et al.* 1972; Neligan *et al.* 1976; Friedman and Sigman 1981). Werner and colleagues (1968) found that the prediction of intelligence and achievement at 10 years was improved by combining test scores at 20 months with the paediatrician's rating of intelligence, perinatal stress score, social quotient and social class. Drillien (1970) noted that the effects of being SGA were demonstrable

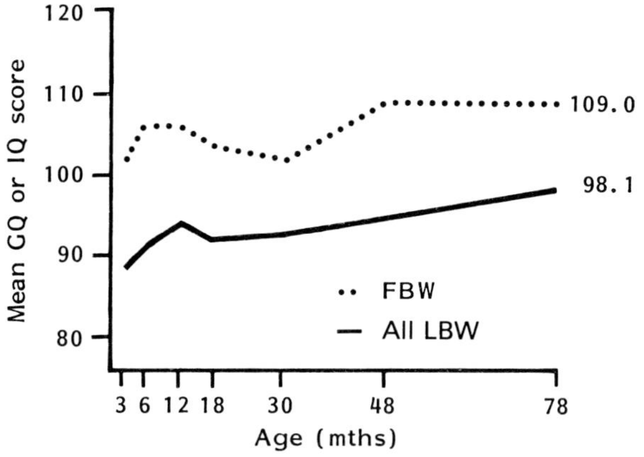

Fig. 4-1. Mean GQ and IQ scores of all LBW *vs.* FBW children. Range of N: FBW controls 114-148, all LBW 165-248.

for lower-class but not upper-class children up to 12 years of age.

Method

The data reported here were collected as part of the longitudinal survey. The ages at examination and the tests used are given in Chapter 2. As also mentioned in Chapter 2, the children's social-class was determined by the Hollingshead scale: five classes were used, with class I representing the highest and class V the lowest socio-economic status (SES). The LBW and control populations did not differ significantly in SES distribution: respectively, 74 and 81 per cent of the children fell into social classes IV and V (see Table 2-VII).

Study sample

The following groups were excluded from the analyses: (1) non-caucasian children; (2) those whose global IQ was below 50; and (3) those with a major cerebral defect or significant hearing or visual problems. The study sample then consisted of 273 LBW children and 148 FBW control children. In the LBW category there remained 140 preterm AGA, 106 SGA and 27 children of unknown gestational age. 58 of the SGA infants had a gestational age of less than 37 weeks and were preterm. For some comparisons we have considered the preterm and fullterm subgroups of SGA children separately.

Since not all children were available at the time of each examination, the numbers in the different comparisons varied. Children included in the longitudinal comparisons were those who had obtained scores on at least two of the Griffiths tests (of which one must have been the 12- or 18-months examination) and on at least two of the three later intelligence tests.

Results

LBW children vs. *FBW controls*

The mean LBW and FBW scores were compared on the Griffiths GQ at three, six, 12 and 18 months, on the Stanford-Binet IQ at 2½ and four years and on the Wechsler

TABLE 4-I
Comparison of GQ and IQ scores of LBW children with FBW controls

		LBW			FBW				
		N	*Mean*	*SD*	*N*	*Mean*	*SD*	*t*	*p*
Griffiths GQ	3 mths	165	88.7	14.0	114	101.6	10.0	8.5	<0.001
	6 mths	200	90.6	14.2	148	106.0	10.5	11.1	<0.001
	12 mths	198	93.7	12.6	132	106.2	8.0	10.1	<0.001
	18 mths	210	91.9	11.9	133	103.3	7.6	9.8	<0.001
Stanford-Binet IQ	2½ yrs	212	92.3	13.4	116	101.9	11.6	6.5	<0.001
	4 yrs	230	94.5	13.9	120	109.0	15.7	8.8	<0.001
WISC Full-scale IQ	6½ yrs	248	98.1	14.6	122	109.0	11.3	7.3	<0.001

Intelligence Scale for Children (Full-scale IQ) at 6½ years (Table 4-I, Fig. 4-1). In each comparison significant differences emerged in favour of FBW children. The magnitude of these differences diminished from 13 to 10.9 IQ points during the period under consideration, the mean difference being 12.5 IQ points.

When the individual Griffiths and WISC subscales were considered, the FBW group again obtained higher scores in all cases. With the exception of the Coding and Mazes subtests, for which differences were not statistically significant, the probability level was less than 0.01. The FBW controls also performed at a higher level on all the remaining psychometric measures. With the exceptions of the Goodenough-Harris test and the Knox Cubes, this was a persistently highly significant finding ($p<0.001$) (Table 4-II).

Sex differences

Within the LBW sample significant differences were found between the sexes on five out of 29 possible comparisons. (Only one or two of these would be expected to be significant by chance.) There were no significant differences until the age of 18 months, when males surpassed females on the Griffiths Locomotor subtest. The Stanford-Binet IQ at four years showed the females scoring significantly higher than the males, but the WISC Full-scale IQ at 6½ years showed no significant differences between the two groups. It is also interesting that the girls had significantly better scores on both administrations of the Vineland Social Maturity Scale, whereas the boys did better in the Block Design subtest of the WISC at 6½ years.

There were also five significant differences among 29 comparisons between boys and girls in the FBW control group. Males showed superiority in several areas at three months, but this must be interpreted with caution in view of the marked effect of birthweight and other factors at this early age. At 18 months the girls were more advanced in the Hearing-Speech subscale. Only one subscale of the WISC (Comprehension) discriminated between the sexes at 6½ years, in favour of the boys.

Birthweight and test performance

To investigate the relationship between weight and performance on cognitive and developmental measures, the LBW children were divided into four categories on the

TABLE 4-II

Comparison of LBW children with FBW controls on all psychometric tests

	LBW			FBW				
	N	*Mean*	*SD*	*N*	*Mean*	*SD*	*t*	*p*
Griffiths—3 mths								
Locomotor	165	8.4	2.6	114	9.3	2.5	3.04	<0.002
Personal-social	165	7.9	2.9	114	9.8	2.2	5.84	<0.001
Hearing-speech	165	6.8	2.6	114	8.8	2.4	6.33	<0.001
Eye-hand	161	6.3	2.5	113	8.6	2.6	7.46	<0.001
Performance	166	6.3	1.9	114	8.2	2.5	7.12	<0.001
General Quotient	165	88.7	14.0	114	101.6	10.0	8.47	<0.001
Griffiths—6 mths								
Locomotor	200	15.8	3.9	148	19.5	4.1	8.62	<0.001
Personal-social	200	15.8	3.9	148	18.3	3.3	6.42	<0.001
Hearing-speech	200	14.2	4.0	148	17.0	2.8	7.25	<0.001
Eye-hand	200	14.1	4.3	148	17.7	2.8	8.76	<0.001
Performance	200	13.6	4.7	148	18.0	3.1	9.85	<0.001
General Quotient	200	90.6	14.2	148	106.0	10.5	11.12	<0.001
Griffiths—12 mths								
Locomotor	198	9.8	2.0	132	11.9	1.7	9.91	<0.001
Personal-social	198	9.6	1.6	132	10.6	1.1	6.11	<0.001
Hearing-speech	198	9.3	1.9	132	10.5	1.3	6.53	<0.001
Eye-hand	198	9.2	1.5	132	10.2	1.2	6.01	<0.001
Performance	198	9.1	1.9	132	10.1	1.3	4.86	<0.001
General Quotient	198	93.7	12.6	132	106.2	8.0	10.06	<0.001
Griffiths—18 mths								
Locomotor	210	15.4	2.5	133	17.2	1.6	7.45	<0.001
Personal-social	210	13.8	2.1	133	15.1	1.6	5.89	<0.001
Hearing-speech	210	13.8	2.6	133	14.7	2.0	3.55	<0.001
Eye-hand	210	14.1	2.3	133	14.9	1.3	4.04	<0.001
Performance	210	14.6	2.9	133	16.0	1.7	5.21	<0.001
General Quotient	210	91.9	11.9	133	103.3	7.6	9.80	<0.001
Stanford-Binet—30 mths	212	92.3	13.4	116	101.9	11.6	6.50	<0.001
Vineland Social Maturity—30 mths	219	112.4	17.4	121	124.5	16.4	6.25	<0.001
Stanford-Binet—48 mths	230	94.6	13.9	120	109.0	15.7	8.84	<0.001
Vineland Social Maturity—48 mths	231	117.7	16.4	118	124.3	11.6	3.91	<0.001
Goodenough-Harris—48 mths	107	90.7	15.3	100	91.3	18.5	0.26	NS
Wechsler—6½ years								
Verbal IQ	246	96.8	14.6	121	108.7	11.9	7.78	<0.001
Performance IQ	245	99.7	14.8	121	108.5	11.8	5.71	<0.001
Full scale IQ	248	98.1	14.6	122	109.0	11.3	7.28	<0.001
Comprehension	245	9.1	3.2	121	11.7	3.1	7.26	<0.001
Arithmetic	244	9.8	3.0	121	12.1	2.4	7.26	<0.001
Digit span	243	9.1	3.0	121	10.7	3.1	4.88	<0.001
Picture completion	243	9.9	2.8	121	11.2	2.5	4.04	<0.001
Block design	244	10.1	3.0	121	11.0	2.4	3.04	<0.003
Coding	242	10.6	5.8	121	11.4	2.9	1.45	NS
Mazes	239	9.9	5.8	121	11.0	2.1	1.97	NS
Goodenough-Harris—6½ yrs								
Man	236	99.2	6.1	121	103.8	8.3	0.59	NS
Woman	234	95.9	6.1	121	100.8	8.3	0.64	NS
Average	239	97.2	6.1	121	102.0	8.3	0.64	NS
Self	231	96.4	6.1	121	101.1	8.3	0.61	NS
Knox cubes	229	8.2	3.3	121	7.9	3.1	0.91	NS
Sentence repetition	236	10.2	2.6	121	11.4	2.4	4.10	<0.001

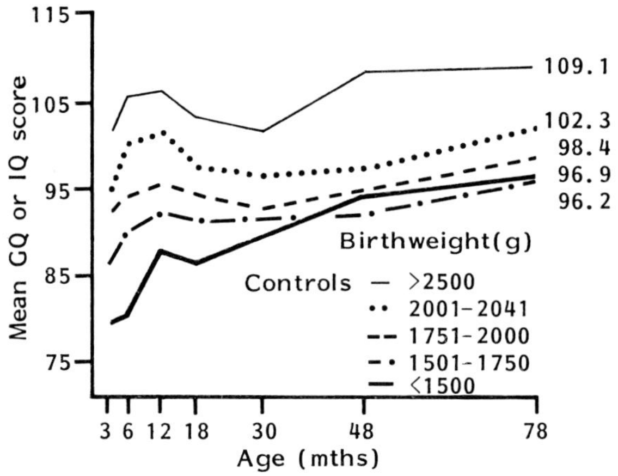

Fig. 4-2. Mean GQ and IQ scores according to birthweight of all LBW and FBW children. Range of N: FBW controls 114-148, 2001-2041g 25-29, 1751-2000g 65-100, 1501-1750g 37-56, ≤1500g 37-61.

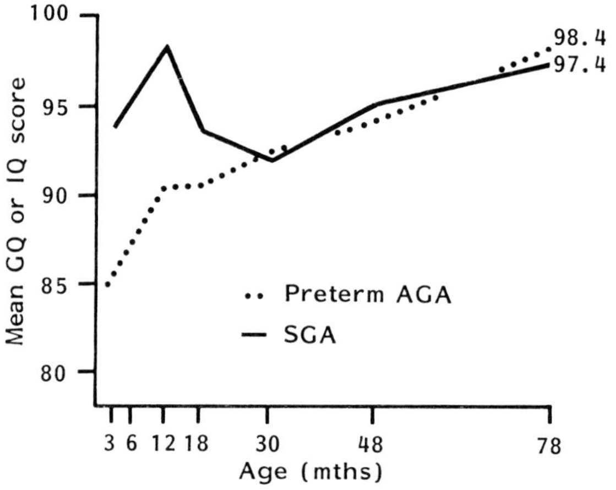

Fig. 4-3. Mean GQ and IQ scores: SGA *vs.* preterm AGA. Range of N: preterm AGA 96-141, SGA 68-105.

basis of birthweight: ≤1500g, 1501 to 1750g, 1751 to 2000g and 2001 to 2041g.

Within the entire group of 273 LBW children there was a consistent trend for the heavier group to have better DQ and IQ scores at all ages (Table 4-IV). Beginning at 18 months there was some convergence of scores, which continued to 6½ years (Fig. 4-2). The mean IQ of these groups remained in the order of their birthweights throughout, except that the lowest weight-group surpassed the second lowest slightly at four and 6½ years. Analyses of variance showed a highly significant ($p<0.001$) interaction between weight category and performance only until the age of 18 months, but the trend continued into the school-years (see Chapter 11).

Similarly, when the LBW children were divided into two groups (≤1750g and >1750g), significant differences were found only up to the age of 18 months, but comparisons continued to favour the higher birthweight category (see Table 4-III).

A comparison of the weight distribution in the SGA and preterm groups

TABLE 4-III

GQ and IQ comparison of lighter and heavier babies within LBW group

	Weight ≤1750g			Weight 1751-2041g				
	N	*Mean*	*SD*	*N*	*Mean*	*SD*	*t*	*p*
Griffiths—								
3 mths	74	83.3	13.0	90	92.9	13.2	4.65	<0.001
6 mths	95	85.1	14.0	103	95.4	12.5	5.44	<0.001
12 mths	91	90.1	12.4	105	96.6	12.1	3.71	<0.001
18 mths	95	88.1	12.5	113	95.0	10.4	4.32	<0.001
Stanford-Binet—								
2½ yrs	93	90.8	12.3	118	93.3	14.1	1.36	NS
4 yrs	104	93.5	13.2	124	95.3	14.4	1.00	NS
WISC Full-scale IQ—6½ yrs	117	96.6	15.3	129	99.2	13.9	1.46	NS

indicated slight differences. The AGA preterm babies included more in the lightest category and fewer in the heaviest group (see Chapter 2).

Significant differences occurred between the two categories in the three lowest weight classifications, the SGA children being consistently superior initially. Again the differences were significant only up to the age of 18 months. This is presented graphically in Figure 4-3. Presumably the SGA children obtained higher scores than those who were preterm during this early period because their nervous systems were more mature. While it might have been possible to correct for gestational age in these comparisons, such correction would not be meaningful after about one year, and Dr. Griffiths, the designer of the developmental scales, advised against it.

A comparison of the weight categories within the group of AGA preterm infants revealed that the heaviest babies were clearly superior at all ages. The three lower weight categories displayed a consistent trend to convergence over time, with the lightest babies improving most markedly. The scores of the SGA children showed more stability within weight classification than did those of the preterm, who tended to have relatively better scores than SGA children at four to 6½ years.

SGA preterm vs. *SGA term infants*

When the SGA group was further subdivided into those with gestational ages <37 weeks and ≥37 weeks it was found that the term SGA babies had significantly superior GQ/IQ scores only at the three- and six-month levels ($p<0.01$) (Fig. 4-4). A similar trend was demonstrable until about the age of 2½ years.

Socio-economic status

The social-class distribution of the preterm, SGA and FBW groups did not differ significantly ($\chi^2 = 6.43$, NS).

The GQ and IQ scores of LBW and control children were compared within the Hollingshead social-class categories. To obtain sufficient numbers for the analyses,

TABLE 4-IV

Mean GQ or global IQ scores and standard deviations, for SGA and AGA preterm children and for FBW controls

Birthweight (g)		*N**	*GQ 3 mths*	*GQ 6 mths*	*GQ 12 mths*	*GQ 18 mths*	*SB IQ 30 mths*	*SB IQ 48 mths*	*WISC IQ 6½ yrs*
≤1500	SGA mean	8-18	91.5±14.6	86.4±14.4	95.5± 6.4	84.5±12.6	84.5± 9.3	92.7± 8.3	94.2±15.4
	Preterm mean	29-43	76.6±10.2	77.7±10.2	85.1±11.4	87.9±13.4	91.8±12.9	94.6±14.5	98.0±15.2
	t		3.34	2.38	3.08	0.85	1.79	0.45	0.88
	p		<0.001	<0.05	<0.01	NS	0.05	NS	NS
1501-1750	SGA mean	21-29	91.1±11.4	95.1±14.4	97.7±12.0	93.8±11.8	92.3± 9.0	93.8±13.1	96.1±16.3
	Preterm mean	16-27	81.2±12.1	85.7±12.4	87.8±12.9	85.3±10.5	91.0±14.7	91.5±13.5	96.3±14.8
	t		2.57	2.39	2.61	2.57	0.35	0.59	0.05
	p		<0.01	<0.05	<0.01	<0.01	NS	NS	NS
1751-2000	SGA mean	26-41	94.2±13.7	96.9±12.7	99.0±11.3	92.4± 9.6	93.7±14.7	96.6±15.4	99.2±14.6
	Preterm mean	39-59	91.1±13.8	92.0±11.6	92.7±12.8	92.7±10.4	91.3±14.0	93.1±14.5	97.8±13.7
	t		0.88	1.81	2.32	1.73	0.82	1.11	0.49
	p		NS	<0.05	<0.05	NS	NS	NS	NS
2001-2041	SGA mean	11-17	98.1±11.5	99.7±13.8	100.2± 8.9	96.2±10.8	92.6± 9.8	95.1±13.4	98.7±12.3
	Preterm mean	10-12	90.4±11.7	101.1±11.6	102.7±10.4	100.4±10.5	100.9±15.0	100.5±11.3	107.3±13.5
	t		1.66	0.26	0.62	0.93	1.65	1.19	1.79
	p		NS	NS	NS	NS	NS	NS	<0.05
>2500	FBW mean	114-148	101.6±10.0	106.0±10.5	106.2± 8.0	103.3± 7.6	101.9±11.6	109.0±15.7	109.0±11.3

*Numbers varied at each testing.

TABLE 4-V

Comparison of GQ & IQ means for LBW children *vs.* FBW controls within social-class groups

Hollingshead social class		*N*	*GQ* 3 mths	*GQ* 5 mths	*GQ* 12 mths	*GQ* 18 mths	*SB IQ* 30 mths	*SB IQ* 48 mths	*WISC IQ* 6½ yrs
I, II & III	LBW mean	48-67	91.8±14.4	91.3±13.4	93.9±11.0	91.9±11.7	97.0±15.1	99.5±13.7	105.1±13.2
	FBW mean	19-26	102.2±11.2	108.3± 8.3	110.4± 7.0	107.4± 6.1	108.8± 8.2	118.3±11.4	114.0±10.2
	t		2.84	6.00	6.77	6.19	3.65	6.04	3.02
	p		<0.01	<0.001	<0.001	<0.001	<0.001	<0.001	<0.01
IV	LBW mean	59-100	86.8±13.2	90.7±13.7	94.3±10.0	92.9±10.1	91.7±10.7	94.3±11.3	98.0±11.2
	FBW mean	43-58	102.1±11.6	107.1±12.1	107.0± 7.2	104.4± 7.8	102.9±12.6	110.0±16.8	110.1±11.7
	t		6.06	6.93	7.69	6.75	5.54	6.75	6.45
	p		<0.001	<0.001	<0.001	<0.001	<0.001	<0.001	<0.001
V	LBW mean	52-79	87.5±13.9	89.0±15.6	91.8±14.9	90.4±14.1	89.5±13.9	90.6±15.8	91.9±16.8
	FBW mean	32-42	102.1± 6.8	104.0± 8.8	103.4± 8.1	100.3± 5.8	96.0± 9.7	102.3±12.9	104.8± 9.8
	t		5.58	5.58	4.67	4.32	2.50	3.98	4.55
	p		<0.001	<0.001	<0.001	<0.001	<0.01	<0.001	<0.001

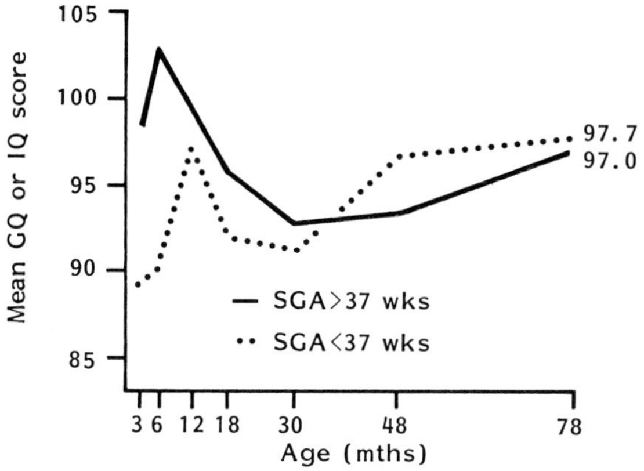

Fig. 4-4. Mean GQ and IQ scores for SGA infants <37 weeks gestation *vs.* SGA infants >37 weeks gestation. Range of N: SGA >37 weeks 35-58, SGA <37 weeks 33-47.

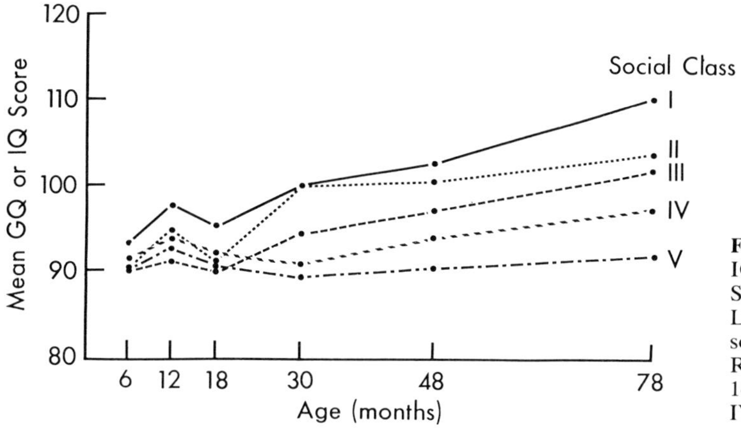

Fig. 4-5. Mean GQ and IQ scores of combined SGA and preterm AGA LBW children within socio-economic classes. Range of N: social class I 14-20, II 7-15, III 21-23, IV 58-100, V 52-79.

social classes I, II and III were combined. It was found that the controls performed significantly better than LBW children of the same social grouping (Table 4-V). Further analysis of covariance with social class as covariate showed significant differences in GQ and IQ scores ($p<0.001$) in favour of the FBW controls at each age. Similar results were obtained in the comparison of AGA preterm and control children. This trend persisted when SGA and control children were compared, except in the case of social class V, where the differences were not significant at 12, 18 and 30 months. However, a highly significant difference was seen again at four and 6½ years.

When the AGA preterm were compared to the SGA children within each of the three social-class categories, no significant differences appeared in the highest grouping. However, the SGA children showed a significant superiority in social class IV up to the age of 12 months, and in social class V this difference was maintained until the age of 30 months. In relation to this observation, it was noted that within

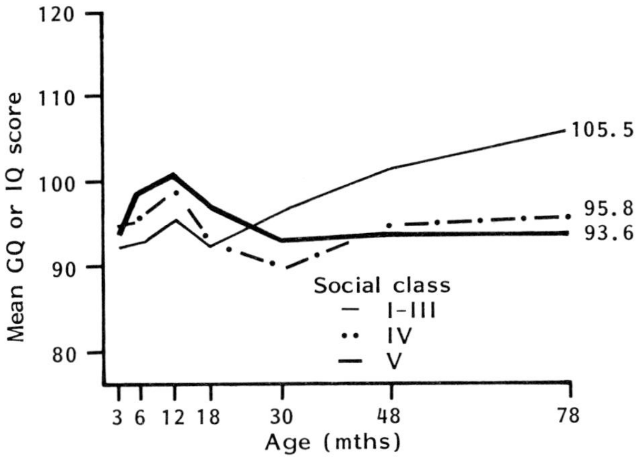

Fig. 4-6. Mean GQ and IQ scores within socio-economic classes for SGA infants. Range of N: social classes I-III 15-26, IV 23-43, V 23-36.

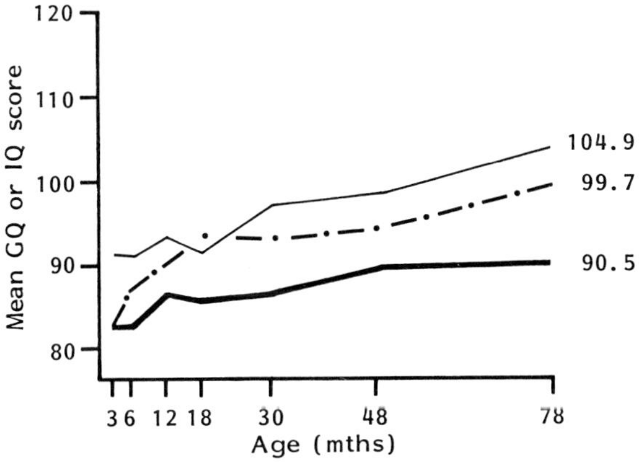

Fig. 4-7. Comparison of mean GQ or IQ score within socio-economic class for AGA preterm babies. Range of N: social classes I-III 27-42, IV 35-57, V 29-43.

the SGA category, children of the two lower social-classes showed a mean decrease or levelling in score with age, while children in the combined top three social-classes improved (Fig. 4-6).

The relative positions of the AGA preterm and control groups remained constant (Fig. 4-7), with the exception of the 18-month scores, when there was a slight blurring of the trend.

For all groups there was a tendency (although not a significant one) for scores to diverge according to social class with increasing age. This phenomenon is illustrated in Figure 4-5, which shows the GQ and IQ scores at each age for the combined SGA and preterm AGA LBW groups. The difference in mean GQ score between the highest and lowest social-classes was 3.1 GQ points at six months of age. The figure increased gradually over time to 18.3 IQ points at 6½ years.

Longitudinal findings

Correlation coefficients were calculated between each pair of scores for all children in the LBW group (Table 4-VI). As would be expected, more significant correlations were found with shorter test-retest intervals. Of all possible correlations, approximately 75 per cent were significant at the 1 per cent level of confidence.

The LBW group tended more to vary in performance, particularly reflecting improvement in the first 2½ years of development. Scores obtained on the Griffiths test at 12 and 18 months showed the least amount of change between testings for both groups. The scores of half the FBW children increased by 10 points or more between 2½ and 6½ years, while those of only 36 per cent of the LBW sample did so. Approximately 40 to 60 per cent of the LBW group showed a variation of 10 points or more in IQ and GQ scores between any two testings, and 10 to 30 per cent changed 20 points or more.

Discussion

The results of the psychological assessments in this sample were consistent with the findings of other researchers. The LBW children performed below the control group at all ages. When the LBW group was considered as a whole, the infants at three months were below average (GQ 88.7) and gradually increased in performance until at 6½ years they were scoring in the average range, but 11 points below the FBW control infants. The chief contributors to the below-average scores at earlier ages

TABLE 4-VI

Correlation matrix of developmental and intelligence test scores of LBW children at various ages

	GQ 3 mths	*GQ 6 mths*	*GQ 12 mths*	*GQ 18 mths*	*SB 2½ yrs*	*VINE 2½ yrs*	*SB 4 yrs*	*VINE 4 yrs*	*GE 4 yrs*	*BEND 6½ yrs*	*WISC VIQ*	*WISC PIQ*
GQ 3 mths												
GQ 6 mths	0.64*											
GQ 12 mths	0.53*	0.58*										
GQ 18 mths	0.38*	0.42*	0.63*									
SB 2½ yrs	0.07	0.17	0.29*	0.54*								
VINE 2½ yrs	0.06	0.07	0.38*	0.51*	0.34*							
SB 4 yrs	0.09	0.23*	0.26*	0.43*	0.66*	0.32*						
VINE 4 yrs	0.19	0.23*	0.27*	0.36*	0.19*	0.43*	0.17					
GE 4 yrs	−0.09	−0.08	−0.15	−0.18	−0.36*	−0.13	−0.48*	−0.62				
BEND 6½ yrs	−0.03	−0.06	−0.17	−0.25*	−0.33*	−0.09	0.34*	−0.11	0.32			
WISC VIQ	0.25*	0.20*	0.24*	0.39*	0.49*	0.09	0.54*	0.16	−0.33*	−0.45*		
WISC PIQ	0.10	0.13	0.28*	0.44*	0.41*	0.25*	0.46*	0.18*	−0.34*	−0.45*	0.62*	
WISC FSIQ	0.21*	0.18	0.28*	0.45*	0.49*	0.19*	0.56*	0.19*	−0.39*	−0.50*	0.91*	0.88*
WISC C	0.24*	0.19	0.15	0.23*	0.23*	−0.03	0.39*	0.06	−0.25*	−0.33*	0.72*	0.37*
WISC A	0.22*	0.13	0.18	0.25*	0.39*	0.11	0.43*	0.21*	−0.22*	−0.35*	0.68*	0.53*
WISC DS	0.12	0.11	0.23*	0.34*	0.39*	0.11	0.46*	0.12	−0.39*	−0.44*	0.76*	0.51*
WISC PC	0.09	0.15	0.24	0.35*	0.26*	0.21*	0.39*	0.14*	−0.30*	−0.31*	0.48*	0.71*
WISC BD	0.08	0.04	0.18*	0.31*	0.26*	0.12*	0.28*	0.12	−0.18	−0.30*	0.44*	0.63*
WISC CD	0.12	0.14	0.24*	0.30*	0.29*	0.24*	0.28*	0.23*	−0.16	−0.30*	0.36*	0.67*
WISC M	0.07	0.07	0.16	0.29*	0.35*	0.14	0.35*	0.17*	−0.23*	−0.35*	0.47*	0.77*
G-H M	0.11	0.06	0.10	0.21*	0.26*	−0.01	0.35*	0.05	−0.18	−0.23*	0.39*	0.41*
G-H W	0.04	0.00	0.11	0.21*	0.20*	0.00	0.25*	0.07	−0.19	−0.28*	0.37*	0.38*
G-H A	0.08	0.03	0.11	0.21*	0.25*	0.01	0.32*	0.06	−0.19	−0.27*	0.40*	0.40*
G-H S	0.06	0.09	0.08	0.25*	0.22*	−0.02	0.27*	0.03	−0.15	−0.24*	0.33*	0.37*
KNOX	0.25*	0.20*	0.28*	0.36*	0.19*	0.14	0.27*	0.22*	−0.12	−0.34*	0.40*	0.43*
VOC ENC	0.03	0.03	0.12	0.26*	0.37*	0.08	0.31*	−0.01	−0.11	−0.30*	0.43*	0.34*
SEN REP	0.11	0.02	0.06	0.19*	0.40*	0.13	0.51*	0.05	−0.23*	−0.28*	0.57*	0.37*

*Significant at $p<0.01$ level. BEND = Bender Visual Motor Gestalt Test; G-H = Goodenough-Harris Draw-a-Person test (M = man, W = woman, A = average, S = self); GE = Graham Ernhart Block Sort Test; GQ = Griffiths Mental Development Scale; KNOX = Knox Cubes Test; SEN REP = Benton Sentence Repetition Test; SB = Stanford-Binet Intelligence Scale; VINE = Vineland Social Maturity Scale; VOC ENC = Vocal

were those in the LBW group weighing ≤1750g. Up to 18 months they were from six to 10 points below the heavier LBW children, but by 6½ years had almost caught up.

When a distinction was made between the preterm AGA and those who were SGA, the results showed that the preterm AGA children scored significantly higher than did those SGA children in the highest LBW category (2001 to 2041g) at age 6½ years. While initially the preterm AGA children were at a disadvantage, after four years of age they reached the level of the SGA children. The scores for the SGA children changed very little from three months to 6½ years, with increases of five points or less. The preterm AGA children, however, showed substantial increases of over 20 points for the smallest, to 17 for the largest. These changes occurred, of course, within the context of family and environment. It has been shown again in this work that the effects of high social-class compensated to some extent for the effects of being born too soon or too small.

How socio-economic status contributes is not completely clear. Factors such as education of the mother, genetic endowment, less stress on the family because of adequate income and nutrition, fewer children and hence more individual attention for each one, and more support for family life, may all be important (see Birch and Gussow 1970). The relationship between social class and IQ was important. Both the preterm AGA and SGA children in the top three social-classes were well into the

TABLE 4-VI

(Contd.)

WISC FSIQ	*WISC C*	*WISC A*	*WISC DS*	*WISC PC*	*WISC BD*	*WISC CD*	*WISC M*	*G-H M*	*G-H W*	*G-H A*	*G-H S*	*KNOX*	*VOC ENC*	*SEN REP*
0.61*														
0.66*	0.30*													
0.71*	0.40	0.51*												
0.65*	0.35*	0.36*	0.40*											
0.58*	0.27*	0.44*	0.41	0.35*										
0.55*	0.15*	0.36*	0.30*	0.28*	0.21*									
0.64*	0.31*	0.41*	0.34*	0.41*	0.47*	0.39*								
0.43*	0.22*	0.36*	0.33*	0.27*	0.41*	0.23*	0.33*							
0.40*	0.27*	0.34*	0.31*	0.25*	0.36*	0.23*	0.30*	0.79*						
0.43*	0.26*	0.37*	0.33*	0.26*	0.40*	0.24*	0.32*	0.95*	0.93*					
0.38*	0.18*	0.32*	0.28*	0.25*	0.33*	0.23*	0.27*	0.81*	0.85*	0.87*				
0.45*	0.19	0.44*	0.36*	0.26*	0.35*	0.33*	0.28*	0.25*	0.27*	0.25*	0.28*			
0.42*	0.25*	0.27*	0.35*	0.24*	0.34*	0.17	0.27*	0.26*	0.23*	0.27*	0.18*	0.21*		
0.53*	0.39*	0.36*	0.55*	0.30*	0.24*	0.17*	0.27*	0.23*	0.14	0.18*	0.15	0.27	0.21*	

Encoding Test; WISC (Wechsler Intelligence Scale for Children)—FSIQ = Full-scale IQ, VIQ = Verbal IQ, PIQ = Performance IQ; WISC subtests—A = Arithmetic, BD = Block Design, C = Comprehension, DS = Digit Span, M = Mazes, PC = Picture Completion.

average range (mean IQ 105) by age 6½ years. However, the average IQ for the FBW in social classes I, II and III was 114, so those born too soon or too small were still at a disadvantage.

In examining IQ results, LBW status cannot be considered apart from social class. However, the interaction with neurological abnormalities was also a factor in the outcome: although IQ increased with increasing socio-economic status, number of years of education of the mother and increasing birthweight, it decreased with an increase in neurological abnormalities assessed at any age. Since the very smallest babies had more neurological abnormalities, it seemed likely that the lower IQ scores associated with lower birthweight were partly a function of the neurological problems rather than of weight alone. The use of a multiple regression model allowed for comparison of these factors simultaneously (see p. 247).

The fact that many LBW children do remain at a disadvantage may be as much the result of how their parents see them as of any innate handicap. Sameroff and Chandler (1975) convincingly argued that the parents' perception of the child played a major rôle in deviant development. The lack of 'bonding', and the anxiety and stress associated with caring for a tiny, possibly sick, infant may affect parent-child interaction. Since the children did develop at a slower rate (in the present study the smallest babies did not catch up in terms of IQ scores until four years of age), reduced expectations for them could have led to self-fulfilling prophecies of lower performance. Drillien (1964) found 'maternal efficiency' to be at least as important as social class as a force affecting development. How this concept is related to parents' perceptions and social class is unknown, but it deserves further attention.

There is much evidence that with changing techniques in the neonatal nursery and support for the families of LBW babies, the outlook for them has improved (see Chapter 1). Reports on children born in the late 1960s indicated fewer neurological problems and a higher level of mental development than in our sample (Rawlings *et al.* 1971, Stewart and Reynolds 1974, Taub *et al.* 1977), but this requires further confirmation.

The average IQ in our LBW sample, born from 1959 to 1965, was 98. Others have had similar findings for babies of even lower birthweight born between 1960 and 1966: Fitzhardinge and Ramsay (1973) reported an average IQ of 90 and Francis-Williams and Davies (1974) an average of 95 to 96. An important difference between our sample and that of Stewart and Reynolds (1974) was in the proportion of low-IQ (≤80) children. They found only 5.3 per cent with an IQ below 80 at a mean age of 5 years 2 months in a sample of children with birthweights ≤1500g born between 1966 and 1970. In the present sample, with birthweights ≤2041g, the proportion was 15 per cent.

Even in studies in which IQ was not found to be significantly lower in the LBW sample there was evidence for a relationship between birthweight and perceptual-motor problems (Lyle 1970, Lee 1977, Taub *et al.* 1977). Taub and co-workers, comparing only 38 LBW and 26 'naturally born' children at seven to 9½ years, found no significant difference in Verbal IQ scores, but significantly lower mean Performance IQs on the WISC-R in the LBW group, with subtests requiring visually mediated behaviour being particularly affected. The notion that LBW children show a relative deficit in the area of perceptual organization and visually mediated function was also supported by the fact that scores on the Bender Visual Motor Gestalt test were significantly poorer for the LBW group. In the experience of Wiener *et al.* (1968), and in our own study, no such particular reduction in WISC Performance IQ was demonstrated in the LBW cohort. However, we noted significantly higher error scores on the Bender Gestalt test for LBW as compared to FBW control children, and we found a close association between these scores, neurological abnormalities and the behaviour syndrome of 'attention deficit disorder' in the LBW group. So, while the frequency of severe intellectual and neurological sequelae in LBW populations may be declining, the presence of subtle difficulties which do not become clearly evident until school age may continue to make the prognosis for LBW children less optimistic.

Summary

FBW children scored significantly higher than LBW children on developmental and psychological tests at all ages from three months to six years. The average difference over all ages was 12.5 IQ points. These differences held for all subtests, with the exception of the Coding and Mazes subtests of the WISC, the Goodenough-Harris test and the Knox Cubes at 6½ years.

A few sex differences were found in both the LBW and FBW samples. These did not form a consistent pattern, nor did the same differences appear in both groups.

Within the LBW sample there was a consistent trend for the heavier babies to score higher at all ages, but the differences between the heavier and lighter babies were not significant after 2½ years. The significant differences were due to the lightest babies (≤2000g) in the AGA preterm group obtaining the lowest scores (unaccounted for by gestational age), and the SGA group scoring higher until 2½ years (uncorrected for gestational age).

Gestational age of 37 weeks or more within the SGA group was an advantage in terms of higher uncorrected developmental test scores only at three and six months. By 12 months those with a gestational age of less than 37 weeks had caught-up and differences between age-groups within the SFD sample were not significant after that age.

The social-class distribution was not significantly different for the LBW and FBW control groups. In each case the controls performed better than the LBW children of the same social grouping. The SGA children had a slight advantage over the preterm AGA children in the lower social-classes until 2½ years of age, when their scores levelled off and those in the top three classes improved.

The social-class differences within the LBW group were remarkable. At six months the difference between the highest and lowest classes was 3.1 IQ points, which increased gradually to 18.3 IQ points at 6½ years. While the effect of birthweight on IQ scores appeared to diminish with age, the relationship of IQ to social class became more marked.

5

Clinical Outcome: Neurological Sequelae and their Evolution

Henry G. Dunn, Ann-Marie Robertson and John U. Crichton

Table 5-I lists the neurological and ophthalmic disorders among the LBW children. 140 (41.8 per cent) of the 335 LBW children had a total of 181 abnormalities (not including strabismus) at 6½ years.

Among 139 FBW control children followed beyond the same age, only 15 (10.8 per cent) were found to have a neurological abnormality, namely minimal brain dysfunctions in nine, more than minimal dysfunctions (IQ 70 to 79) in two, mental retardation in two, and epilepsy (idiopathic) in two.

The proportion of affected children in the main diagnostic categories at various ages is shown in Figure 5-1. The increasing frequency of neurological defects at successive age-levels among LBW children is largely due to the emergence of 'minimal brain dysfunctions' after the age of 2½ years.

Table 5-II provides a further analysis of neurological status at 6½ years for boys *vs.* girls, single *vs.* multiple births, and different birthweight-gestation categories (according to the norms of Naeye *et al.* 1966 and Babson *et al.* 1970). The frequency of neurological abnormalities in boys (51.5 per cent) is significantly higher than in girls (32.6 per cent, $p<0.001$), whereas the proportions of abnormal children among singletons *vs.* twins, and in truly premature infants of appropriate gestational age (AGA) *vs.* 'small for gestational age' (SGA) children are not significantly different.

The prevalence of the various types of neurological defects in AGA preterm and SGA children is listed in Table 5-III. Mental retardation is somewhat more common among the SGA children, whereas cerebral palsy occurred more frequently among the preterm AGA children. However, the differences are not significant. These details are shown in Figure 5-2.

As will be seen later, there is a marked predominance of preterm AGA children among those with spastic diplegia, retrolental fibroplasia and sensorineural deafness.

The SGA children delivered prematurely did not differ significantly from those born at term; if singletons are added to twins in Table 5-II, 28 of 69 (40.6 per cent) preterm SGA and 27 of 61 (44.3 per cent) term SGA children were neurologically abnormal at 6½ years. Since this was surprising and others have stressed the poor outcome for preterm SGA children (Commey and Fitzhardinge 1979, Hack *et al.* 1979), we analyzed the actual abnormalities and mean IQ in each group (Table 5-IV). It appears that preterm SGA children may have a slightly higher frequency of cerebral palsy, but there is little difference between the groups in intellectual level. Somewhat similar, relatively encouraging neurological findings on follow-up of

TABLE 5-I

Neurological and ophthalmic disorders in 140 of 335 LBW children followed to 6½ years

		N	*% of total cohort*
Minimal brain dysfunctions (WISC Full-scale IQ ≥80)		61	18.2
Mental retardation* (global IQ <70)		30	9.0
With cerebral palsy	9		
With epilepsy	6		
With chromosomal defect (2 Down's, 1 XXX)	3		
With severe visual defect	4		
With severe hearing defect	1		
With fetal alcohol syndrome	3		
With multiple congenital defects	3		
Other	8		
Cerebral palsy		27	8.1
Spastic diplegia (2 mixed with extrapyramidal features)	13		
Spastic quadriplegia	3		
Spastic hemiplegia	6		
Spastic crural monoplegia	4		
Ataxia	1		
Visual defects (excluding strabismus and refractive errors)		16	4.8
Congenital optic atrophy	1		
Congenital glaucoma	1		
Retrolental fibroplasia	12		
Cortical blindness	2		
Epilepsy*		14	4.2
With mental retardation	6		
With cerebral palsy	2		
With other brain dysfunctions	2		
Idiopathic	6		
Post-hypoglycaemic	1		
Sensorineural hearing-defect		12	3.6
Bilateral	8		
Unilateral	4		
Miscellaneous cerebral dysfunctions more than minimal, *e.g.* borderline low-normal intelligence (IQ 70-79), autism, dysphasia		21	6.3
Total disorders		181	

140 with abnormalities among 335 followed survivors = 41.8 per cent.
*Some children had more than one disorder.

preterm SGA infants have been reported by Lubchenco *et al.* (1972*b*), Vohr *et al.* (1979) and Vohr and Oh (1983).

Evolution of neurological findings

The methods used for assessing neurological abnormality and the ages at which the various examinations were carried out are given in Chapter 2.

In the nursery, the infants were classified into four categories after clinical examination: N = normal—no abnormal neurological findings at any time; A =

TABLE 5-II

Neurological status of LBW children at 6½ years

	Singletons						*Twins*								*Triplets*								
	AGA preterm		*SGA*				*AGA preterm*		*SGA*				*LGA*				*Gest. age uncertain*			*Total*			
			<37 wks		*≥37 wks*				*<37 wks*		*≥37 wks*												
	N	*A*	*N*	*A*	*N*	*A*	*N*	*A*	*N*	*A*	*N*	*A*	*N*	*A*	*N*	*A*	*N*	*A*		*N*	*A*	%	
Male	31	31	16	10	7	16	16	17	1	2	4	1	1				3	7	163	79	84	51.5	$\chi^2 = 12.38$
Female	40	20	22	15	18	8	19	9	2	1	5	2	2		3		5	1	172	116	56	32.6	$p < 0.001$
Total normal	71		38		25		35		3		9		3		3		8			195			
Total abnormal		51		25		24		26		3		3						8			140		
% abnormal		41.8		39.7		49.0		42.6		50.0		25.0						50.0			41.8		
Total	122		63		49		61		6		12		3		3		16		335				
			112 (43.75% abnormal)						18 (33.3% abnormal)														

N = normal, A = abnormal.

TABLE 5-III

Main neurological defects in LBW children at least 6½ years of age

	Preterm AGA (N = 189)		*SGA (N = 130)*			
	N	%	*N*	%	χ^2	*p*
Minimal brain dysfunctions	39	20.6	21	16.1	1.013	NS
Mental retardation	12	6.3	14	10.8	2.010	NS
Cerebral palsy	18	9.5	7	5.4	1.824	NS
Miscellaneous	17	9.0	16	12.3	0.911	NS
Total defects	77*	40.7	55*	42.3	0.078	NS

*Several children had more than one defect, hence total less than sum. (Children with uncertain gestational age not included.)

TABLE 5-IV

Neurological sequelae among 28 preterm and 27 term SGA LBW children

	Preterm SGA (<37 wks)	*Term SGA (≥37 wks)*
Minimal brain dysfunctions	9	15
Mental retardation (global IQ <70)	4	8
More than minimal brain dysfunctions	8	2
Cerebral palsy	5	1
Epilepsy	1	1
Sensorineural hearing-loss	1	—
Total	28	27
Mean WISC Full-scale IQ	83.4	74.5
Mean WISC Full-scale IQ, excluding cases with IQ <50	84.8	83.0

TABLE 5-V

Neonatal neurological abnormalities in relation to later neurological status

Neonatal findings	*N*	*Neurol. status at 1 yr* *Normal*	*Suspect*	*Abnormal*		*Neurol. status at 6½ yrs* *Normal*	*Abnormal*	
Normal throughout	59	50	7	2 (15%)	$\chi^2 = 17.1$, $p < 0.0005$	39	20 (34%)	$\chi^2 = 5.3$, $p < 0.05$
Early or late abnormality only	92	66	19	7 (28%)		54	38 (41%)	
Abnormal throughout	100	54	30	16 (46%)		48	52 (52%)	

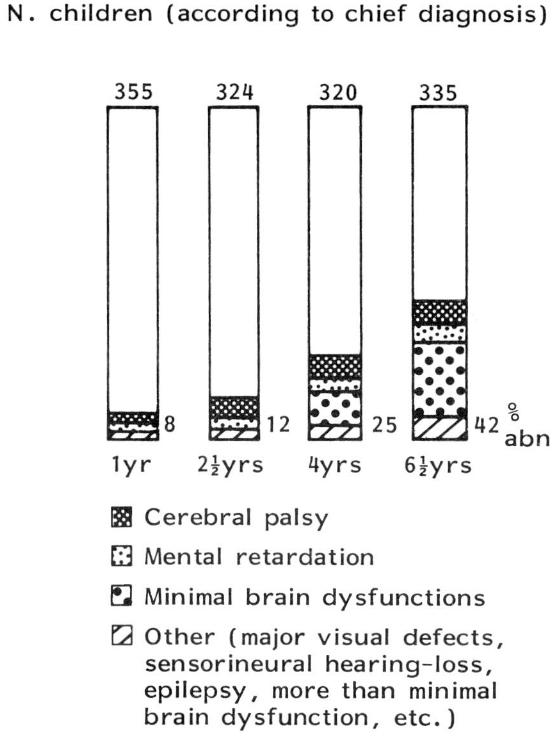

Fig. 5-1. Evoltuion of neurological sequelae in low-birthweight children.

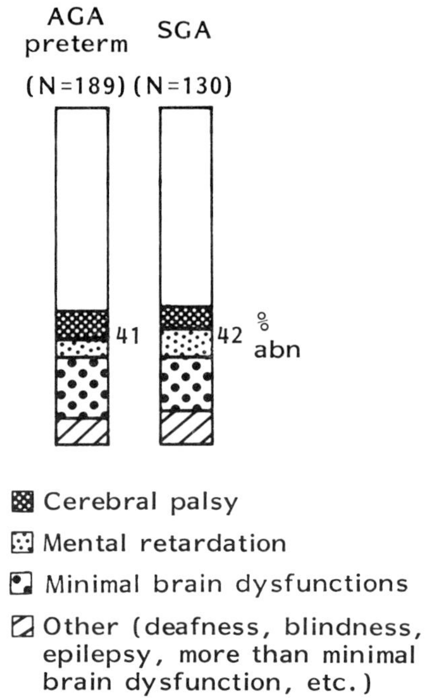

Fig. 5-2. Neurological abnormalities of low-birthweight children followed to at least 6½ years of age.

abnormal neurological findings in the first two weeks only; B = abnormal neurological findings at discharge examination only; and C = abnormal neurological findings all through stay in nursery. When 197 LBW survivors had reached the age of one year, neurological abnormality was considered definite or was suspected in the following proportions of infants: N seven of 54 (13 per cent); A 25 of 82 (30 per cent); B two of nine (22 per cent); and C 25 of 52 (48 per cent). Since the B group contained only nine infants, this was combined with group A, and in the final analysis of LBW infants the outcome was as shown in Table 5-V.

The persistence of abnormal neurological findings through the newborn period indicated the highest probability of abnormality at one year, whereas the group without any neonatal abnormal signs had the lowest rate of subsequent abnormality. The third group with only early or late abnormality in the nursery were in an intermediate position. These differences were highly significant. They persisted at 6½ years, but then were only just statistically significant.

The analysis also showed that the frequency of neurological abnormality was inversely related to birthweight. Already at one year the frequency of definite or suspected abnormality rose significantly from 24 per cent in the birthweight group 1801 to 2041g to 45 per cent in the group below 1361g (Table 5-VI). Further, in view of the relationship between neurological status and intellectual development,

TABLE 5-VI

Neurological abnormality after 1 year negatively correlated with birthweight

Birthweight (g)		N	Normal	Neurol. status at 1 yr: Definite or suspected abnormal N	%
(1)	<1360	42	23	19	45
(2)	1361-1600	55	37	18	33
(3)	1601-1800	74	52	22	29
(4)	1801-2041	123	93	30	24

(1), (2), (3) *vs.* (4): $\chi^2 = 3.47$, NS.
(1), (2) *vs.* (3), (4): $\chi^2 = 4.25$, $p < 0.05$.
(1) *vs.* (2), (3), (4): $\chi^2 = 5.20$, $p < 0.025$.

TABLE 5-VII

Neonatal neurological abnormalities in relation to Griffiths GQ at 1 year and WISC Full-scale IQ at 6½ years

Neonatal findings	*N*	*GQ at 1 yr Mean*	*N*	*IQ at 6½ yrs Mean*
Normal throughout	54	98.6± 8.9	69	99.8±14.4
Early or late abnormality only	74	91.3±13.7	109	96.7±15.4
Abnormal throughout	87	91.5±13.1	90	93.7±15.8

t tests indicate a highly significant difference ($p < 0.001$) between scores for first and second groups and between first and third groups at 1 year, and a significant difference ($p < 0.05$) between the first and third groups at 6½ years.

it is of interest to show the correlation between neurological status in the nursery and psychological test scores later. Table 5-VII lists the mean Griffiths GQ scores at the age of one year and the mean Full-scale WISC IQ scores at 6½ years in relation to neurological findings in the neonatal period, analyzed as in Table 5-VI. Non-caucasian children and those with scores below 50 have been excluded, and only LBW children with valid scores at either age-level are considered. It can be concluded that the neurological findings in the nursery have considerable prognostic significance, and can be expected to make a major contribution to the prediction of neurological and intellectual development (see Chapter 14).

Postural and plantar responses

We studied the postural responses of LBW infants as possible early indicators of neurological sequelae, in a similar manner to that described for fullterm infants (Paine *et al.* 1964). We were particularly interested in the Moro, parachute and plantar responses. We also investigated the asymmetrical tonic neck responses, but found them less helpful.

Moro response

The Moro response should be able to be elicited from a conceptional age of about 28 weeks onward. We distinguished whether it was complete and obtained with ease by dropping the head backward about 30° in relation to the trunk; whether it was obtained only with difficulty (often without flexion of the arms, asymmetrical or without leg movements); whether it had no consistent pattern; or whether there was no response at all.

Seven of the 335 LBW infants (2 per cent) followed to 6½ years had no response at first testing, and all were neurologically abnormal at follow-up. Another 45 (13 per cent) of the infants' responses showed no constant pattern or were obtained only with difficulty; 30 (67 per cent) of these were found later to be neurologically abnormal. The initial Moro response could always be elicited in the 138 FBW control children: in 131 (95 per cent) it was obtained with ease and in the other seven there was some difficulty, but these were all neurologically normal at 6½ years.

At the time of discharge from the nursery all the LBW infants had a response, but in five it was obtained only with difficulty: four of these later were found to be neurologically abnormal.

School placement was recorded for 258 children in their third year in school, with the following categories: (1) at grade level; (2) in ordinary school-class but having remedial teaching and/or placement in lower grade; and (3) special class or school. There was a statistically significant relationship between placement in third year at school and ease of obtaining the first neonatal Moro response ($\chi^2 = 10.78$, $p<0.005$). Five children who had not had a Moro response at first testing were all below grade level. Of another 36 who had no constant pattern or in whom the response was obtained only with difficulty, 21 (58 per cent) performed below grade level or were in a special class or school. Four of the five children whose response was obtained only with difficulty on discharge from the nursery had school problems.

Paine *et al.* (1964) found that at three months about 40 per cent of normal FBW infants still had the response, with both extension and flexion of the upper extremities. In our series, this degree of response was still present at three months in 86 per cent of 104 preterm AGA infants and in 84 per cent of 81 SGA infants (including 89 per cent of 35 *term* SGA infants), but in only 33 per cent of 102 FBW control children.

Paine and colleagues also reported that *none* of their normal FBW infants had persistence of extension or flexion of the upper extremities at six months. In our series at six months *chronological* age the following proportions still had a response with both extension and flexion of the upper limbs: 32 per cent of 118 preterm AGA children; 26 per cent of 82 SGA infants (including 27 per cent of 37 *term* SGA infants); but only 4 per cent of 125 FBW controls. The difference between each LBW category and the FBW controls is significant ($p<0.001$). A Moro response at six months in LBW children did not carry a more serious prognosis for neurological outcome at 6½ years than its absence. However, among the five FBW control children who still had a distinct Moro response at six months two subsequently were neurologically abnormal, compared with the total frequency of neurological

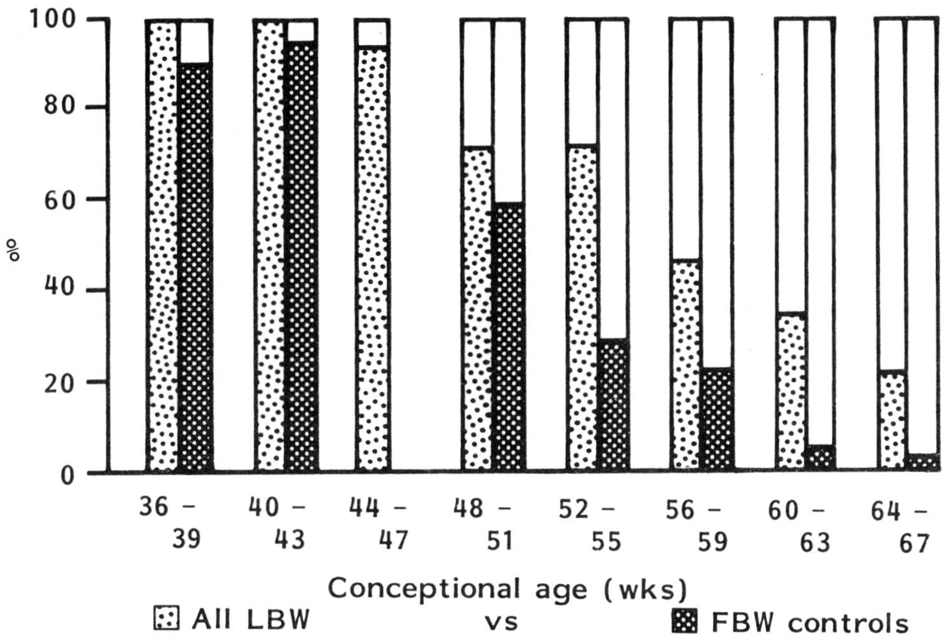

Fig. 5-3. Dissolution of Moro response with extension and flexion of upper limbs at increasing conceptional ages.

sequelae in the control group of 11 out of 125 (9 per cent).

When the dissolution of the Moro response was analyzed according to *conceptional* age (gestational plus chronological age), it tended to occur later during the period from 36 to 64 weeks conceptional age among LBW compared to FBW infants (Fig. 5-3), but the difference was significant only at 52 weeks.

At 12 months chronological age only five (6 per cent) of 78 preterm AGA infants still exhibited the Moro response: four responded with both extension and flexion of the upper limbs and the fifth had an abnormal response, elicited with difficulty. At 6½ years all five were neurologically abnormal; four had spastic cerebral palsy (two diplegia, one quadriplegia, one crural monoplegia) and the fifth had more than minimal brain dysfunction. Of 57 SGA infants, three still had the response at 12 months (one with extension and flexion of the arms, two abnormal and obtained with difficulty), and again all three were abnormal at 6½ years: two had spastic cerebral palsy (one quadriplegia, one monoplegia) and the third had more than minimal brain dysfunction. None of the 117 FBW control children had a residual Moro response.

We may conclude that:

(1) an *absent* Moro response after birth in an LBW infant with a gestational age of ⩾28 weeks heralds neurological sequelae and educational backwardness; if it is difficult to elicit and/or shows no constant pattern the prognosis is only slightly less serious, being associated with subsequent neurological abnormality in about

two-thirds of cases;
(2) an *incomplete* response on discharge from the nursery is also of serious significance; and
(3) the response takes longer to disappear in LBW than FBW infants, and its persistence at six months chronological age is of no concern, but if it still occurs at 12 months a neurological defect is certain and cerebral palsy is likely.

Parachute reponse
This movement is also described as protective extension of the arms. To elicit it, the infant is suspended horizontally in space in the prone position and plunged towards a table-top or other flat surface. The arms extend and separate somewhat, and the fingers spread as if to break the fall. Paine *et al.* (1964) found that healthy FBW infants sometimes responded with incomplete extension of the arms at as early as two months, but the response was not present universally until the age of nine months. The complete response, with full extension of the arms and spreading of the fingers, was elicited in 100 per cent only at 12 months. Asymmetrical participation of the arms is abnormal.

At three months 12 of 101 of our FBW controls already had a distinct response, compared to only two of 109 LBW babies ($\chi^2 = 3.86$, $p<0.05$). The 12 FBW infants who acquired the response early did not differ significantly from the rest in neurological status at 6½ years.

At six months the response had been acquired by 14 of 85 preterm AGA infants (16.5 per cent), 19 of 61 SGA infants (31.1 per cent) and 65 of 124 FBW controls (52.4 per cent). The difference between the AGA and SGA infants just failed to reach significance, but a significantly higher proportion of FBW children had a positive response than either LBW group alone, or both together. It was interesting that only one of the 65 FBW controls with a parachute response at six months was neurologically abnormal at 6½ years, whereas nine of the 52 FBW controls who did not respond at six months were subsequently abnormal ($\chi^2 = 9.19$, $p\leq0.005$).

At 12 months full-blown responses had been acquired by 79 of 99 preterm AGA infants (79.8 per cent), 59 of 65 SGA infants (90.8 per cent) and 118 of 119 FBW control children (99.2 per cent). Again the difference between the AGA and SGA just failed to reach significance, but a significantly higher proportion of FBW than LBW children had acquired the response. Further, of the 20 preterm AGA children with an abnormal or absent response at one year, 16 were neurologically abnormal at follow-up, whereas only 29 of 79 who had acquired the response were similarly abnormal ($\chi^2 = 10.3$, $p<0.001$). Of the six SGA infants with an abnormal or no response, four were neurologically abnormal at follow-up, as was the one FBW control baby who did not have the response.

For 157 LBW children the presence of the parachute response at one year was significantly related to performance in the third year at school ($\chi^2 = 9.28$, $p<0.01$). Of 27 children with absent or abnormal response at 12 months, 17 had school problems.

It was also interesting that 11 of 36 LBW infants with no Moro response or an abnormal one at either the first or second nursery examination did not have a normal parachute response at one year. 10 of these 11 were followed to Grade 3 in school: they were all neurologically abnormal and only two were performing at grade level (one with visual handicap, the other with MBD). Two had failed at least one grade and six were in a special class or a special school.

It may be concluded that:

(1) at three to 12 months chronological age the FBW control children were significantly ahead of the LBW infants—and particularly the preterm AGA infants—in acquiring the parachute response;

(2) the neurological outcome at 6½ years was significantly better for FBW controls who had acquired the parachute response at six months than for those who had not;

(3) the neurological outcome at 6½ years was significantly better for preterm AGA infants who had acquired the response by the age of one year than for those who had not;

(4) for LBW children generally, the presence of the parachute response at one year was significantly related to performance in the third year in school; and

(5) the absence of a normal parachute response at one year after an abnormal neonatal Moro response is an ominous predictor of neurological abnormality and school failure among LBW children.

Plantar responses

At 12 months definite extensor plantar responses were still obtained from 31 of 124 preterm AGA infants (25 per cent), 23 of 88 SGA infants (26 per cent) and 29 of 118 FBW infants (25 per cent). Thus there was little difference between the groups. However, among the 60 preterm AGA infants who had a definite flexor response, 20 (33 per cent) subsequently had a neurological abnormality, whereas among the 64 preterm AGA who had a definite extensor or an equivocal response, 37 (58 per cent) subsequently developed such an abnormality. This difference is significant (χ^2 = 7.47, $p<0.01$). No such significant difference could be established for the SGA or FBW groups. It is concluded that a definite flexor response in the plantar reflex at 12 months is a significantly favourable sign for neurological development of preterm AGA infants, but this could not be demonstrated for the SGA or FBW infants.

At 18 months definite extensor responses were elicited from 24 of 125 preterm AGA children (19 per cent), 19 of 97 SGA children (19 per cent) and 15 of the 118 FBW controls (13 per cent). Again there was little difference between the groups, but it was of interest that of the 64 preterm AGA infants with a definite flexor response, only 18 (28 per cent) subsequently developed a neurological abnormality, whereas of the 61 with extensor or equivocal plantar responses, 32 (52 per cent) did so (χ^2 = 7.7, $p<0.01$). Also, while there was no significant difference among the SGA and FBW infants in this respect, a significant difference was demonstrable when all LBW infants were analyzed together. Of 118 LBW infants with a definite flexor plantar response at 18 months, 14 (34 per cent) later developed a neurological abnormality, compared to 54 of 104 LBW infants (52 per cent) with extensor or equivocal plantar responses (χ^2 = 7.35, $p<0.01$).

A definite flexor plantar response at 18 months appears to be significantly favourable for neurological development of LBW infants, and for the subgroup of preterm AGA such a response was favourable even at the chronological age of 12 months.

Asymmetrical tonic neck reflex
Paine *et al.* (1964) considered an imposable asymmetrical tonic neck reflex (ATNR) to be quite rare in the neonatal period, even in abnormal infants. By the age of one month 60 per cent of babies exhibited the reflex, and by two months imposable and more equivocal responses were obtained in 80 per cent. After that the frequency declined and imposable ATNR could not be demonstrated after the age of six months, and not even an equivocal one after about seven months. Gesell and Amatruda (1947) considered the response to be abnormal from 24 weeks onward, and Paine (1961) thought that retention of ATNR was an important early sign of cerebral palsy and generally inconsistent with acquisition of free standing.

We recorded extension or flexion of the 'jaw' arm and leg and of the 'occiput' arm and leg in each case and documented the ATNR as being imposable with ease, obtainable with difficulty, showing no constant pattern, no response or 'other'. During their stay in the nursery it was obtained with ease in 64 per cent of 149 preterm AGA infants, 56 per cent of 50 term SGA babies and 49 per cent of 137 FBW controls. It was inconsistent or unimposable in 19 per cent of the preterm AGA group, 22 per cent of the term SGA and 27 per cent of the FBW controls.

By the age of three months ATNR was obtained with ease in 28 of 95 preterm AGA infants (29 per cent), 11 of 35 term SGA (31 per cent) and 26 of the total 78 SGA infants (33 per cent), compared to only four of 104 FBW controls (4 per cent). The difference between the first three groups (*i.e.* each LBW category) and the FBW group was statistically significant ($p<0.001$). Conversely, the ATNR was inconstant or not imposable in 76 of 104 FBW controls (73 per cent), but in only 85 of 173 LBW infants (49 per cent) ($\chi^2 = 15.3$, $p<0.001$). It is recognized, of course, that a brisk easily imposable ATNR is unusual in normal FBW infants at any age, and may cause concern as an early manifestation of cerebral palsy. However, it evidently occurs more commonly among LBW infants, even when there are no neurological sequelae.

The persistence of the response at six months (usually obtained with difficulty) in 12 per cent of preterm AGA and 6 per cent of term SGA infants did not appear to be of definite significance. The two term SGA babies who still had an ATNR at six months were both abnormal subsequently, but of the 13 preterm AGA infants who still showed it, only six (46 per cent) later were abnormal. However, 44 per cent of the infants who no longer showed the response also were abnormal, so there was little difference.

Persistence of the ATNR at 12 months may be more ominous. This occurred in three of 80 preterm AGA infants, but in no others, and two of these three proved to have spastic cerebral palsy. Conversely, among the 27 infants who did develop cerebral palsy, the ATNR persisted at one year significantly more often than in other LBW children, as will be shown later.

Head circumference
In Chapter 1 it was pointed out that post-haemorrhagic hydrocephalus has become

one of the major complications for VLBW survivors of intraventricular haemorrhage (Larroche 1972, Lorber and Bhat 1974, Korobkin 1975, Wise and Ballard 1976, Volpe *et al.* 1977, Pape and Wigglesworth 1979, Chaplin *et al.* 1980). Using CT scanning, Ahmann *et al.* (1980) found severe, progressive hydrocephalus in 12 of 55 survivors of subependymal or intraventricular haemorrhage (IVH) who had been born at less than 35 weeks gestation. Ventricular dilatation is thought to begin within a week of the haemorrhage and to precede a period of rapid head-growth and signs of increased intracranial pressure by an average of one to three days. A high proportion of affected infants have severe neurological defects at follow-up. It may seem surprising, therefore, that we did not recognize a single case in our series.

Six of the 275 children with satisfactory follow-up and whose head circumference was measured at one year did have a head size more than 2SD above the mean. Five of these were preterm AGA and one was SGA. However, none had a clinical course suggestive of neonatal IVH or hydrocephalus. Similarly, McDonald (1967) encountered only a single case of hydrocephalus among 1081 children with birthweights ≤1800g, and Saint-Anne Dargassies (1977) also diagnosed only a single case (considered antenatal) when following 286 LBW infants born before 1962. One reason for the difference between those reports and more recent ones may be that the great majority of VLBW infants with IVH used to die before modern methods of intensive care were introduced. However, even more recently, Camfield *et al.* (1981) encountered only one case of post-haemorrhagic hydrocephalus among 341 infants with birthweights ≤1500g born in Nova Scotia between 1976 and 1978. Also, Flodmark *et al.* (1981) argue strongly that 'ventriculomegaly' occurs commonly on CT scans of asphyxiated neonates, with or without IVH, and that the diagnosis of progressive hydrocephalus should be made with caution and with clinical correlation. Another reason why we did not encounter such a case may be that we had only 55 singletons and 10 twins with birthweights <1251g among the 501 infants taken into the study between 1959 and 1965.

In contrast, we encountered 46 children with a significantly *small* head-circumference (more than 2 SD below the mean) among the 275 with head measurements at one year (*i.e.* 16.7 per cent). The prognostic significance of small head-size has been discussed in Chapter 3: the intellectual and neurological outcome was significantly worse for the newborn SGA infants with a head circumference below the 10th percentile for gestational age, and the situation remained serious if catch-up growth during the first year did not bring the head circumference above the 10th percentile.

Of the 46 LBW infants in our series whose head circumference was still below the third percentile at one year, 22 were preterm AGA, 20 were SGA, and the length of gestation was unknown for the other four. At the age of 6½ years 11 of the 46 were mentally retarded (including three with cerebral palsy, one with blindness and one with epilepsy); one had cerebral palsy alone, one epilepsy alone and one sensorineural hearing-loss; six had more than minimal brain dysfunctions; and 10 had minimal brain dysfunctions: only 16 were neurologically normal. Therefore the neurological prognosis for this group with small heads at one year was significantly worse than for the total cohort ($\chi^2 = 8.9827$, $p<0.005$).

It was also shown in Chapter 3 that increasing head-circumference tended to have a linear relationship with increasing IQ at 6½ years, though for boys this did not continue after a certain maximum size had been reached. Certainly the six infants who had a significantly large head at one year did relatively well compared to those with significantly small heads. One girl who had been preterm AGA developed spastic diplegia, but with normal intelligence; two other children (one preterm AGA, the other SGA) were finally considered to have minimal brain dysfunctions and the remaining three were all thought to be neurologically normal at 6½ years or older. One of the last three appeared to have benign familial megalencephaly.

Mental retardation

It has long been recognized that there is an excessive proportion of LBW children in institutions and ambulatory facilities for the retarded (Asher and Roberts 1949, Pasamanick and Lilienfeld 1955, Moore 1965, Katz and Taylor 1967). As noted in Chapter 1, also the mean IQ scores of LBW children have been found to be lower than those of normal FBW controls, even when socio-economic status was taken into account (Harper *et al.* 1959, Douglas 1960, Drillien 1961*a*). Below the birthweight of 2000g there is an increasing proportion of LBW children with intellectual defects (see Chapter 4). With the recent improvement in outcome for LBW children, the prevalence of mental retardation among survivors has fallen. Mental retardation, as defined by the World Health Organization in 1954 (*i.e.* global IQ below 70) used to occur in about 8 to 10 per cent of LBW children. More marked mental retardation (IQ below 50) was found in 2.7 per cent of LBW survivors in the comprehensive survey by McDonald (1967), compared to approximately 0.4 per cent in the general population. When VLBW infants (birthweight ≤1500g) were considered the outlook was even worse, and from 11 to 27 per cent of survivors have been reported to be retarded (Knobloch *et al.* 1956, Lubchenco *et al.* 1963*b*, Bacola *et al.* 1966, Drillien 1967, Wright *et al.* 1972).

Since 1965, prevalence figures for subsequent mental retardation among LBW survivors have been claimed to be only in the range encountered in the general population, *e.g.* 2.2 per cent by Bjerre (1975*b*), and among VLBW infants only about 3 to 10 per cent (Rawlings *et al.* 1971, Stewart and Reynolds 1974, Jones *et al.* 1979). However, Drillien (1972) and her associates (1980) warned that major neurological handicaps in LBW children may arise early in gestation, particularly for SGA infants, and would not be likely to be affected by improved perinatal management. In this connection McDonald (1967) noted that an IQ below 70 occurred in 2.6 per cent of 905 children with birthweights ≤1800g who did not have cerebral palsy, blindness or deafness. Hagberg (1979) drew attention to the fact that the main causative factors of severe mental retardation differ greatly from those for cerebral palsy and that no less than some two-thirds of all such severe retardation is caused by very early prenatal factors, for which preventive measures are more limited. He also commented that the 10 per cent of severe mental retardation due to perinatal brain-damage is nearly always combined with cerebral palsy. The increased prevalence of mental retardation among the lower social-classes must also be considered (Willerman *et al.* 1970, Eaves *et al.* 1970, Francis-Williams and Davies 1974). Moreover, Drillien (1964) noted that, except for those who were smallest at birth, more boys than girls were considered to be making unsatisfactory progress in school.

As shown in Table 5-I, there were 30 children whose global IQ was less than 70 among the 335 LBW children in our study who were followed to the age of 6½ years. The retarded children fall into two main categories: at least 10 (3 per cent) whose retardation was due to factors operating in early gestation and probably at least 17 (5.1 per cent) whose brain damage occurred late in pregnancy or during the perinatal course. The latter may be largely avoidable by improved perinatal management, while the former are more difficult to prevent. In three other cases causation was less clear, and possibly was mixed, with both gestational (or genetic) and perinatal factors.

Among the 10 children whose retardation was thought to be due to gestational or genetic causes, eight had been SGA and only one had been born preterm AGA. The length of gestation was uncertain for the remaining child. Among the 17 children with probable perinatal causation, 11 had been preterm AGA, only four SGA, and in two cases the length of gestation was uncertain. The degree of mental retardation in the 10 cases caused early in gestation was mild in six, moderate in two and severe in two, so genetic and early gestational factors do not necessarily cause more severe retardation than perinatal hypoxic-ischaemic encephalopathy, haemorrhage or other damaging factors.

Certain items in the history or examination during infancy were significantly correlated with mental retardation compared to the antecedents of 27 LBW children with cerebral palsy (see Table 5 X). Since 32 interdependent variables were analyzed, a p value of 0.0015 would be equivalent to the usual critical value of $p = 0.05$, according to the Bonferroni rules for inequality. Since the interdependence clearly is not complete, one may claim significant relationships when p is less than 0.005. Mental retardation is highly significantly correlated with a lower mean social-class than the average for the LBW group as a whole. It is also highly significantly correlated with an abnormal Moro response in the nursery, abnormal neurological examination at one year and at 1½ years, abnormal posture or delayed walking at 18 months, and a low mean Griffiths GQ score at 12 and 18 months. Further, there is a just-significant correlation with low birthweight and an abnormal head-circumference (usually significantly small) at one year. There are also non-significant trends towards a correlation with maternal neurological or psychiatric disease (evident during pregnancy) and neonatal abnormalities like poor sucking or excessive need for oxygen and intravenous therapy in the nursery, as well as abnormality of the EEG at one year. It is also noteworthy that there is no more significant correlation with shorter gestation than for the rest of the cohort, with neonatal haemorrhage or respiratory abnormality, with abnormal neurological status on discharge from the nursery, with persistence of the Moro or asymmetrical tonic neck reflex at one year, or a variable or extensor plantar response at 18 months. In these respects the situation is quite different from that for cerebral palsy (Dunn *et al.* 1982*b*).

Cerebral palsy

Before 1965 the incidence of cerebral palsy in European surveys was found to range from about one to three per 1000 livebirths (Asher and Schonell 1950, Woods 1957, Hansen 1960, Ingram 1964). It was also a universal finding that a high proportion of affected children had birthweights ≤2500g. While about 5 to 7 per cent of caucasian children have such a low birthweight, the frequency among children with cerebral palsy has ranged from about 22 to 40 per cent (Childs and Evans 1954, Eastman and De Leon 1955, Fuldner 1957, Crothers and Paine 1959, Ingram 1964, Ellenberg and Nelson 1979). Further, it was shown that the characteristic form of cerebral palsy for LBW children was spastic diplegia, in which the legs are affected more severely than the arms. Occasional cases presented as cerebral spastic paraplegia, with the upper limbs appearing to be normal. For both diplegia and paraplegia a bimodal birthweight distribution has been reported, showing peaks around 1800g and 3200g (Childs and Evans 1954, Fuldner 1957, Stanley 1981). Childs and Evans suggested that this might indicate two different aetiological patterns. The recent evidence from CT scans and ultrasonograms shows that for LBW children, and particularly those with VLBW, neonatal intracranial haemorrhage often may be at least a partial cause of the cerebral palsy, whereas for FBW infants periventricular leucomalacia appears to be the predominant causative lesion. Drillien *et al.* (1962) also noted that the mothers of a group of FBW diplegic children tended to be of superior social-class, older and less fertile than the mothers of a group weighing ≤2000g.

In the introductory chapter we presented some evidence that the incidence of cerebral palsy fell with the advent of improved perinatal care in the 1960s, particularly in Sweden and in Britain. Since then no further fall appears to have occurred. Kiely *et al.* (1981*b*) calculated that the frequency of cerebral palsy among VLBW infants still ranged from 2 to 12 per cent, and mostly from 6 to 9 per cent. In 1952 the aetiology of cerebral palsy was reviewed by Perlstein, who concluded that in 30 per cent the causes were prenatal, in 60 per cent natal and in 10 per cent postnatal. Similarly, Brown (1980) found in eastern Scotland in the early 1970s that in a series of 92 consecutive children referred with cerebral palsy, the condition appeared to be due to perinatal abnormalities in two-thirds; and in a follow-up study from the newborn nursery about 35 per cent of those who emerged with cerebral palsy had a low birthweight. He considered that the proportion of cerebral-palsied patients attributable to perinatal causes had diminished in the second half of the decade. Holm (1982) retrospectively investigated the causes of cerebral palsy in 142 children born after 1st January 1970 and living in the north-western United States. She concluded that the causes were prenatal in 50 per cent, perinatal in 33 per cent, postnatal in 10 per cent and mixed in 7 per cent. These resembled the findings in Sweden, where the proportion of cerebral palsy due to perinatal factors was thought to have diminished from more than 50 per cent between 1945 and 1959 to 40 per cent between 1967 and 1970 (Hagberg *et al.* 1975*a*). However, the interplay between prenatal and perinatal factors may be

TABLE 5-VIII
Analysis of 27 LBW children with cerebral palsy

	N	*AGA preterm*	*SGA*	*Gest. age uncertain*	*Mentally retarded (IQ <70)*
Spastic diplegia*	13	9*	2	2	4*
Spastic quadriplegia	3	2	1	—	3
Spastic crural monoplegia	4	1	3	—	—
Spastic hemiplegia	6	5	1	—	1
Ataxia	1	1	—	—	—
Total	27	18	7	2	8

*Including two mixed with extrapyramidal features.

complex and requires further study (Bennett *et al.* 1981, Kudrjavcev *et al.* 1983).

The prevalence of spastic diplegia, which in the past has represented approximately one-third of cases of cerebral palsy in childhood, ranged from 9 to 32 per cent in three surveys of surviving VLBW infants who were born before 1965. McDonald (1962, 1967) found cerebral palsy in 6.5 per cent of children with birthweights ≤1800g born between 1951 and 1953, and 81 per cent of these were included in the syndrome of spastic diplegia (which also comprised cerebral spastic paraplegia). That investigator also showed that spastic diplegia was more common in single than in multiple births, and in singletons it was most frequent among those with short gestation, reaching its maximum in pregnancies lasting 31 weeks. In other words, these findings suggested that spastic diplegia tends to occur most often in VLBW preterm infants. McDonald also noted that cyanotic attacks in the early postnatal period were associated with diplegia, and she suggested that the cerebral damage might occur during these episodes. Other types of cerebral palsy differed in that they showed a significant association with convulsions or signs suggestive of cerebral pathology in the early postnatal period.

Results

In our study there were 27 cases of cerebral palsy among the 335 LBW children followed to school-age (see Table 5-I). This represents the expected high prevalence (8.1 per cent) among children with birthweights ≤2041g in the years 1959 to 1965, when our intake occurred. It contrasts with no cases of cerebral palsy at all among the 139 FBW control children, and also with the usual estimate of about 0.2 per cent among the general population at that time. Among our cases there was also the expected predominance of spastic diplegia (13 of 27), as shown in Table 5-VIII.

The mean WISC Full-scale IQ at 6½ years was only 82.65 ± 22.74 for 26 children with cerebral palsy in whom it had been measured, while it was 96.12 ± 16.89 for 277 other LBW children in whom it had been ascertained ($p = 0.000$). It will be noted that only eight of the 27 LBW children with cerebral palsy were retarded

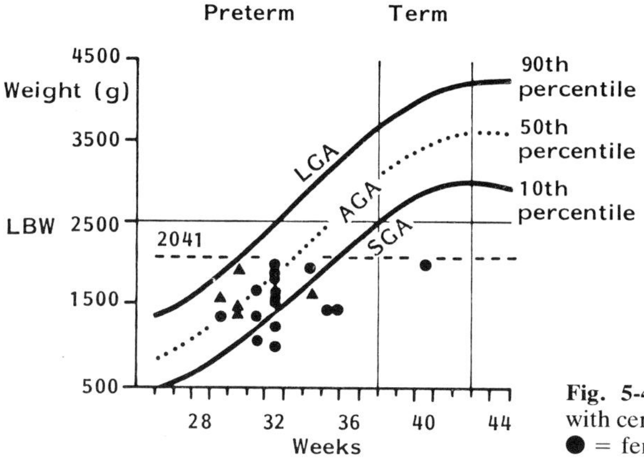

Fig. 5-4. Birthweights of 21 LBW singletons with cerebral palsy (and known gestational age). ● = female, ▲ = male

(IQ<70). Further, nine of the 11 children with spastic diplegia for whom the length of gestation was known, and five of the six with spastic hemiplegia, were preterm AGA.

There is a predominance of AGA preterm over SGA infants among the LBW patients with cerebral palsy, but the higher ratio fails to reach significance compared to other LBW children in the study. Nelson and Ellenberg (1982) noted that most preterm babies who developed cerebral palsy were concentrated between the 10th and 50th percentiles on growth curves, so they were somewhat undergrown. This is also true of our LBW group, though there is considerable scatter (Fig. 5-4). Bennett *et al.* (1981) had similar findings in relation to spastic diplegia.

In our series of 27 LBW children with cerebral palsy there were also six with spastic hemiplegia, and five of these were preterm AGA. While this has been considered a less common type among LBW infants, Brown (1980) found it in three (12 per cent) of 25 children with cerebral palsy who had had birthweights ≤2000g. Conversely, it is recognized that about 20 to 25 per cent of children with congenital hemiplegia are LBW (Woods 1957, Hansen 1960). Armstrong and Norman (1974) demonstrated that unilateral secondary haemorrhage, and even cavitation, may occur in periventricular leucomalacia and form an anatomical substrate for spastic hemiparesis.

Of our 27 cases of cerebral palsy, 23 were singletons and four were twins; this proportion did not differ significantly from that of the other LBW children. The mean birthweight of the 27 children was 1515g and thus significantly lower than the mean birthweight of 1719g of all other LBW infants ($p = 0.000$). The length of gestation was known in 25 cases and their mean was 31.60 weeks, while 280 other LBW children with known length of gestation had a mean gestational age of 33.96 weeks at birth ($p = 0.000$). Thus cerebral palsy in LBW children tends to occur particularly in association with a relatively brief length of gestation and with low birthweight, compared to the means for other LBW children in our study. It is interesting that the social-class distribution with cerebral palsy does not differ significantly from the rest of the LBW group, whereas there was an impressively significant correlation between mental retardation and very low social-class.

Antecedents

All 27 children with cerebral palsy had some abnormal neurological signs in the nursery, as was previously reported by Brown (1980) with respect to palsied infants who had had perinatal asphyxia. Like the mentally retarded children, those with cerebral palsy tended to have an abnormal or absent Moro response in the nursery, and their mean birthweight was even more significantly reduced compared to the rest of the LBW group. There was also an increased trend towards poor sucking and the need for intravenous therapy. They differed from the retarded children in having a significantly lower mean gestational age compared to other LBW children, more respiratory abnormalities and prolonged oxygen therapy, frequent persistence of the Moro and asymmetrical tonic neck responses at one year, and of extensor or equivocal plantar responses at 18 months. There was also a trend towards *clinical* bleeding in the nursery among the infants who subsequently developed cerebral palsy, and this was not noted as a group phenomenon among the 30 babies who later were found to have mental retardation. No doubt this point will be proved more definitively in the future with CT-scan and ultrasound studies. It may even become possible to use periventricular low-density on CT scan as a predictor of neurobehavioral outcome for LBW infants (Daum *et al.* 1981), though the radiological demonstration of leucomalacia still appears to be less reliable than that of cerebral haemorrhages (Flodmark *et al.* 1980). The frequent abnormal neonatal findings as predictors of cerebral palsy were also noted by Nelson and Ellenberg (1979).

Evolution

Ingram (1955, 1964) described a characteristic evolution of neurological findings in 79 cases of spastic diplegia. He recognized three stages in the gradual development of paresis with spasticity and flexion contractures of the limbs: hypotonic, dystonic, and rigid or spastic, in varying proportions. In the dystonic phase the child stiffens and extends the neck and back when there is a sudden change in position, as in being bathed or dressed. The limbs are liable to be adducted, extended and internally rotated for only a few seconds at a time. They remain hypotonic at rest. The grasp reflexes are brisk, and the Moro response may be retained longer than normally. Such generalized dystonic attacks are present at two to 12 months, and as they wane the limbs become hypertonic, particularly the hip adductors and calf muscles. Paine (1961) and colleagues (1964), and Brown *et al.* (1974), described various sequences in the evolution of muscle tone, but agreed that infants who later developed diplegia or tetraplegia often were hypotonic in the first year, especially in the neck and trunk. Hyperreflexia, prolongation of adductor spread of knee jerk, ankle clonus and delayed retention of an imposable asymmetrical tonic neck response were early clues to spasticity. Brown and colleagues followed 93 severely asphyxiated neonates and found that infants with prolonged hypotonia or with hypotonia progressing to extensor hypertonus had a very bad prognosis, in contrast to those with normal flexor tone.

These sequences were also observed in the infants in the present series. The 26 children with spastic forms of cerebral palsy may be divided into the four categories of diplegia, quadriplegia, hemiplegia and crural monoplegia.

In *spastic diplegia*, all but one of the 13 affected infants initially had abnormally depressed muscle-tone—seven were assessed as flaccid, five as significantly hypotonic (in comparison with other LBW babies), and only one was considered to have normal tone after birth. The reduced muscle-tone and associated inertia were accompanied by tremulous or 'jittery' movements in eight of the 12 LBW neonates, and nine of the 12 were unable to suck or could do so only weakly. Usually muscle tone improved progressively while they were in the nursery; by the time of discharge from hospital (usually in the second to third month) it had become normal in seven of the 12 infants. Three still exhibited some hypotonia, particularly in neck and trunk muscles, one had already entered the dystonic phase in the second month and one had become hypertonic. The tremulous movements also usually subsided in the nursery; they were accompanied by twitching in three infants and persisted beyond discharge in only two cases. A distinct dystonic phase was recognized in only four of the 13 infants with spastic diplegia; its onset varied from the second month to one year. Two of the 13 children had a residual movement disorder (*e.g.* static tremor, athetoid hand-movements) which indicated that the spasticity was mixed, with extrapyramidal features.

By the age of 12 to 18 months some hypertonus of the legs was usually evident, which often led on to spasticity. Sometimes knee jerks were absent initially, but usually they could be demonstrated to be normal in the nursery and did not become increased until the second year. Sustained ankle clonus (*i.e.* more than 10 beats in neonates: Paine *et al.* 1964) was found in only one of the 13 infants before discharge from the nursery (in that case at 10 weeks), but was encountered later in four others, mainly between the ages of 1½ and four years. *Both plantar responses remained extensor in the second year and throughout the period of observation in all cases* (except one, who changed from extensor to equivocal responses at 6½ years).

The Moro response was depressed to varying degrees after birth in seven of the 13 infants, but in all cases was elicited with ease on discharge from the nursery; it persisted beyond six months in three instances. While this was a warning sign of cerebral palsy, other postural responses were often helpful in the diagnosis, namely: abnormal Collis test for leg position in inverted suspension (seven) (Collis 1954); poor traction response at end of stay in the nursery (four); inability to raise the chin in the prone position at end of stay in the nursery (four); absence or asymmetry of placing or stepping responses in the first six months (three); delayed appearance or asymmetry of parachute response (four); and delay in adopting Landau posture (two). In addition, locomotor development was delayed in all cases; *e.g.* free sitting and creeping were still impossible at one year. Two of the 13 children never learned to walk freely; the others began to walk at ages ranging from 14 months to seven years, with a mean of 33 months. Strabismus occurred in no fewer than eight of these 13 children with spastic diplegia.

The diagnosis of *spastic quadriplegia* was made for three children. Their clinical course at first resembled that of the diplegic infants, but the Moro response persisted to at least one year in all three cases, and the postural responses tended to be more consistently abnormal. As one might expect from the involvement of the arms, this also applied to the parachute response. In view of the marked impairment of function in the arms and the asymmetrical involvement of the limbs in the first two patients, they may be considered to have double hemiplegia and hemiparesis, respectively. Only one of the three children learned to walk, and all three are mentally retarded, with strabismus. The third case, one of the VLBW infants in the series, represents a clinical picture which may have become more common with increased survival of VLBW infants (Teberg *et al.* 1982).

Spastic hemiplegia affected six of the LBW children. Unfortunately, follow-up was interrupted for three of these, so the information is incomplete for this group, particularly as to the evolution of postural responses. Two had normal muscle-tone after delivery and no major disorder during their neonatal course, but the other four had neonatal problems similar to those of the spastic diplegic infants. It is generally agreed that congenital hemiplegia takes several months to evolve and, like diplegia, may pass through a hypotonic to a hypertonic phase, and often finally a spastic one. In the present cases the age at onset of clinical unilateral weakness and impaired function varied from five months to the fourth year. Early clues to the diagnosis were provided by *asymmetries*, not only in placing and stepping responses, in hip flexion on suspension of the infant and in the Collis test, but also somewhat later in early unilateral hand-preference, and in asymmetrical parachute responses and Landau posture. Like Ingram (1964), we also found persistence of the grasp and asymmetrical tonic neck reflexes on the affected side when they had disappeared on the contralateral side.

Interestingly, the knee jerk and other tendon reflexes did not become noticeably brisk on the affected side until the age of one year or later, and often the reflexes on the contralateral side were also somewhat increased. Ankle clonus was not found in any of our cases of hemiplegia. The plantar responses did not become distinctly different until they had reached ages between 1½ and 6½ years. These children walked freely from between 11 months and two years, with a mean of 18.6 months. Only one had a seizure (with abnormal EEG), and strabismus occurred in two cases. Asymmetry of limb size was already detectable at one year in two of these patients.

The four cases of *spastic crural monoplegia* were challenging diagnostically. They resemble the group with spastic diplegia in having had a somewhat stormy neonatal course, with initial hypotonia. However, three of the four were preterm SGA, and at least two had the type of congenital stigmata often found in SGA LBW children (Crichton *et al.* 1972*b*), *i.e.* hypertelorism, koilonychia, absent upper lateral incisors and wide-open fontanelle at 1½ years in one, and abnormal dermatoglyphics and asymmetrical refractive errors, with astigmatism, in another. Again the initial hypotonia changed gradually to hypertonus, and in at least one case a dystonic phase intervened. Between one and 2½ years the knee jerks were found to be brisk *bilaterally* in three of the four children and the plantar responses appeared to be extensor on both sides, so that early spastic diplegia was often suspected. When asymmetries were noted at one to four years (such as asymmetrical postural responses, more marked tip-toeing on one side or better hopping on the other, early hand-preference, dragging of one leg, or inversion and reduced growth of one leg) the examiner might wonder if these were cases of asymmetrical spastic diplegia. Ultimately, however, the plantar responses on the contralateral side became flexor in three of the four cases and the upper limb on the affected side tended to be somewhat hypertonic, swinging less on walking or showing motor impersistence. Thus the clinical features were intermediate between spastic diplegia and hemiparesis. These children walked freely at the ages of 18 to 20 months, the mean of 19 months being close to that for the hemiplegic patients. Two of these four children had strabismus.

The frequent finding of strabismus should be emphasized. As discussed in Chapter 8, strabismus in LBW infants should always lead to a careful neurological and behavioural assessment, with particular attention to muscle tone, postural responses, co-ordination and involuntary movements (Ingram 1955, Paine 1961, Twitchell 1963, Paine *et al.* 1964).

The diagnosis of cerebral palsy had been made by the age of one year in 11 of the 27 cases in this series. The relevant physical findings at that time (often in combination) were: persistent Moro response (seven), strabismus (usually esotropia) (seven), leg hypertonus and abnormal Collis response (five), abnormal or asymmetrical parachute response (four), persistent asymmetrical tonic neck reflex (three), ankle clonus (three), asymmetrical muscle tone (one) and asymmetrical plantar responses (one).

Our data show that abnormal neurological findings at one year are a highly significant predictor of cerebral palsy, and it would appear that this is also true at four months (Ellenberg and Nelson 1981). Abnormal neurological status on discharge from the nursery was of borderline significance as a predictor, but with the newer refined techniques of neurological examination, CT scan and ultrasound examination, a more accurate early diagnosis should become possible (Howard *et al.* 1976, Kurtzberg *et al.* 1979, Bejar *et al.* 1980, Graziani *et al.* 1980, Njiokiktjien and Kurver 1980, Dubowitz and Dubowitz 1981, Flodmark *et al.* 1981, Thorburn *et al.* 1981, Harvey *et al.* 1982).

Intellectual outcome

The mean global IQ (mostly WISC Full-scale) of the children with cerebral palsy was about 83, and thus significantly lower than that for the LBW group as a whole. However, the range was from 31 to 124. As can be seen in Table 5-VIII, only eight of the 27 children had an IQ below 70. The mean final WISC Full-scale IQs at 6½ years were 83.1 for the 13 with diplegia, 83.5 for the six with hemiplegia, 50 for the three with quadriplegia and 91 for the four with crural monoplegia. One girl with congenital ataxia had a Full-scale IQ of 117.

Other investigators have reported that LBW children with spastic diplegia more often are of average intelligence than those of full birthweight (Childs and Evans 1954, Russell 1960, Scherzer and Miké 1974). It has also been noted that spastic diplegic children of full birthweight include a larger proportion who are SGA, implying prenatal causation (Alberman 1963, Scherzer and Miké 1974). Among the LBW children with cerebral palsy in the present study, the mean global IQ at 6½ years was 85.1 for the 14 AGA preterm singletons, and thus not significantly higher than the mean of 81 for the seven who were SGA. We had no FBW children with cerebral palsy with whom we could make comparisons.

Epilepsy

In 1942 Thom collected information from 914 working-class families in Boston and found that 67 children per 1000 had had convulsions in the first five years of life. In the prospective study of 1000 consecutive births in Newcastle upon Tyne, Miller and colleagues (1960) similarly found that one in every 14 of more than 800 children (*i.e.* 72 per 1000) had had one convulsion or more during the first five years. The frequency of at least one febrile convulsion in childhood has been calculated in six surveys to range from 1.9 to 3.6 per cent of all children, with a mean of 2.7. Lennox-Buchthal (1974) estimated that febrile convulsions accounted for about one-half of all convulsions under the age of five years. In the British National Child Development Study, 1043 children (6.7 per cent) had a history of episodes of loss of consciousness by the age of 11 years, and 322 (20.8 per 1000) had a history of febrile convulsions without other epileptic problems. A clear-cut diagnosis of non-febrile epilepsy was established for only 64 children (4.1 per 1000); a further 39 (2.6 per 1000) were reported as having epilepsy but did not fulfil the study criteria (Ross *et al.* 1980).

Several authors have demonstrated an excess of LBW children among those who had recurrent fits after the age of two years (McDonald 1964, Cooper 1965, van den Berg and Yerushalmy 1969). In the British National Study, 10 of the 64 children with established epilepsy were LBW singletons but, surprisingly, this was not a statistically significant excess (Ross *et al.* 1980). McDonald (1964), who followed 1081 children with birthweights ≤1800g to the age of six to eight years, found that 102 (9.4 per cent) had a history of one or more fits. 12 of these (11.8 per cent) had cerebral palsy, with or without mental retardation, and a further six (5.9 per cent) had mental retardation alone. When these subgroups were excluded, the residual prevalence of 8.1 per cent still exceeded that of about 5.1 per cent for the general population. In contrast to spastic diplegia, there was no negative correlation between prevalence and birthweight in singletons; the history of fits was more common with a gestational age of ≥35 weeks than with shorter gestation. In other words, fits were more common in SGA children born approaching term.

Van den Berg and Yerushalmy (1969) distinguished between febrile and non-febrile convulsions in a cohort of some 18,500 children in California: they found that the risk of a convulsive disorder by the age of five years was about 2 per cent for febrile seizures and 1 per cent for non-febrile seizures. Nearly one-third of children in the febrile and two-thirds in the non-febrile groups had multiple seizures. The risk of febrile seizures was approximately equal for boys and girls, but more boys than girls had non-febrile seizures. In the febrile group the relative frequency of LBW children was similar to that in the total cohort, whereas the non-febrile group had an excess of LBW children, particularly those born at term (*i.e.* with gestational ages ⩾37 weeks). The frequency of severe congenital anomalies was 7 per cent in the febrile group and 31 per cent in the non-febrile, contrasting with only 3 per cent for the entire cohort. The majority of severe anomalies in the non-febrile group affected the central nervous system, especially in the form of mental retardation or cerebral palsy. In the Collaborative Perinatal Project in the United States, Nelson and Ellenberg (1982) also found that disorders in the groups with non-febrile seizures were slightly more frequent among SGA children at term than in other categories, but the difference was not statistically significant. Those authors concluded that VLBW and immaturity did not represent risk factors for epilepsy, unless the children had cerebral palsy.

With respect to EEGS, Dreyfus-Brisac and Monod (1966) studied consecutive records from birth onward for 1020 children and encountered 88 cases with focal spikes between the ages of four months and 12 years. Of these 88, 45 had been born as 'prematures'. Epilepsy occurred in only 18 of the 88, but 37 had serious neurological defects, and for most of these the spike discharges had appeared before the age of two years.

Results

Epilepsy (excluding idiopathic generalized febrile convulsions)

There were 14 LBW children (4.2 per cent) among the 335 followed to the age of 6½ years who had recurrent seizures, other than idiopathic 'benign' febrile convulsions. The epilepsy could be classified* as follows: primary generalized, often familial (five); secondary (lesional, symptomatic) generalized, *i.e.* superimposed on other marked cerebral dysfunctions (six); undetermined generalized (one); and partial with secondary generalization (two). Admittedly the distinction between primary and secondary generalized epilepsies is somewhat arbitrary, and it is agreed that in so-called secondary, symptomatic or lesional forms often there may be an underlying hereditary predisposition to seizures. We assumed that the epilepsy was likely to be primary if children had a family history of epilepsy and evidence of, at most, minimal brain dysfunctions. On the other hand, we termed the epilepsy secondary if there were major neurological deficits. One child had attacks of staring and syncope with urinary incontinence beginning in infancy, but with a normal EEG, and we preferred to label this epilepsy undetermined generalized.

These 14 epileptic LBW children included only one with distinct cerebral palsy, but five were more than mildly retarded, with a global IQ below 50. For all the cases regarded as secondary (or lesional) generalized epilepsy there had been significant abnormal neurological findings in the newborn period.

The birthweights of these epileptic children in relation to gestational age were known for 11 singletons and were evenly distributed (Fig. 5-5), *i.e.* they were not so much confined to the low gestational age of the preterm AGA children as in cerebral palsy. Six of the epileptic children were SGA, six were preterm AGA and two were of unknown gestation. Three were twins. 10 of the 14 were male.

*According to the proposed *International Classification of the Epilepsies* (*Epilepsia*, 1970, **11,** 114-119).

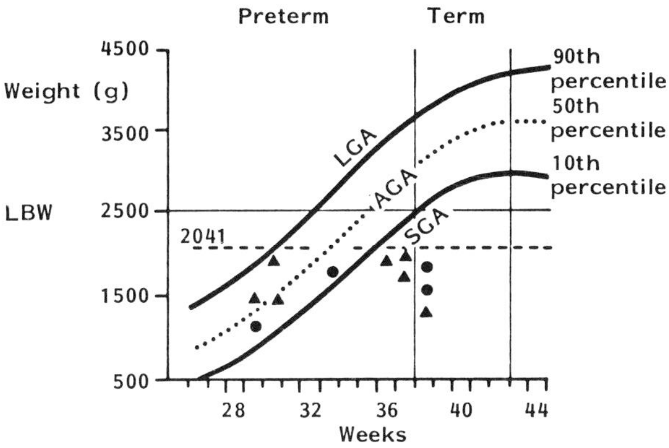

Fig. 5-5. Birthweights of 11 LBW singletons with epilepsy (and known gestational age). ● = female, ▲ = male

Among the 139 FBW control children followed to the age of 6½ years, one girl developed idiopathic 'absence' seizures (so-called 'true petit mal') at school-age, and one boy with Duane's retraction syndrome had febrile convulsions at the ages of nine, 12 and 19 months, and again at seven years, when his EEG showed discharges. Another boy was considered neurologically normal but had enuresis and aggressive behaviour at seven years after febrile convulsions in infancy, and his EEG at seven years showed an excess of 2 to 5 Hz slow-wave activity posteriorly, often with sharp forms, and also episodic generalized slow and sharp activity during sleep. If he is included, the prevalence of epilepsy in the FBW control group was three out of 139 (2.2 per cent).

Idiopathic febrile convulsions

Among the 335 LBW children followed to school-age, eight (2.4 per cent) were diagnosed as having febrile convulsions, mostly recurrent with infections and not associated with any EEG evidence of seizure discharges. Among the 139 FBW control children, five (3.6 per cent) had febrile convulsions which appeared to be idiopathic. An EEG was refused for one of these, was normal in three cases and showed only asymmetries for the fifth child. All five were considered to be neurologically normal at 6½ years.

Thus, from this small sample, we can confirm that the frequency of epilepsy among LBW children appears to be higher than among the FBW controls, *i.e.* 4.2 *vs.* 2.2 per cent, whereas the prevalence of idiopathic febrile convulsions is not increased in the LBW group (2.4 per cent in LBW *vs.* 3.6 per cent in FBW controls). However, these differences are not statistically significant.

Survivors lost from the study

Eighty-four (20 per cent) of the 419 LBW and 62 (31 per cent) of the 203 FBW survivors were lost to follow-up. Their characteristics were analyzed to see whether they differed from those of the children who remained, in case this might bias the results. 29 (35 per cent) of the LBW and 25 (40 per cent) of the FBW children lost to follow-up were last seen in the nursery. The remaining 55 of the LBW were last examined at a mean age of 14.8 months (median 12 months), whereas the remaining 37 FBW children were last seen at a mean age of 28.7 months (median 18 months). Only 19 per cent of the LBW infants and 27 per cent of the FBW children who were lost to follow-up defaulted as a result of the parents' or physicians' refusal to co-operate. Most became difficult to follow after adoption, or moved away.

The children lost to follow-up are compared to those followed to school-age in Table 5-IX. The following points will be noted:

(1) When the LGA and the infants of unknown gestational age are omitted, the distribution of the main birthweight categories (SGA, preterm AGA and FBW) among those lost to follow-up is significantly different from that for the study cohort. It appears that this difference is largely due to a relatively greater proportion of FBW children in the group lost to follow-up. As might be expected, parents of LBW (SGA and preterm AGA) infants had more incentive to continue with the study than the parents of FBW control infants because they had more reason to be concerned about the possible ill-health or abnormal development of their child.

(2) The sex composition of the LBW infants lost to follow-up and those who were followed differs significantly. The difference seems to reflect the loss of a larger proportion of female LBW singletons from the study. The reasons for this are obscure, except that parents may have been more concerned about their boys in view of the higher prevalence of MBD and other problems. The group of FBW infants lost and followed-up do not have a significantly different sex composition.

(3) As to social class, not all the infants lost could be included because the social class of those seen only in the nursery could not be determined with certainty from available information. The social-class distribution of LBW infants lost subsequently was not significantly different from that of the remaining LBW group. However, the social-class distribution of the FBW controls lost to follow-up differed significantly from the remaining FBW children. A larger proportion of FBW children in social-classes I-III and V were lost or refused to co-operate than those in social-class IV.

(4) Often knowledge of the lost children's neurological outcome was based on limited information. As more than one-third of the LBW infants lost were last seen in the nursery and the remainder at a mean age of 14.8 months, their neurological outcome was compared to that of the remaining LBW children at one year. There was no significant difference. In the case of the FBW children, we attempted to compare the ultimate outcome at 6½ years, often on the basis of school reports, and again there did not appear to be any significant difference.

Summary

On follow-up to the age of 6½ years, 140 (41.8 per cent) of 335 LBW children who mostly had weighed ≤2041g at birth had a total of 181 neurological or ophthalmological abnormalities (not including strabismus). In contrast, only 15 (10.8 per cent) of 139 FBW control children had such abnormalities. The most common neurological abnormality were minimal brain dysfunctions (61 or 18.2 per cent LBW; nine or 6.5 per cent FBW). In the LBW cohort, other abnormalities were mental retardation (global IQ <70) (9 per cent), cerebral palsy (8.1 per cent), visual

TABLE 5-IX

Surviving children lost to follow-up compared to those followed to 6½ years

BIRTHWEIGHT CATEGORIES					
Both sexes	*SGA*	*Preterm AGA*	*FBW*	*Total*	*p*
Lost to follow-up	28 (21%)	46 (34%)	62 (45%)	136	<0.005
Followed to 6½ yrs	130 (29%)	183 (40%)	139 (31%)	452	
Follow-up rate %	82.3	79.9	69.2	76.9	
Singletons					
Lost to follow-up	26 (21%)	37 (29%)	62 (50%)	125	<0.01
Followed to 6½ yrs	112 (32%)	122 (34%)	135 (34%)	369	
Follow-up rate %	81.2	76.7	68.5	74.7	
Multiple births					
Lost to follow-up	2 (18%)	9 (82%)	—	11	NS
Followed to 6½ yrs	18 (23%)	61 (72%)	4 (5%)	83	
Follow-up rate %	90.0	87.1	100	88.3	
SEX DISTRIBUTION					
LBW	*Female*	*Male*	*Total*		
Lost to follow-up	55 (66%)	28 (34%)	83		<0.02
Followed to 6½ yrs	172 (51%)	163 (49%)	335		
Follow-up rate %	75.8	85.3	80.1		
FBW					
Lost to follow-up	33 (33%)	29 (47%)	62		NS
Followed to 6½ yrs	67 (48%)	72 (52%)	139		
Follow-up rate %	67.0	71.3	69.2		
*SOCIAL-CLASS DISTRIBUTION**					
LBW	*I-III*	*IV*	*V*	*Total*	
Followed beyond nursery but subsequently lost	12 (39%)	12 (39%)	7 (22%)	31	NS
Followed to 6½ yrs	83 (26%)	118 (36%)	124 (38%)	325	
FBW					
Followed beyond nursery but subsequently lost	10 (33%)	5 (17%)	15 (50%)	30	<0.025
Followed to 6½ yrs	29 (20%)	62 (43%)	54 (37%)	145	
NEUROLOGICAL OUTCOME					
LBW		*Normal*	*Abnormal*		
Recognized or presumed neurological status at 1 yr of infants lost to follow-up		56 (87.5%)	8 (12.5%)		NS
Neurological status at 1 yr of infants followed		327 (92%)	28 (8%)		
FBW					
Recognized or presumed neurological status at 6½ yrs of children lost to follow-up		54 (95%)	3 (5%)		NS
Neurological status at 6½ yrs of children followed		124 (89%)	15 (11%)		

*Social class could not be determined for many children who were lost soon after leaving the nursery.

TABLE 5-X

Correlated variables in mental retardation (MR) and cerebral palsy (CP) in comparison with LBW cohort

	MR (N = 29) *p*	*CP (N = 27)* *p*
Maternal neurological or psychiatric disease during pregnancy	NS (0.043)	NS
Lower mean social class than other LBW*	0.0000	NS
Lower mean gestational age than other LBW	NS	0.0000
Lower mean birthweight than other LBW	0.002	0.000
Abnormal Moro response in nursery	0.0000	0.0008
Moro response still present at 1 yr	NS	0.0000
Baby bleeding in nursery	NS	NS (0.0146)
Baby sucking poorly in nursery	NS (0.0536)	NS (0.0195)
Oxygen therapy in nursery	NS (0.0264)	0.0032
Intravenous therapy in nursery	NS (0.0066)	NS (0.0108)
Respiratory abnormalities in nursery	NS	0.0031
Abnormal neurological status at discharge	NS	NS (0.0127)
Abnormal neurological exam. at 1 yr	0.0000	0.0000
Abnormal neurological exam. at 1½ yrs	0.0000	0.0000
ATNR† still present at 1 yr	NS	0.0003
Abnormal head circumference (± >2SD) at 1 yr	0.0012	NS
EEG abnormal or borderline at 1 yr	NS (0.0104)	NS
Low mean Griffiths GQ at 1 yr	0.000	0.000
Low mean Griffiths GQ at 1½ yrs	0.000	0.000
Abnormal posture or gait at 1½ yrs	0.0000	0.0000
Plantar response still variable or extensor at 1½ yrs	NS	0.0000

Not significantly correlated with MR or CP:
Sex, plurality, weight-for-gestational-age category, maternal toxaemia, neonatal seizures or twitching, involuntary movements in nursery, type of delivery, presence of fetal distress, need for resuscitation, antepartum bleeding.

*Low birthweight; † asymmetrical tonic neck reflex.

defects, excluding strabismus and refractive errors (4.8 per cent), epilepsy (4.2 per cent) and sensorineural hearing-loss (3.6 per cent).

The frequency of neurological abnormalities among the LBW children increased from 8 per cent at one year and 12 per cent at 2½ years to 41.8 per cent at 6½ years, largely because of the emergence of MBD after the age of 2½ years. Neurological abnormalities at 6½ years were significantly more common among LBW boys (51.5 per cent) than girls (32 per cent). There was no significant difference between singletons *vs.* twins, or SGA *vs.* preterm AGA children. Mental retardation was somewhat more common among SGA children, as was cerebral palsy in the preterm AGA group, but the differences were not significant. Outcome for preterm and term SGA children was surprisingly similar.

The infants were classified in the nursery according to whether they had *(a)* no abormal neurological signs at any time, *(b)* abnormal signs only in the first two weeks or at discharge, or *(c)* abnormal signs all through their stay in the nursery. At one year 15 per cent of the first group had suspect or abnormal neurological status, compared to 28 per cent of the second and 46 per cent of the third groups ($p<0.0005$). The difference continued to be significant at 6½ years (34 *vs.* 41 *vs.* 52 per cent; $p<0.05$).

At one year the prevalence of neurological abnormality was inversely correlated with birthweight. Neonatal neurological abnormality was also negatively related to mean Griffiths GQ at one year and to WISC Full-scale IQ at 6½ years for the LBW children.

Seven LBW children had no Moro response after birth and this always heralded neurological sequelae and educational backwardness. If the response was difficult to obtain and/or showed no constant pattern it was associated with later neurological abnormality in about two-thirds of cases. An incomplete response on discharge from the nursery was associated with neurological abnormality and school problems in four of five cases. The response took longer to dissolve in LBW than FBW children, but if it could still be elicited at 12 months a neurological defect was certain and cerebral palsy was likely.

Between three and 12 months chronological age the FBW infants were significantly ahead of the LBW group in acquiring the parachute response. Neurological outcome was significantly better at 6½ years for FBW infants if they had acquired the response by six months rather than later, and for preterm AGA infants if they had acquired it by one year rather than later. The combination of an abnormal neonatal Moro response and absence of a normal parachute response at one year was a predictor of neurological abnormality in all cases, and of educational handicap in eight of 10 LBW children.

A definite plantar flexor response was neurologically favourable at 18 months for all LBW infants, and even at 12 months for preterm AGA infants.

At the age of three months the asymmetrical tonic neck reflex was elicited with ease in 29 per cent of preterm AGA and 33 per cent of SGA infants, but in only 4 per cent of FBW controls ($p<0.001$). Its persistence at six months in some LBW babies did not appear to be of significance. It persisted at 12 months in three preterm AGA infants, two of whom subsequently were found to have spastic cerebral palsy.

Only six LBW infants had a head circumference more than 2SD *above* the mean at one year, and none had a history of intraventricular haemorrhage or hydrocephalus. In contrast, 46 LBW infants had a head circumference more than 2SD *below* the mean, of whom 30 had neurological defects by 6½ years, so their prognosis was significantly worse than that for the total group ($p<0.005$).

At 6½ years 30 children were mentally retarded (global IQ <70). Their mean birthweight of 1554g was lower than that of the other LBW children ($p = 0.002$), and their lower social-class was even more significant ($p = 0.0000$). Mental retardation was also significantly correlated with an abnormal Moro response in the nursery, with abnormal neurological findings at 12 and 18 months, with abnormal (plus or minus more than 2SD) head-circumference at one year, low mean Griffiths GQ at 12 and 18 months, and abnormal posture or gait at 18 months.

Cerebral palsy ensued in 27 LBW infants, but in none of the FBW controls.

Among the antecedents of cerebral palsy were a significantly shorter mean gestation and lower mean birthweight than for the rest of the LBW cohort. All the affected children had had abnormal neurological signs in the nursery. There were also significant correlations with abnormal or absent Moro response in the nursery, persistent Moro and asymmetrical tonic neck responses at one year, oxygen therapy and respiratory abnormalities in the nursery, abnormal neurological examination and low Griffiths GQ at 12 and 18 months, abnormal posture or gait at 18 months and variable or extensor plantar responses at 18 months. These children's social class did not differ significantly from that of the LBW group in general.

Of the 14 LBW children (4.2 per cent) with epilepsy, five were classified as primary generalized (often familial), six as secondary generalized (lesional), one as undetermined generalized and two as partial epilepsy with secondary generalization. At most, the figure for the FBW controls was 2.2 per cent. The difference was not statistically significant, but it does appear that the frequency of seizure disorders is increased in LBW infants. On the other hand, idiopathic febrile convulsions were diagnosed in 2.4 per cent of LBW children and 3.6 per cent of FBW controls, so these were not increased for the LBW group.

6
Minimal Brain Dysfunctions

Henry G. Dunn, Helena H. Ho and Michael Schulzer

> *The idea of a continuum of reproductive casualty now appears to be unequivocal. One can only be uncharitable and suggest that those who cannot find children with minor degrees of handicap must not be able to perform an adequate neurological assessment* (Brown 1980).

In the introductory chapter we discussed the somewhat controversial concept of minimal brain dysfunction (MBD) and its behavioural component, the so-called hyperkinetic or 'organic' behaviour syndrome (OBS) or attention deficit disorder (ADD). Although MBD is a very diffuse syndrome, we find it useful as a unitary concept of mild brain dysfunction with an organic component. This applies particularly to young children when the different features of the syndrome are still evolving and cannot yet be ascertained completely (*e.g.* reading disability, dyscalculia, finger agnosia).

Kessler (1980) has described the history of the MBD concept. Following the earlier publications by Kahn and Cohen (1934) and by Bradley (1937), Strauss and colleagues thought that 'brain injury' was associated with a characteristic form of behaviour, and that its diagnosis could be based on the presence of faulty perception and conceptual thinking alone, for which they devised a system of corrective perceptual-motor training (Strauss and Werner 1942, Strauss and Lehtinen 1947, Strauss and Kephart 1955). These views have been criticized considerably (*e.g.* Herbert 1964, Hallahan and Cruickshank 1973). Schulman and colleagues (1965) found that the neurological examination did not relate significantly to any other measures and that distractability was the only reliable behavioural correlate of brain damage. In 1971 Dykman and co-workers shifted the emphasis from hyperkinesis to faulty attention-span. The term 'attention deficit disorder' was made official by the American Psychiatric Association (1978); according to that terminology, hyperkinesis may or may not be associated. Another study found disinhibition to be the only significant behavioural correlate of brain injury. The problem is discussed by Rutter and colleagues (1980), who reaffirm that brain injury is followed by behaviour disorders but do not concede the existence of a 'brain-damage syndrome', though they allow that pervasive severe hyperkinesis may represent a rare but distinct entity. Kalverboer (1978) allows that the concept of a continuum of degrees of damage may be valid, as aetiological studies show relationships between behaviour disorders of the type described in MBD and risk factors early in development, but he maintains that such behaviour disorders are not sufficient evidence for brain damage or dysfunction. Wolff and Hurwitz (1973) did demonstrate behavioural differences between groups distinguished solely on a neurological basis, as shown by correlation between choreiform dyskinesia and teachers' behaviour ratings.

With respect to longitudinal studies, Kalverboer *et al.* (1973) found little neurobehavioural correlation at five years with neonatal apathy, hyperexcitability or other features indicating a risk of MBD. Shaffer (1978) argued that, in any case, perinatal complications are common and not independent of social and family disadvantages. He suggested prospective studies using direct neurological data and the Prechtl (1965) scores of optimality. The results of such a follow-up study in Groningen, carried out only to the age of 18 months, were published by Bierman-van Eendenburg *et al.* (1981). It confirmed the sensitivity of the neonatal neurological examination among 80 abnormal newborns and 80 normal controls. However, 66 of the abnormal infants appeared to have recovered, which indicates a high frequency of what the authors considered to be transient neonatal morbidity. It might be useful to follow such a group of children longer to check for MBD at school-age.

The value of the psychological criteria for MBD has also been criticized. Yule (1978) pointed out, for instance, that 10 per cent of the population have a difference in Verbal and Performance IQ scores as large as 22 points on the WISC (Field 1960), so even big differences may not be clinically relevant.

Criteria and findings in present study

In our study MBD was the most common neurological sequel for LBW children. It was diagnosed in 61 of the 335 LBW children (18 per cent) at the age of 6½ years, compared to only nine out of the 139 FBW control children (6.5 per cent). In making this diagnosis we have accepted the views of the International Study Group on Minimal Cerebral Dysfunction, in which the Project Director participated (Mac Keith 1963). As mentioned in Chapter 1, we also accept the definition by Clements (1966) of the 'minimal brain dysfunction syndrome', which refers to 'children of near average, average or above average general intelligence with certain learning or behavioural disabilities ranging from mild to severe, which are associated with deviations of function of the central nervous system'.

It is agreed that similar symptoms may complicate the problems of children with cerebral palsy, epilepsy, mental retardation, blindness or deafness, but we have not used the term 'minimal brain dysfunction' in such cases because the brain dysfunction is then certainly more than minimal. Like Paine *et al.* (1968), we excluded children with a global IQ <80. Those authors had as minimum criteria for inclusion only *one* of the following: (1) abnormal neurological signs (beyond mere clumsiness); (2) abnormal EEG; or (3) psychological findings of the type seen in organic encephalopathies, *plus* either excessive clumsiness or abnormal EEG. It seemed to us somewhat hazardous to base the diagnosis solely on an abnormal EEG (depending on how this is defined), or a few 'soft' neurological signs which may also be encountered in healthy children (Kennard 1960, Hertzig *et al.* 1969, Rutter *et al.* 1970, Peters *et al.* 1975, Erickson 1977, Hertzig 1981). Therefore we established the minimum requirement that at least two out of a possible four points should be scored in the following areas: (1) abnormal neurological signs; (2) abnormal behavioural findings of the type encountered in the so-called 'organic behaviour syndrome' (brief attention-span, hyperkinesis, distractability, low tolerance of frustration, temper tantrums, mood swings, unpredictability, perseveration, impulsiveness, irritability, variability of performance); (3) psychological findings of the type seen in organic encephalopathies; and (4) abnormal EEG.

We also established a rule that diagnosis could not be based on behavioural and psychological findings alone, since both are somewhat controversial; there also had to be some neurological or EEG abnormalities. On the other hand, we permitted half-points for borderline abnormal findings in these four areas, provided a total of at least two full points was obtained. For many children we also used the more elaborate 50-point scoring-system, in which 15 possible points are allotted for neurological abnormalities, 10 each for psychological and EEG abnormalities, and five each for 'organic behaviour syndrome', speech and hearing abnormalities, and learning problems (Crichton *et al.* 1971). On this system a score of 15 points or more coincided closely with a clinical diagnosis of MBD and with two or more points on the above simpler scale.

The psychological criteria for the diagnosis of MBD at 6½ years were as follows: (1) on the WISC a half-point was given for a difference of 20 or more between the Verbal and Performance scores; (2) on the Goodenough-Harris Draw-a-Person test a half-point was given for a total score <80 (averaging the scores for drawing a man and a woman) *or* for a score 15 or more points below the WISC Full-scale IQ score; (3) on the Bender Visual-Motor Gestalt test a half-point was given for a borderline error score of more than 1SD and a full point for an abnormal error score of more than 2SD, *or* a half-point for the presence of certain qualitative errors indicating 'brain injury'. The maximum total score for 'organic' psychological findings was one point.

With respect to the 'organic behaviour syndrome', the components were listed and the child was given one point if all or nearly all (at least seven) of the above features had been witnessed by mother and physician; a half-point was given for only three to six of these 11 features.

In this way 61 LBW children (41 boys, 20 girls) were diagnosed as having MBD syndrome at 6½ years. 39 were AGA preterm, 21 were SGA, and one was of uncertain gestational age. 46 were singletons, 15 were twins. Individual features were tabulated as follows:

(1) *Abnormal neurological signs* (53 points in 59 of the 61 patients).

(a) Motor findings

poor fine co-ordination	35
hypertonus and/or unusually brisk tendon reflexes	25
involuntary movements or motor impersistence	21
apraxia, *e.g.* of tongue	21
poor balance or tandem gait	21
poor gross co-ordination	18
crossed laterality (excluding eyedness)	9
fluctuating dystonia	7
hypotonia and/or depressed tendon reflexes	5

(b) Sensory findings	
poor finger localization*	38
right-left confusion*	36
poor visual and/or auditory perception	16
astereognosis and/or poor graphaesthesia	8
poor body-image	6
impaired two-point discrimination	2
(c) Speech	
mildly impaired articulation	18
delayed speech development	11
articulatory apraxia	7
dysphasia	7
dysarthria	6
cluttering or stuttering	5
poor auditory comprehension	4
echolalia	1
(d) Eye signs	
strabismus	16
saccadic eye-movements	2
nystagmus	1
(e) Others	
impaired visual-motor co-ordination	24
reading and/or spelling disability*	11
difficulty with number concepts*	10

(2) *Abnormal behavioural findings*—'organic behaviour syndrome' (OBS) or attention deficit disorder (ADD) (39½ points in 56 of the 61 patients).

brief attention-span, distractability	53
excessive motor activity	45
irritability, low frustration threshold	31
tantrums	25
perseveration	22
unpredictability	19
mood swings	17
impulsiveness	14
destructiveness	6

(3) *Abnormal psychological findings* (29 points in 39 of the 61 patients).

WISC difference of 20 or more points between Verbal and Performance scores	14
Goodenough-Harris total score <80	9
Goodenough-Harris score 15 or more points below WISC Full-scale IQ score	10

*At 6½ years these skills are only just being acquired. While the figures for poor finger localization and right-left confusion on the child himself therefore may be somewhat high (particularly for those with low-normal intelligence), the difficulties in reading, spelling and arithmetic may be underestimated in Grade 1. In tests of finger localization, one error was permitted for 10 digits.

Bender Visual-Motor Gestalt Test error score 1-2	14
Bender Visual-Motor Gestalt Test error score >2	13
Bender Visual-Motor Gestalt error score not high but with significant 'brain injury indicator'	3

(4) *EEGs* (these were available only for 55 cases, yielding 26 points for abnormality in 30 of the 55 records at about 6¾ years).

abnormal	22
borderline (mildly dysrhythmic or asymmetrical)	8
normal	25

Further details about these EEGS will be found in Chapter 13.

Thus the neurological and behavioural features made greater numerical contributions to the diagnosis than the psychological and EEG findings at this age. In addition to the features of OBS (or ADD), 55 of the 61 children had other behavioural abnormalities commonly indicative of insecurity (shyness, thumb-sucking, enuresis, rocking, sibling rivalry, nightmares), and accompanied the ADD in 52 (93 per cent) of the 56 children in whom it was present in complete or partial form.

Correlations between psychological test scores and the presence of MBD and its behavioural component, ADD, and other variables, are explored in Tables 6-I to IV. For this purpose we graded the ADD (or OBS) into: 1 = no or few (up to two) features; 2 = some (three to six) features; 3 = seven or more features. In Tables 6-I and II we analyze all LBW children at 6½ years of age, excluding only those with a WISC Full-scale IQ <50 and those with unknown or suspicious neurological findings. The neurological examination was graded into: 1 = normal; 2 = minor abnormality; 3 = major abnormality. Socio-economic status was classified into five grades, according to the Hollingshead Two-factor Index (1957).

Table 6-I shows that the mean WISC Full-scale IQ scores are significantly higher for the FBW controls than for the LBW children, and for the neurologically normal FBW as compared to normal LBW subjects, while the last have significantly higher scores than the LBW children with MBD. These differences are significant, even when the effects of social class and sex are taken into consideration. Children with LBW who have major abnormal signs on neurological examination have a mean WISC Full-scale IQ significantly lower than that for children with minor abnormal signs, and the latter again have lower mean WISC IQ than those who are considered to have no neurological abnormality. In the FBW controls, the number of children with abnormal neurological signs is small and the IQ difference between normal children and those with minor abnormalities is not significant, but those with major abnormality have a significantly lower mean IQ. LBW children with no, some or all features of ADD have signifcantly lower global IQ scores, in that order. For FBW controls, cases with some, nearly all and all features, respectively, were pooled and then have a significantly lower mean IQ than those with no or few (less than three) features, even when social class is partialled out. Mean global IQ scores in general are highly correlated with social class.

TABLE 6-I

Comparison of adjusted mean WISC-R Full-scale IQs at 6½ years for LBW children and FBW controls (exluding IQ <50)

		N	*Adjusted mean IQ*	*Significance*	*Duncan analysis*	*Covariates**
Birthweight	1 LBW ≤2041g	305	96.0	F = 87.17 p = 0.000	2 >1	Social class p = 0.000; sex NS
	2 FBW >2500g	139	108.7			
Neurological status	1 LBW MBD	58	95.3	F = 50.31 p = 0.000	3 >2 >1	Social class p = 0.000; Sex p = 0.008
	2 LBW neurologically normal	183	102.3			
	3 FBW normal	125	110.1			
Neurological examination: LBW	1 Normal	159	102.0	F = 58.67 p = 0.000	1 >2 >3	Social class p = 0.000; sex NS
	2 Minor abnormality	71	93.4			
	3 Major abnormality	55	74.1			
FBW	1 Normal	120	109.9	F = 18.34 p = 0.000	1,2>3	Social class p = 0.000; sex NS
	2 Minor abnormality	5	107.0			
	2 Major abnormality	4	80.7			
Attention deficit disorder: LBW	1 No or few (0–2) features	159	99.8	F = 19.97 p = 0.000	1 >2 >3	Social class p = 0.000; sex NS
	2 Some (3–6) features	119	91.3			
	3 All or nearly all (7–11) features	33	79.3			
FBW	1 No or few (0–2) features	111	109.7	F = 7.975 p = 0.005	1 >2,3	Social class p = 0.000; sex NS
	2 + 3 Some (3–6), all or nearly all (7–11) features**	27	103.0			
Social class: LBW	I	23	109.8	F = 12.32 p = 0.000	1 >3,4 >5 2 >5	Sex NS
	II	18	103.8			
	III	38	99.5			
	IV	117	96.8			
	V	115	85.8			
FBW	I	9	119.8	F 6.969 p = 0.000	1,2 >4 >5 1,2 >3	Sex NS
	II	7	119.9			
	III	11	106.7			
	IV	61	109.4			
	V	51	103.9			

*Age at testing also included as covariate but not significant in this analysis.
**Only one child had all or nearly all features; this case was added to the 26 with some features.

WISC Verbal-Performance IQ scores

Table 6-II tests the hypothesis that a large difference between WISC Verbal and Performance IQ scores at 6½ years may be related to brain dysfunction. It is interesting that the mean Verbal and Performance IQ scores are not significantly correlated with birthweight category, social class or ADD. Among LBW children those with major abnormal neurological findings even have a significantly smaller score difference than those who are neurologically normal or have only minor

TABLE 6-II

Mean WISC Verbal-Performance IQ score difference at 6½ years for LBW children and FBW controls

		N	*Adjusted IQ score difference*	*Significance*	*Covariates*	*p*
Birthweight category:	LBW ≤2041g	303	10.2±7.6	F = 0.70	Social class	NS
	FBW >2500g	138	9.5±8.0	NS	Sex	NS
					Age at testing	NS
Neurological examination: LBW	1 Normal	157	10.8±8.1	F = 5.328	Social class	NS
	2 Minor abn.	71	11.0±7.1	p = 0.005	Sex	NS
	3 Major abn.	47	6.4±5.5	Duncan 1, 2 >3	Age at testing	NS
Social class	I	31	9.8±7.7			
	II	25	9.7±5.6	F = 0.226	Sex	NS
	III	47	9.1±5.8	NS	Age at testing	NS
	IV	177	10.3±8.5			
	V	161	9.9±7.7			
Attention deficit disorder (LBW + FBW)	1 0–2 features	267	9.8±8.1	F = 0.768	Social class	NS
	2 3–6 features	141	10.6±7.4	NS	Sex	NS
	3 7–11 features	32	8.9±6.3		Age at testing	NS

abnormal findings. All this would suggest that the difference between verbal and performance skills is a poor indicator of cerebral dysfunction at this age.

Bender Visual-Motor Gestalt Test

Table 6-III analyzes Bender Visual-Motor Gestalt error scores (according to the Koppitz system) at 6½ years in relation to birthweight category, neurological signs and degrees of ADD. It will be seen that LBW children as a whole obtained significantly higher mean error scores on this test than the FBW control group, even when the effect of IQ (which is highly significant) is taken into consideration. Further, LBW children with abnormal neurological findings tended to obtain higher Bender error scores than those whose neurological examination was normal. When the total group of LBW plus FBW control children was analyzed similarly, the difference in Bender scores between children with normal and abnormal neurological findings was more highly significant. Thus the Bender Gestalt Test scores appear to vary in a direct relationship to abnormal neurological findings, as one might expect in associated components of MBD. Further, such Bender test scores are also significantly associated with increasing numbers of features of ADD in the combined LBW and FBW groups, even when these scores are controlled for IQ differences. The analysis of Bender scores in relation to neurological findings in the FBW control group alone did not show significant differences, largely because there were only five children with minor and four with major abnormal neurological findings, as compared to 120 with no abnormal neurological signs. The analysis of Bender scores in relation to the number of features of ADD in the LBW and FBW groups alone also failed to reach statistical significance when IQ was taken into consideration, though the trend was evident in the LBW group.

Goodenough-Harris Draw-a-Person Test

Table 6-IV explores the correlation of Goodenough-Harris drawing scores with birthweight category, neurological signs, ADD and social class. In this analysis the

Table 6-III

Mean Bender Visual-Motor Gestalt error scores at 6½ years for LBW children and FBW controls

		N	*Raw mean score*	*Adjusted mean score*	*Significance*	*Covariates*	*p*
Birthweight category:	1 LBW ≤2041g	293	0.624	0.540	F = 12.409	Social class	NS
					p = 0.0005	Sex	NS
	2 FBW >2500g	138	−0.241	0.150	Duncan 1 >2	Age at testing	NS
						WISC FS IQ	0.000
Neurological examination: LBW	1 Normal	155	0.244	0.566	F = 2.666	Social class	0.012
	2 Minor abn.	71	0.987	0.892	p = 0.071	Sex	NS
	3 Major abn.	42	1.293	0.826	Duncan 1 <3,2	Age at testing	NS
						WISC FS IQ	0.000
LBW + FBW	1 Normal	275	−0.0003	0.264	F = 5.938	Social class	NS
	2 Minor abn.	76	0.893	0.699	p = 0.003	Sex	NS
	3 Major abn.	46	1.29	0.605	Duncan 1 <3,2	Age at testing	NS
						WISC FS IQ	0.000
Attention deficit disorder LBW + FBW	1 0–2 features	263	−0.090	0.345	F = 4.592	Social class	NS
	2 3–6 features	136	0.653	0.489	p = 0.011	Sex	NS
	3 7–11 features	27	1.401	0.966	Duncan 1,2 <3	Age at testing	NS
						WISC FS IQ	0.000

TABLE 6-IV

Mean Goodenough-Harris Draw-a-Person Test scores (with age adjustment) at about 6½ years for LBW children and FBW controls

		N	*Adjusted mean score*	*Significance*	*Covariates**	*p*
Birthweight category	1 LBW ≤2041g	295	92.87	F = 2.450	Social Class	0.001
	2 FBW >2500g	137	94.71	NS		
Neurological examination: LBW	1 Normal	155	96.47	F = 14.07	Social class	0.015
	2 Minor abn.	71	90.25	p = 0.000		
	3 Major abn.	43	85.19			
FBW	1 Normal	120	95.39	F = 1.96	Social class	NS
	2 Minor abn.	5	90.77	NS		
	3 Major abn.	3	85.86			
Attention deficit disorder: LBW	1 0–2 features	155	94.60	F = 4.514	Social class	0.005
	2 3–6 features	112	92.11	p = 0.012		
	3 7–11 features	28	86.40			
FBW	1 0–2 features	111	95.40	F = 2.874	Social class	NS
	2 3–6 features	25	91.84	NS		
	3 7–11 features	0				
Social class: LBW	I	22	98.56			
	II	18	97.07	F = 2.403		
	III	37	94.24	p = 0.050		
	IV	115	93.00			
	V	102	90.16			
FBW	I	9	95.34			
	II	7	98.26	F = 0.947		
	III	11	93.78	NS		
	IV	59	95.89			
	V	51	92.93			

*Age at testing adjusted individually for all children.

mean raw drawing-scores of LBW children were slightly lower than those of the FBW controls, as one might expect. When age at testing was taken into consideration, the Goodenough-Harris scores of the FBW control children were not statistically related to age. Evidently the scores were adjusted satisfactorily for age in the calculation used for the test, as they are expected to be. On the other hand, in the LBW children there was a significant ($p = 0.03$) relationship of Goodenough-Harris (G-H) score with age, with a negative coefficient: G-H score = 122–0.366A, where A is age in months.

In Table 6-IV mean scores have been adjusted for age according to the above equation. The somewhat low mean scores of the FBW control children for the Goodenough-Harris drawing test will be noted again in Chapter 7.

With respect to the neurological findings, it will be noted that children with minor and major abnormal neurological signs tend to obtain lower scores on the Draw-a-Person Test, both in the LBW and the FBW groups, as might be expected. However, when WISC Full-scale IQ was taken into consideration the differences in the mean scores in relation to neurological examination and ADD in the LBW groups became less significant. In general, it would appear that the Goodenough-Harris Test yields mean scores which do not correlate with birthweight categories, abnormal neurological findings or features of ADD as significantly as error scores in the Bender Gestalt Test shown in the previous Table. Also, social class appears to have little correlation with drawing scores when controlled for IQ. Intelligence may be correlated with drawing skills to a more significant extent than neurological and 'organic' behavioural findings or social class. In addition, the age at testing was a significant covariate for the LBW children in this test, while it was not found to be so critical in relation to other tasks.

Interaction of variables related to IQ

In order to study further the interaction of the behavioural and neurological components of MBD, the relationship of abnormal neurological findings, degrees of ADD and social class to WISC Full-scale IQ was then analyzed for the LBW children (Table 6-V). These data indicate that the mean WISC Full-scale IQ of LBW children at 6½ years varied just significantly inversely with the extent of ADD (usually including hyperkinesis) by itself, varied very significantly inversely with the degree of neurological abnormality, and also varied very significantly directly with social class when the other variables were controlled. There was also marked interaction in the effect of low social-class with both ADD and abnormal neurological signs in lowering mean IQ, but interestingly there was no significant interaction between attention deficit and abnormal neurological signs in this respect. Thus both abnormal neurological findings and ADD are associated with lower IQ, even after adjustment for social class, but not more than additively.

In a separate analysis it was also shown that the degree of ADD varied very significantly with abnormal neurological findings in LBW children when the effects of sex, intelligence (WISC Full-scale IQ) and social class were controlled. Among FBW children there was a similar trend, but the numbers of neurological abnormalities were too few for meaningful statistical analysis.

TABLE 6-V

WISC Full-scale IQ in relation to attention deficit disorder (ADD), neurological examination and social class and their interactions in LBW children

	F-ratio	*p*	*Duncan analysis at 5% probability*
Variables:			
ADD score*	2.875	0.053	ADD score 3 <score 1
Neurological examination**	51.442	0.000	Neurol. score 3 <neurol 2 <neurol 1
Social class***	9.795	0.000	Class I >II,III,IV,V; III >IV,V
Interactions			
ADD score *vs.* neurological examination	0.416	NS	No significant interaction on IQ
ADD score *vs.* social class	3.852	0.0005	Highly significant interaction on IQ. (1,I) >others, including (3,I)
Neurological examination *vs.* social class	5.152	0.000	Highly significant interaction on IQ (1,I) >(3,I) (3,V) <rest

	*ADD score**			*Neurological examination***			*Social class****				
	1	2	3	1	2	3	I	II	III	IV	V
N	149	105	31	158	71	56	22	14	38	106	105
Adjusted mean IQ	97.1	94.3	90.2	101.6	94.3	78.7	107.4	97.6	100.7	94.6	91.2
SD	12.9	18.65	21.1	11.0	12.6	20.9	17.1	8.9	12.7	13.8	20.2

*ADD score 1 = no or few (0–2) features; 2 = some (3–6) features; 3 = all or nearly all (7–11) features.
**Neurological examination score 1 = normal; 2 = minor abnormality; 3 = major abnormality.
***Social class numbered according to Hollingshead Two-factor Index.

Attention deficit disorder

Table 6-VI explores the controversial ADD further in relation to other variables in LBW children. The mean ADD scores are significantly higher for boys than for girls and also among LBW as compared to FBW children, even when controlled for IQ. The association between ADD scores and social class is less highly significant, and there is no linear relationship. ADD scores are significantly highest in social-class III. In a separate analysis of covariance, it was shown that if social-classes I and II and classes IV and V, respectively, are combined, the probability of class III being different, with higher ADD scores, rises to $p = 0.013$ on Duncan's analysis. In FBW control children, social-class III also has the highest mean score for ADD, but the differences from other classes are not significant, partly because the numbers are too small.

In another analysis it was shown that interaction of sex and social class on ADD scores is non-significant, *i.e.* the effects are not more than additive.

There is a highly significant negative relationship of ADD scores to IQ, and the mildy retarded children (IQ 50 to 69) had a significantly higher mean ADD score than those within the normal range (IQ ⩾80). There is also a very significant

TABLE 6-VI

Attention deficit disorder (ADD) scores* for LBW children at 6½ years in relation to sex, FBW controls, social class and WISC Full-scale IQ (excluding IQ <50)

		N	*Adjusted mean ADD score**	*Significance*	*Duncan analysis at 5% probability*	*Covariates*	*p*
Sex	1 Male	154	1.759	F = 21.094	1 >2	WISC FS IQ	0.000
	2 Female	157	1.440	p = 0.000		Social class	NS
Birthweight category	1 LBW ≤2041g	311	1.543	F = 12.139	1 >2	WISC FS IQ	0.000
	2 FBW >2500g	138	1.327	p = 0.001		Social class	NS
						Sex	0.000
Social class	I	23	1.616				
	II	18	1.487	F = 2.709	III>II, IV, V	WISC FS IQ	0.000
	III	38	1.869	p = 0.030		Sex	0.000
	IV	118	1.509				
	V	114	1.613				
WISC Full-scale IQ (LBW)	1 50–69	22	2.244				
	2 70–79	29	1.959				
	3 80–89	53	1.692	F = 9.485	1 >3 >6	Social class	NS
	4 90–99	64	1.592	p = 0.000	2 >4 >5	Sex	0.000
	5 100–109	84	1.381		1,2 >5,6		
	6 ≥110	59	1.412		3,4 >5,6		
Neurological examination (LBW)	1 Normal	158	1.309			WISC FS IQ	0.025
	2 Minor abn.	71	1.905	F = 31.180	2,3 >1	Social class	NS
	3 Major abn.	56	1.962	p = 0.000		Sex	0.001

*ADD scores: 1 = no or few (0–2) features; 2 = some (3–6) features; 3 = all or nearly all (7–11) features.

relationship between ADD and minor or major neurological findings.

Relationship of ADD to EEG abnormalities

Among the LBW children, an abnormal EEG and increase in mean ADD score at 6½ years are not significantly correlated when it is taken into consideration that WISC Full-scale IQ is significantly lower (p = 0.000) and sex significantly more often male (p = 0.00001) with EEG abnormality. The findings for the FBW control children are similar.

In summary, ADD emerges as an entity significantly related to abnormal neurological findings and negatively related to global IQ, occurring most often in social-class III and more commonly in boys than in girls, and also more commonly in LBW children with birthweights ≤2041g than in FBW control children. In its relationship to IQ it shows significant interaction with social class but not with abnormal neurological signs. ADD scores are also related significantly to the error scores on the Bender Visual-Motor Gestalt Test at 6½ years but not to differences in mean WISC Verbal and Performance IQ scores or to Goodenough-Harris Draw-a-Person Test scores at about 6½ years. ADD is not significantly correlated with EEG abnormalities. In the context of MBD, it was accompanied by other behavioural abnormalities, possibly secondary and commonly suggestive of insecurity, in more than 90 per cent of affected children.

TABLE 6-VII

Correlated variables in histories of 61 LBW children with minimal brain dysfunction

	p
Initial neonatal Moro response not obtained with ease	0.0002
Hypothermia (<35.6°C) on admission to nursery	0.0051
Plantar response not yet distinctly flexor at 18 mths	0.0058
Abnormal movements on initial examination in nursery, chiefly tremulous or 'jittery'	0.0062
Abnormal truncal tone (chiefly flaccid)	0.0090
Male sex	0.0110
Maternal toxaemia	0.0237
Neck flexor tone abnormal (chiefly flaccid)	0.0271
Maternal hypertension in pregnancy	0.0369
Neck extensor tone abnormal (chiefly flaccid)	0.0401
Neonatal twitching in nursery	0.0443
Birthweight lower than mean LBW (t test with pooled variance)	0.0450
Weak palmar grasp in nursery	0.0560

No significant relationship was found with 75 other variables concerning the mother, pregnancy, delivery, newborn period or infancy.

Antecedents

In Chapter 5 we explored the antecedents of mental retardation and cerebral palsy in LBW children and showed considerable differences between them. Since MBD is clearly a milder disorder, we expected to find fewer abnormalities in the histories of the children, but we thought it would be interesting to comb through a large number of variables in order to detect any possible associations (Table 6-VII).

It will be seen that there is a significant relationship to some early neonatal variables, particularly the initial Moro response, hypothermia on admission to the nursery, and abnormal movements on initial examination there. There is also a significant relationship with delayed appearance of flexor plantar responses. Naturally there was also a significant relationship to poor class-placement in Grade 3 and to teachers' reports of academic difficulties, but this is only to be expected in a condition which includes learning disabilities. MBD syndrome occurred in both AGA preterm and SGA children, without significant difference. Since many of these variables are interdependent, a significant correlation presumably should exist at a probability of less than 0.005, as calculated in Chapter 5.

Cerebral dysfunction, more than minimal

In the analysis of neurological or ophthalmic disorders among LBW children (Table 6-I), a final group emerged with miscellaneous cerebral dysfunctions more than minimal. This includes 21 children (13 boys, eight girls) with borderline low-normal intelligence (global IQ 70 to 79). 11 were AGA preterm and 10 were SGA. Of the latter, seven were born preterm and three at term. 14 were singletons and seven were twins.

The abnormal neurological signs were similar to those in MBD, but in view of the lower IQ at the chronological age of about 6½ years, right-left distinction, finger localization, apraxia of tongue-movements, and learning disabilities could not yet be evaluated. The following were the most common features found among the 21 patients: crossed laterality (with respect to hands and feet only and not considering eyedness) and/or ambidexterity (13); poor visual-motor co-ordination and drawing (13); clumsiness and/or poor balance (11); mildly impaired articulation or lisp (eight); delayed or immature speech (four); abnormalities of muscle tone (five); strabismus (three) and gait disorder (three).

It was also noted that five of these patients, all SGA, had congenital stigmata, such as unusual facies (with hypertelorism, blepharophimosis, ptosis, *etc.*), cleft palate or kyphosis. Four had a significantly small stature and three a significantly small head (below 3rd percentile). On psychological testing, four had a Bender Visual-Motor Gestalt error score of more than two. All or nearly all the features of the ADD were found in three, and some features in another six of these 21 children, and at least five exhibited other features of emotional disturbance, often insecurity. EEGs were recorded at about 6¾ years in 20 of these children and were considered normal in nine, abnormal in 10 and borderline in one.

Discussion

In the introductory chapter we noted that the syndrome of MBD is extremely wide, ranging from clumsy children to those with learning disabilities and others with attention deficit and hyperactive behaviour. It is generally agreed that it would be desirable to split this into subsyndromes, but in view of the extensive overlap of neurological, psychological and behavioural features this has been difficult to accomplish (Paine *et al.* 1968, Strother 1973, Peters *et al.* 1975). Another difficulty is that the features of the syndrome merge imperceptibly into the normal. The equivocal character of such features had been noted by Kennard (1960), who compared the neurological signs of 'brain-damaged' children with those of normal controls and found a quantitative rather than a qualitative difference. Adams *et al.* (1974) stated that '9- and 10-year-old learning-disabled children cannot be reliably distinguished from normally achieving children on the basis of the soft neurological signs outlined'. This applied equally to the behavioural features of the syndrome. Accordingly, we thought it wise to establish a simple scoring system whereby the contributions to the diagnosis of the neurological and psychological assessment, the so-called organic behaviour syndrome (now renamed ADD) and the EEG can be quantitated, at least roughly. Also, with respect to ADD itself, we recorded in each case whether no or few (less than three) features, some (three to six) features, or all or nearly all (seven to 11) features were present. We agree with previous authors that the features of this so-called organic behaviour syndrome very frequently are accompanied by other, possibly secondary, behavioural abnormalities which commonly are indicative of insecurity (*e.g.* shyness, enuresis, sibling rivalry, nightmares), but this does not rule out the possibility that a core group of symptoms may have an organic basis. In view of the controversy concerning the psychological criteria and behavioural manifestations of 'brain damage', we insisted that the diagnosis of MBD could not be made on the basis of abnormalities in these areas alone, and required at least a half-point of contribution from the neurological examination or EEG. Moreover, we decided that a suspicious history of events causing possible brain-damage should not be included among the diagnostic criteria, but only the actual findings on examination.

It is interesting to see, then, that the mean WISC Full-scale IQ of LBW children with MBD is significantly lower than the mean for those who were considered neurologically normal at 6½ years, even when social class and sex are taken into consideration. It is also noteworthy that the presence of an increasing number of features of ADD is significantly correlated with an increasing number of abnormal neurological findings, even when controlled for IQ. While both abnormal neurological signs and features of ADD are related inversely to Verbal IQ, even after adjustment for social class, their effects appear to be additive rather than interactive. It is also of interest that the features of ADD are found significantly more often among boys than girls and among LBW children than FBW controls, even when global IQ is controlled.

With respect to social class, we noted in Table 6-VI that ADD is most common in class III rather than in the lowest classes. Here it may be recalled that Werry (1968) studied 103 *hyperactive* children of normal intelligence at a mean age of 8½ years and found (1) a marked predominance of boys (91 per cent); (2) a slight predominance of social-class III (37 per cent); (3) an increased prevalence of abnormal perinatal events (34 per cent); and (4) abnormal neurological status in 64 per cent. Factor analysis showed common variance, evenly distributed among 10 factors, suggesting heterogeneity of dysfunctions in MBD. Socio-economic status, birth order and severity of hyperkinesis did not appear to be loading variables. One possible explanation may be that the irritable, hyperactive child with brief attention-span and mood swings causes more emphatic complaints by middle-class than by working-class parents. The trend for FBW control children was similar, but the differences were not significant, perhaps because the numbers were too small.

Regarding psychological tests, it is interesting that the difference between the Verbal and Performance IQ scores of the WISC was no greater in neurologically normal LBW than in FBW control children, and that it was not significantly correlated with birthweight in general, social class or ADD. Thus our findings support the opinion that this score difference is a poor indicator of cerebral dysfunction, at least at the age of 6½ years (Rutter *et al.* 1970, Rourke *et al.* 1973, Yule 1978). Similarly, the difference between the mean Goodenough-Harris Draw-a-Person Test scores of LBW and FBW control children is not significant when social class and age at testing are controlled. Intelligence, social class and age appear to make a more significant contribution than birthweight to higher scores in this test. A recent publication also indicates that the result of this test is affected by art instruction (Lindsey and Frith 1981). The findings on the Bender Visual-Motor Gestalt Test appear to be more helpful with respect to the presence of MBD. The error scores are lower for FBW controls than for the neurologically normal LBW children, and very significantly lower for FBW than for all LBW children. The scores also correlate significantly with the presence of ADD, even when differences in social class are taken into account.

Since MBD, including learning disabilities, represents only mild disturbances in brain activity, we hardly expected to find significant differences in the family and pregnancy histories and in the perinatal course of these children, as compared to neurologically normal LBW children. Surprisingly, a number of such variables were found to have a significant relationship with the diagnosis for the 61 children with MBD. The most significant relationship was with the neonatal Moro response not being obtained with ease ($p = 0.0002$). More than 100 other variables were analyzed. Since many of them are interdependent, the p figures shown in the variables listed in Table 6-VII may be considered to be of borderline or doubtful significance. Nonetheless, one gains the impression that there might well be a relationship between adverse perinatal factors and subsequent mild dysfunction, and it also seems that the delayed attainment of certain neurological milestones (*e.g.* flexor plantar response at 18 months) may point toward the diagnosis. As might be expected, these antecedents are notably different from those for mental retardation and cerebral palsy (see Chapter 5). They are consistent with some of the neuropathological findings in learning disabilities and MBD which have been documented (Drake 1968, Towbin 1971, Galaburda and Kemper 1979, Fuller *et al.* 1983).

Finally, while MBD appears to merge imperceptibly into characteristics of normal children, its features also appear to be found quite commonly in children of borderline low-normal intelligence (global IQ 70 to 79). In our 21 cases of 'cerebral dysfunction more than minimal' this was evident on clinical examination, and again the EEG was abnormal in approximately one-half of the patients.

Our attempt to investigate subsyndromes of MBD by cluster analysis will be described in the next chapter.

Summary

The study of neurological sequelae in LBW infants and other newborns 'at risk' for cerebral defect or damage should include the examination for minor forms of brain dysfunction. Although MBD represents a diffuse and heterogeneous syndrome with a complex matrix of neurological, psychological, behavioural and EEG aspects, we consider this syndrome a useful unitary concept of brain dysfunctions with an organic component, particularly in young children, provided that details of the dysfunctions are specified in each case. The behavioural aspect is the most controversial, and it is realized that the existence of a specific 'organic' or hyperkinetic behaviour syndrome associated with 'brain damage' is still in doubt. Meanwhile, emphasis has shifted (with some justification) from the overactivity to the attention deficit, which is likely to be more persistent in this syndrome.

In our study MBD was the most common neurological sequel, affecting 61 of the 335 LBW children (18 per cent) at the age of 6½ years, as compared to only nine of the 139 FBW control children (6.5 per cent). The diagnosis was based on minimum criteria of at least two out of a possible total of four points in terms of neurological, behavioural, psychological and EEG abnormalities. It had to include at least one half-point for abnormal neurological or EEG findings, *i.e.* it could not be based on behavioural or psychological features alone, since both are controversial. The global IQ had to be at least 80.

Of the 61 LBW children diagnosed as having MBD at 6½ years, 41 were boys and 20 were girls. Individual features are tabulated in the different spheres. The neurological and behavioural abnormalities made greater numerical (point) contributions to the diagnosis than the psychological and EEG findings. More than two features of the 'organic' behaviour syndrome were present in 56 of the 61 patients, and brief attention-span (or distractability) was noted in 53 of the 56, while excessive motor-activity was recorded in 45. In addition to the 'organic' behaviour syndrome or ADD, other behavioural abnormalities commonly indicative of insecurity were very common.

Analysis showed that the neurologically normal LBW children had significantly higher WISC Full-scale IQ scores at 6½ years than those with MBD, and LBW children with no, some or all features of ADD had significantly lower IQ scores in that order. Mean global IQ scores were also highly correlated with social class and negatively with neurological abnormalities.

The mean difference in WISC Verbal-Performance IQ score and the mean Goodenough-Harris Draw-a-Person Test score were not significantly different for the LBW children and the FBW controls. The WISC Verbal-Performance IQ score difference also was not significantly correlated with social class or ADD; the mean of the score difference was actually lower for LBW children with major abnormal neurological findings than for neurologically normal LBW children, or those with only minor abnormal findings. The Goodenough-Harris scores appeared to be strongly influenced by intelligence and age at testing. Hence both the WISC Verbal-Performance IQ score difference and the Goodenough-Harris Draw-a-Person score appeared to be poor indicators of cerebral dysfunction at this age.

On the other hand, the Bender Visual-Motor Gestalt Test yielded significantly higher error-scores for LBW children than for FBW controls, and the scores were significantly correlated with abnormal neurological signs and with the presence of all or nearly all features of ADD in LBW and FBW children, even when controlled for IQ.

The mean WISC Full-scale IQ of LBW children at 6½ years varied inversely with the extent of ADD at a just-significant level, with the degree of abnormal neurological signs to a more significant degree, and also directly and very significantly with social class, when the other variables were held constant. There was also a marked interaction in the effect of low social-class with both attention deficit and abnormal neurological signs in relation to low IQ, but there was no significant interaction between attention deficit and abnormal neurological signs.

Features of the 'organic' behaviour syndrome (or ADD) with hyperkinesis were significantly more common among boys than girls and among LBW than FBW children, even when the effect of IQ was taken into consideration. This behaviour syndrome was encountered most frequently in social-class III, just as Werry (1968) had noted with respect to hyperactive children. It was also related inversely and very significantly to global IQ ranges.

Abnormality of EEG and mean ADD score of LBW children at 6½ years were not significantly correlated after sex and IQ had been partialled out.

The antecedents of MBD in LBW children included a significantly high frequency of abnormal initial Moro response, hypothermia on admission to the nursery, abnormal movements on initial examination in the nursery, and delayed emergence of flexor plantar responses at 18 months.

The clinical and EEG features of 21 LBW children with 'cerebral dysfunction more than minimal' (mostly with global IQ within the 70 to 79 range) were not greatly different from those of MBD.

7
Statistical Analysis of Mild Brain Dysfunctions

Martin L. Puterman and Henry G. Dunn

In the introductory chapter we noted that the concept of 'minimal brain dysfunction' (MBD) had been criticized on the grounds that it was too diffuse and that more specific neurological and psychiatric diagnoses should be made so that specific treatment could be carried out (Gomez 1967, Rutter *et al.* 1970, Kalverboer *et al.* 1978, Rie 1980). Clements (1966) stated that the 10 characteristics most often cited were, in order of frequency: (1) hyperactivity; (2) perceptual-motor impairments; (3) emotional lability; (4) general co-ordination deficits; (5) disorders of attention (short attention-span, distractability, perseveration); (6) impulsivity; (7) disorders of memory and thinking; (8) specific learning disabilities—*(a)* reading, *(b)* arithmetic, *(c)* writing, *(d)* spelling; (9) disorders of speech and hearing; and (10) equivocal neurological signs and EEG irregularities. One could group these characteristics into three main clinical presentations: (1) attention deficit disorders, often including hyperactivity, perseveration and other features of the so-called 'organic behaviour syndrome'; (2) learning disabilities; and (3) clumsy children.

Attempts to separate these subsyndromes have not been very successful, partly because the pattern of abnormalities in MBD 'reflects a complex matrix of underlying dimensions, some innate, some traumatic and some psycho-social' (Paine *et al.* 1968, Werry 1968). In practice, we are liable to encounter a considerable overlap between different aspects of MBD. For instance in our study 61 LBW children were diagnosed as having MBD at 6½ years. 45 of them were considered hyperactive by parents and physicians. Of the 45, 29 also had poor co-ordination of fine movements and 11 also had reading disabilities (including six of those with poor co-ordination), leaving only 11 who were purely hyperactive.

Similarly, attempts have been made to classify children with specific dyslexia into three subgroups on the basis of their type of errors in reading—audiophonic, visuospatial or mixed (Ingram *et al.* 1970). The errors of the majority were found to be mixed. Denckla (1977) has gone further and defined five subsyndromes: (1) articulatory-graphomotor; (2) visuospatial perceptual; (3) language disorder—*(a)* mixed, *(b)* anomic and *(c)* dysphonemic sequencing; (4) verbal memorization (learning) disorder; and (5) right hemisyndrome with mixed language disorder. However, Denckla found that purity of complaint and homogeneity of syndrome were not strongly associated with either definitely abnormal or the 'developmental delay' type of neurological signs, nor with one type of presumptive aetiology. An implication of that study was that one must take into account multiple aetiologies of brain dysfunction in any one individual. The advantage of proceeding within the concept of MBD thus proved to be that it frees the investigator from the pursuit of the elusive 'pure' syndrome.

The use of factor analysis (Werry 1968, Crinella 1973) and cluster analysis (Schulman *et al.* 1965, Conners 1973) in subdividing the MBD syndrome did not lead to clinically meaningful subgroups, but cluster analysis apparently has been more successful when applied to psychiatric diagnoses (Paykel 1971, Strauss *et al.* 1973). Accordingly we thought it worthwhile to attempt a subdivision of our whole LBW population by cluster analysis (Anderberg 1973, Sneath and Sokal 1973, Everitt 1974), excluding children with mental retardation or severe neurological defects. We hoped to discover groups of children at 6½ years with common abnormal traits, corresponding to clinically meaningful syndromes. In contrast to earlier studies, we did not subdivide a population which had been preselected because of the presence of specified MBD abnormalities; we chose to analyze the entire cohort of LBW children in order to see what groupings of mild brain dysfunction might emerge. One specific goal was to find out how these groups would relate to our clinical diagnosis of MBD.

Comparison of LBW and control groups

Method

For analysis we excluded all children with cerebral palsy, epilepsy, visual and sensorineural hearing-defects, and all those with a WISC Full-scale IQ below 80. The last exclusion was consistent with our definition of MBD requiring a global IQ of at least 80. The resulting population contained 237 LBW children and 133 FBW controls.

Factors were selected from the 6½-year examination form, with emphasis on those used for the clinical diagnosis of MBD, as described in the previous chapter. From each factor a single binary variable was formed (coded 0 for normal, 1 for abnormal) by determining a suitable set of normal *vs.* abnormal scores or signs. The resulting 32 variables and their codings are described in the Appendix to this chapter.

Just as children with MBD were required to have normal intelligence, individual variables were allowed a similar range of 'normal'. For instance in the category for drawing at the age of 6½ years, children were considered normal and received a code of 0 if they could copy a diamond (seven-year skill), or at least a triangle (five-year skill). On the other hand, they were classified as abnormal (code 1) if they were able to copy only a simpler figure such as square, cross or circle, but not a triangle.

The clustering method used is based on a measure of disparity between subjects. By choosing binary variables for each factor, we felt it would be easier to obtain a comprehensible measure of difference, one that was not biased by the use of unequal scales or a mixture of quantitative and qualitative variables. For instance instead of considering the actual weight as a variable, a child was coded as abnormally low if weight was below the third percentile for age. The use of actual weight in combination with other binary or quantitative variables would have distorted the distance measure between cases, unless an arbitrary scaling of the weight variable had been introduced. Naturally some information is lost through this coding, since several gradations are lumped into the categories normal or abnormal and often it is difficult to determine which symptoms, signs or scores should indicate abnormality. However, this method of coding produced results which could be interpreted more easily. The use of binary coding in analyses of the type considered here is recommended by Sneath and Sokal (1973, p. 157).

Results
Table 7-I shows the proportions of children with each abnormality in the LBW and control groups. The third column gives the p-values from testing the hypothesis that each group has an equal proportion of abnormalities for each factor*.

As expected, the LBW group had a significantly higher proportion of abnormal responses than the control group in many categories. At an over-all 0.05 significance level†, the LBW group had higher proportions of children who had had diseases possibly affecting the central nervous system, or who had any of the following features: ADD, other behavioural abnormalities, low weight for age, small head-circumference for age, impaired right-left discrimination (on themselves), finger agnosia, increased or decreased tendon reflexes, abnormal plantar or Chaddock responses, or poor performance on the Bender Visual-Motor Gestalt Test. Peculiarly, the control group contained a significantly higher proportion of children with articulation difficulties and with score differences of more than 20 points between the WISC Full-scale IQ and the Goodenough-Harris drawing test. Also it is interesting that both groups contained a similarly high proportion with crossed laterality and with differences exceeding 20 points between the WISC Verbal and Performance IQ scores.

Cluster analysis of LBW subgroups
Method
The object of cluster analysis is described by Anderberg (1973, p. 3) as 'to sort the observations into groups such that the degree of 'natural association' is high among members of the same group and low between members of different groups'. Here we attempt to classify the children in the LBW subgroup into categories based on the presence or absence of abnormalities in the factors described above. Only 31 variables were used; the variable corresponding to a *history* of disease affecting the nervous system was excluded since it was not used for the clinical diagnosis of MBD and therefore was not considered suitable as a basis for grouping the children. However, the relationship of this variable to the derived clustering was analyzed. It was our intent to produce distinct clusters possessing characteristics in agreement with interpretable and clinically observable syndromes.

*Calculations were performed using the BMD P3D Programme. Tests were based on a pooled estimate of the population variance.

†For all statements to hold simultaneously at the 0.05 level, Bonferroni's rule for inequality (Miller 1966) requires that each statement hold at the 0.05/33 or 0.0016 level. In this study we considered a hypothesis rejected at the 0.002 level to be significant.

Methods tried were the k-means algorithm (Anderberg 1973), using the BMD PKM programme, and a variety of hierarchical techniques, including nearest neighbour, farthest neighbour, centroid and median methods available in the MIDAS computer programme. Results in closest agreement with our objectives were obtained using the Ward method of hierarchical clustering (Anderberg 1973), which was also used successfully on similar data by Everitt (1974).

This method works as follows. Initially each subject is considered to be a cluster. At each stage of this iterative procedure two clusters are merged to form a new one. These two clusters are selected in such a manner that their merger contributes least to the total within-group error sum of squares (ESS), a measure of cluster homogeneity. This process is continued until all subjects are merged into a single cluster. A tree or dendrogram showing the pattern of clustering is the result of this process. Working upwards through the tree one can then select a suitable number of clusters for analysis. Large changes in ESS at some step in the procedure indicate that two disparate clusters have been merged. This measure gives considerable guidance in determining the number of clusters within the population.

The above procedure was applied to data from the LBW group. Because cases with missing data were excluded, only 148 children for whom all data were available were used. The ESS with various numbers of clusters is tabulated as:

Number of clusters	1	2	3	4	5	6
Total error sum of squares (ESS)	76.166	51.104	42.948	29.695	25.635	25.446
% decreases in ESS by subdividing to create an additional cluster	30.4	15.7	30.9	13.6	0.7	10.0

Note that there are large percentage decreases in ESS when the number of clusters is increased from one to two, two to three, and three to four. There is a smaller decrease with the creation of five clusters from four, and almost no change when we increase the number of clusters from five to six. This preliminary analysis suggests the presence of four or more distinct clusters in the data (see Discussion).

Results

Table 7-II is a quantitative description of the four clusters produced by the above procedure. Each column gives the percentage of abnormalities for each variable in the particular cluster. p-values from a χ^2 test for lack of association of each factor across the clusters are given in the final column. Small values (<0.002)* suggest that the factors differed significantly between clusters[†]. The history of diseases affecting the nervous system and the clinical diagnosis of MBD were not used for clustering, but were cross-tabulated with the cluster pattern. These results appear in two separate rows. The final row is the number of children in each cluster.

*See footnote [†] on opposite page.

[†]These p-values are approximate, since the results were not based on random sampling from separate populations but on groups derived from clustering.

TABLE 7-I

Proportions of LBW and FBW control children with various abnormalities at 6½ years

Variable showing abnormality	*LBW (N = 237)*	*FBW (N = 133)*	*p*
'Organic behaviour syndrome' (ADD)	0.4051	0.1742	0.000
Other behaviour abnormalities	0.4810	0.2857	0.000
Affective responses	0.0464	0.0677	0.387
Response to parental direction	0.0563	0.0458	0.669
Low weight	0.1288	0.0301	0.002
Small head-circumference	0.0684	0.0000	0.002
Abnormal facies or bruit	0.1350	0.0827	0.133
Alertness and co-operation	0.0211	0.0075	0.322
Articulation	0.1139	0.3258	0.000
Motor integration	0.0717	0.0301	0.097
Tongue movement	0.0549	0.0150	0.063
Muscle tone	0.0759	0.0075	0.004
Maintenance of extended arms	0.0591	0.0303	0.220
Involuntary movements	0.0464	0.0606	0.556
Tendon reflexes	0.2425	0.0451	0.000
Plantar and Chaddock responses	0.2137	0.0758	0.001
Arm co-ordination	0.0802	0.0601	0.479
Leg co-ordination	0.0808	0.0451	0.192
Line walk	0.0258	0.0000	0.062
Incomplete handedness	0.0691	0.0236	0.068
Crossed laterality	0.3924	0.3759	0.756
Cortical sensory interpretation	0.0169	0.0000	0.133
Right-left discrimination	0.2415	0.0677	0.000
Finger localization	0.3707	0.1298	0.000
Language ability	0.0135	0.0000	0.184
Drawing ability	0.0356	0.0000	0.028
Hearing ability	0.0633	0.0303	0.170
EEG	0.3819	0.2636	0.036
Bender Gestalt score	0.2456	0.0752	0.000
WISC Verbal/Performance difference	0.1350	0.1128	0.539
Full-scale WISC/Goodenough difference	0.2575	0.5338	0.000
Clinically diagnosed MBD	0.2574	0.0601	0.000
History of diseases possibly affecting CNS	0.3207	0.1053	0.000

TABLE 7-II

Quantitative features of clusters

Variable showing abnormality	*Cluster* *1*	*2*	*3*	*4*	*p*
'Organic behaviour syndrome' (ADD)	9.1	35.7	76.6	100.0	0.000
Other behaviour abnormalities	12.7	47.1	93.6	83.3	0.000
Affective responses	0	0	2.1	16.7	0.001
Response to parental direction	0	10.7	6.4	16.7	0.043
Low weight	10.9	3.6	17.0	0	0.120
Small head-circumference	10.9	3.6	2.1	0	0.141
Abnormal facies or bruit	14.5	14.3	4.3	38.9	0.005
Alertness and co-operation	1.8	0	0	11.1	0.020
Articulation	7.3	3.6	2.1	55.6	0.000
Motor integration	1.8	10.7	4.3	27.8	0.002
Tongue movement	5.5	0	0	27.8	0.000
Muscle tone	3.6	3.6	8.5	27.8	0.009
Maintenance of extended arms	0	0	4.3	44.4	0.000
Involuntary movements	0	3.6	4.3	38.9	0.000
Tendon reflexes	29.0	7.1	19.1	33.3	0.082
Plantar and Chaddock responses	12.7	28.6	19.1	27.8	0.278
Arm co-ordination	1.8	0	4.3	38.9	0.000
Leg co-ordination	3.6	3.6	6.4	33.3	0.001
Line walk	0	7.1	2.1	5.6	0.236
Incomplete handedness	3.6	10.7	2.1	16.7	0.092
Crossed laterality	20.0	100.0	25.5	38.9	0.000
Cortical sensory interpretation	0	0	4.3	11.1	0.056
Right left discrimination	30.9	10.7	23.4	38.9	0.119
Finger localization	34.5	17.9	44.7	72.2	0.002
Language ability	0	0	2.1	11.1	0.027
Drawing ability	7.3	3.6	0	5.6	0.312
Hearing ability	5.5	7.1	2.1	11.1	0.513
EEG	50.9	7.1	40.4	44.4	0.001
Bender Gestalt score	27.3	35.7	6.4	55.6	0.000
WISC Verbal/Performance difference	14.5	7.1	17.0	27.8	0.298
Full-scale WISC/Goodenough difference	30.9	3.6	23.4	11.1	0.022
Clinically diagnosed MBD	18.2	21.4	29.8	77.8	0.000
History of diseases possibly affecting CNS	23.6	21.4	40.4	50.0	0.059
Number in cluster	55	28	47	18	

TABLE 7-III
Qualitative features of clusters

Category	*Cluster* 1	2	3	4
'Organic behaviour syndrome' (ADD)	Uncommon	Frequent	Very frequent	Constant
Other behaviour abnormalities	Uncommon	Frequent	Almost constant	Very frequent
Physical characteristics	Normal	Normal	Normal	Abnormal facies frequent
Motor	Normal	Crossed laterality constant	Normal	Frequently abnormal
Sensory	Poor finger localization	Normal	Poor finger localization	Frequently abnormal
Other neurological findings	Normal	Normal	Normal	Frequently abnormal
EEG	Abnormal in half	Normal	Frequently abnormal	Frequently abnormal
Psychological	Frequently abnormal	Abnormal Bender Gestalt	Normal	Abnormal
Proportion of MBD	Low	Low	Moderate	High

Table 7-III is a qualitative summary of Table 7-II, and the main features in each category are indicated. It is noteworthy that cluster four, containing 18 children, is characterized by a comparatively high proportion of abnormalities in most categories. In particular, all possess at least two features of ADD, while 85 per cent show other behavioural abnormalities. This group also has a large proportion with motor difficulties and with high error scores on the Bender Gestalt Test. 14 of the 18 members of this group (77.8 per cent) had been diagnosed clinically as having MBD. In group 3, which contains 47 children, 76.6 per cent had ADD, while 93.6 per cent showed other behavioural abnormalities. This group also has the highest proportion of underweight children, and was characterized by frequent poor finger-localization (though less often than in group 4) and by 40 per cent abnormal EEGs. Only 29.8 per cent of this group had been diagnosed clinically as having MBD. Clusters 1 and 2 contained higher proportions of normal children. In cluster 2 there are 28 children, of whom 35.7 per cent were diagnosed as having ADD, while 47.1 per cent had other behavioural problems. All children in this cluster had crossed laterality, and there was a high proportion with abnormal Bender Gestalt scores. Cluster 1 was the largest, containing 55 children, and included few with behavioural abnormalities. It was characterized by a larger than normal proportion with poor finger-localization, abnormal EEGs, poor Bender scores and a difference exceeding 20 points between the Full-scale WISC and Goodenough-Harris test scores.

In short, cluster 1 might be labelled as a group expected to range from normal to some learning disabilities, and cluster 2 as a group that is grossly normal but has crossed laterality, some behavioural abnormalities and difficulty with visual perception, and might also exhibit learning disabilities in some cases. Cluster 3 presents as a group with behaviour difficulties, whom a child psychiatrist might be likely to encounter, and cluster 4 as an 'organically abnormal' group with 'organic' and frequent other emotional disturbance, possibly secondary, whom a child neurologist might be likely to see. The relatively high proportion with poor finger-localization in cluster 1 might well be due to immaturity or delayed cognitive development rather than neurological abnormalities, since these skills are acquired around the age of 6½ years. The large differences between the scores on the WISC Full-scale IQ and the Goodenough-Harris Draw-a-Person Test for nearly one-third are hard to evaluate, since they appear to be less common in the LBW than in the FBW control subjects (Table 7-I), and the latter were shown in the previous chapter to have similar Draw-a-Person scores to the neurologically normal LBW children.

Clusters 3 and 4 show an interesting difference with respect to behavioural abnormalities. All members of group 4 have the so-called 'organic behaviour syndrome' (ADD) and 83 per cent have other behavioural abnormalities, largely indicative of insecurity. This cluster shows abnormal signs in most other categories. In particular, a large proportion of motor, sensory and other neurological characteristics are abnormal. In contrast, group 3 shows approximately inverse proportions of the behavioural abnormalities, with relatively fewer of the 'organic' type. In this cluster most of the neurological findings are normal, though 40 per cent of the EEGs were abnormal (or borderline). Thus the 'organic behaviour syndrome' and the other emotional difficulties, though frequently linked, appear to be somewhat independent in their prevalence.

We next explored the relationship of the above clusters to the 44 clinically diagnosed MBD cases for whom all data were available. There were 10 in the first cluster, six in the second, 14 in the third and 14 in the fourth. If MBD could not be broken down into subsyndromes, we would expect the MBD cases to be spread evenly across the clusters in proportion to cluster size. The hypothesis of independence of MBD and cluster patterns was tested. As indicated in Table 7-II, the p value was 0.000, and we conclude that there is an association between MBD and the derived clustering; and further, that the MBD categorization includes groups of children with predominant 'organic' defects, other (perhaps secondary) behavioural problems, and 'developmental' learning disabilities, respectively.

If we consider cluster 1 and 2 as 'normal' and clusters 3 and 4 as 'abnormal', we obtain the following two-way table:

	'Normal clusters 1 and 2	*'Abnormal' clusters 3 and 4*	
MBD	16	28	$\chi^2 = 9.84$
No MBD	67	37	$p = 0.000$

This indicates a highly significant relationship between the normal-abnormal cluster dichotomy and the clinical diagnosis of MBD. Thus the systematic procedure is in agreement with the clinical diagnoses.

TABLE 7-IV
Additional features of clusters

Characteristics	*Cluster* 1	2	3	4	p^{**}
Mean WISC Full-scale IQ	101.1	101.6	103.4	93.9	0.015
Percentage male	47.3	39.3	55.3	83.3	0.023
Percentage SGA*	50.9	50.0	31.1	33.3	0.132

*In each of groups 1, 2 and 3 classification as SGA or preterm AGA was unknown for two children.
**Values are based on the appropriate test for lack of homogeneity across the four clusters (see text).

Since it had been decided that the variable corresponding to previous diseases possibly affecting the central nervous system should not be used as a criterion for *diagnosis* of MBD, that variable was not used as a basis for clustering. Table 7-II shows that there is a marginally significant ($p = 0.059$) degree of association between the derived clustering and the presence of such previous diseases. In particular, the 'abnormal' groups 3 and 4 had had considerably more such diseases (40.4 and 50.0 per cent) than the 'normal' groups 1 and 2 (23.6 and 21.4 per cent), respectively. This suggests that some of these abnormalities might be the result of those earlier illnesses.

Discussion

The p values in the last column of Table 7-II are a rough indication of which variables differed significantly across clusters. Interestingly, the proportion of abnormalities was somewhat different for 23 of the 31 variables ($p < 0.10$). Items which did *not* differ significantly were line walking, drawing ability, hearing, abnormal plantar and Chaddock responses, and WISC Verbal *vs.* Performance IQ-score differences. The lack of disparity between clusters on the first three items might be accounted for by the small numbers with abnormal performance (four, six and eight, respectively), while in the previous chapter the difference between Verbal and Performance skills on the WISC had already appeared to be a poor indicator of cerebral dysfunction at this age. It is harder to explain why the plantar and Chaddock responses, which are significantly more often abnormal among LBW children than among FBW controls, did not differ significantly in the various clusters.

An attempt was made to divide the cases further into five clusters. Because of the hierarchical method employed, one of the existing groups (cluster 1) was split into subclusters of 41 and 14 members. These groups were similar on most factors, except that all the children in the smaller subgroup had abnormal EEGs and 85.6 per cent had abnormal Bender scores, while in the larger fragment 31.7 per cent had abnormal tendon reflexes and 39 per cent had WISC Full-scale *vs.* Goodenough-Harris drawing score differences exceeding 20 points. In the larger cluster there were four MBD cases (9.7 per cent), compared to six (42.9 per cent) in the smaller fragment. Since no meaningful groups were formed we felt that this and any further subdivisions would be of little practical value.

In Table 7-IV we tabulate additional characteristics of the sample that were not used to derive the clustering. They are the WISC Full-scale IQ, the percentage of males and the percentage of LBW SGA (as opposed to preterm AGA) children in each group. Based on a one-way analysis of variance, we can conclude that there is a difference in mean IQ among the four clusters ($p = 0.015$). Groups 1, 2 and 3 had approximately equal IQs, while group 4, the organically abnormal group, had a considerably lower mean IQ. χ^2 tests for association indicated that there was a relationship between sex and the derived clustering ($p = 0.023$), with group 4 having a considerably higher percentage of males than the other three groups. The percentage of SGA children did not appear to vary significantly across groups ($p = 0.132$). Not surprisingly, the most abnormal group also had the lowest mean IQ. Since the proportion of SGA children was not significantly different across groups, we might conclude that this dichotomy (SGA *vs.* preterm AGA) is not useful for determining the presence of organic or other behavioural abnormalities.

In general, cluster analysis is liable to yield groups of variables which do not correspond to recognizable clinical syndromes and appear somewhat artificial. However, when the technique is used in the way illustrated here it does seem to yield some interesting data concerning the validity of diagnostic criteria and of clinical concepts. As mentioned in the introductory chapter, there is particular diversity of opinion in the literature concerning ADD. Many authorities consider this to be characteristic of children with 'brain damage' or MBD (Strauss and Lehtinen 1947, Rosenfeld and Bradley 1948, Knobloch and Pasamanick 1959, Paine 1962, Anderson 1963, Clements 1966, Stevens *et al.* 1967, Wender 1971, Gross and Wilson 1974, Laufer 1979). On the other hand, Pond (1961) considered that 'the brain-damaged-child syndrome does not exist in its own right', that the symptoms which bring a brain-damaged child to a psychiatric clinic are very similar to those for which others are brought, and that the age and previous character of the person suffering brain injury and the ways in which he is subsequently handled are the main factors in determining the nature, severity and duration of symptoms. Shaffer *et al.* (1974) tried to measure activity, attention and impulsivity objectively in boys with and without a conduct disorder and with and without associated brain injury and concluded that overactivity is a function of psychiatric disturbance rather than of an abnormality of the central nervous system. Rutter (1977) and colleagues (1980) also concluded that children with brain damage tend to have the usual mixture of behaviour disorders found in others and that there was no stereotyped psychiatric syndrome, though a few exhibited the rare syndrome of hyperkinesis and this was related to low IQ. In our LBW children with MBD, hyperkinesis and brief attention-span were shown to be associated with other symptoms of emotional disturbance in more than 90 per cent of cases (see previous chapter). Nonetheless, the different relative preponderance of 'organic' and other behaviour disorders in clusters 3 and 4 is consistent with the concept that they may be somewhat independent, though commonly associated; or even that the hyperactivity and attention deficit may be the primary disturbance which causes other behavioural symptoms. In future the relationship between these behavioural symptom complexes may well be clarified by quantitative studies of neurotransmitters.

Summary

The concept of MBD in LBW children was investigated by statistical techniques using cluster analysis.

First, the prevalence of 32 abnormal features was compared for 237 LBW children who did not have any serious neurological handicap and for 133 FBW controls. This showed that the following features were significantly more common among the LBW children:

History of diseases possibly affecting the central nervous system
Presence of ADD
Other manifestations of emotional disturbance
Low weight (below 3rd percentile)
Small head-circumference (below 3rd percentile)
Poor right-left distinction
Finger agnosia
Hypotonia or hypertonus
Depressed or brisk tendon reflexes
Extensor plantar or Chaddock responses

On the other hand, a significantly higher proportion of the FBW controls had difficulties with articulation and differences exceeding 20 points between the WISC Full-scale IQ and the Goodenough-Harris Draw-a-Person Test scores.

Cluster analysis was then applied to 148 LBW children without major neurological defects for whom all the relevant data were available. Four clusters were found and the distribution of abnormal features was analyzed in each. Clusters 1 and 2 appeared to be largely 'normal', with a mean WISC Full-scale IQ of 101, though about one-half of these children had abnormal EEGS, about one-third had poor finger localization and other hints of possible learning disabilities, and group 2 was marked by crossed laterality in all and behavioural abnormalities in many. About one-fifth of the members of both clusters 1 and 2 had been diagnosed clinically as having MBD, and a similar proportion had a history of diseases possibly affecting the central nervous system. On the other hand, clusters 3 and 4 appeared more distinctly 'abnormal'. Cluster 3 was marked by a high proportion of behaviour disturbance (76.6 per cent 'organic' or hyperkinetic with attention deficit, 93.6 per cent other behavioural abnormalities) but with a mean WISC Full-scale IQ of 105.8. Finger localization was abnormal in nearly 50 per cent and the EEG was abnormal in about 40 per cent, but they presented few neurological abnormalities, though nearly 30 per cent had been diagnosed clinically as having MBD. The fourth cluster exhibited the highest proportion of both behavioural and neurological abnormalities. All 18 members of this group showed at least two features of the so-called organic or hyperkinetic behaviour syndrome, and 83 per cent had other behavioural abnormalities. The mean WISC Full-scale IQ in this cluster was only 93.9; there was a marked predominance of males (15:3) and 14 of the 18 children had been diagnosed clinically as having MBD.

It was concluded that MBD, as defined by our criteria, primarily includes children with 'organic' problems and learning disabilities. Although ADD is usually associated with other manifestations of emotional disturbance, it appears to be a somewhat independent entity, as shown in clusters 3 and 4. The relative 'normality' of clusters 1 and 2 as compared to 3 and 4 correlates well with the relative infrequency of the clinical diagnosis of MBD.

The difference between the WISC Verbal and Performance scores appears to be of little use in the diagnosis of brain dysfunction at 6½ years, whereas the Bender Visual-Motor Gestalt Test is more helpful, as was noted in the previous chapter.

Acknowledgement: This research was partially supported by Natural Science and Engineering Research Council Grants A3609 and A5527.

APPENDIX

Description and coding of variables

'Organic behaviour syndrome'. At least two of the following features: excessive motor activity, short attention-span, irritability, temper tantrums, mood swings, unpredictability, perseveration.

Other behavioural abnormalities. At least one of the following features: nervousness, fears, undue shyness, disobedience or negativism, hostility, unhappiness, withdrawal, autism, head-banging, rocking, masturbation, finger- or thumb-sucking, encopresis, enuresis, sleep disturbances.

Affective responses. At least one of the following features: excessive tension, shyness, hostility, inappropriate responses, depression, euphoria, sibling rivalry or other abnormal affective response towards family, other persons, animals or objects.

Response to parental direction. Active disobedience, deliberate inattention or over-submission to parent.

Low weight. Below 3rd percentile for age.

Small head-circumference. Below 3rd percentile for age.

Abnormal facies or bruit. Epicanthic folds, hypertelorism, abnormal slope of palpebral fissures, bruit, or other abnormalities.

Alertness and co-operation. Drowsiness, confusion or non-co-operation.

Articulation. Dyslalia, dysarthria, articulatory apraxia or other abnormalities.

Motor integration. Clumsiness or apraxia.

Tongue movement. Deviation to right or left, difficulty in manipulation, apraxia.

Muscle tone. Increased or diminished tone in at least two of the following: both arms, both legs, neck (flexor or extensor), trunk (flexor or extensor).

Maintenance of extended arms. Arms drift, fall away, flex, rise, pronate or adduct when extended forwards (with eyes open or closed).

Involuntary movements. Athetosis, dystonic twisting, choreiform movements, myoclonus, tics, tremors.

Tendon reflexes. Increase or decrease in at least three of biceps, triceps, supinator, knee and ankle jerks.

Plantar and Chaddock responses. Either response extensor or variable or equivocal in one or both feet.

Arm co-ordination. Dyskinesia, intention tremor, dysdiadochokinesia, dysmetria, poor finger opposition.

Leg co-ordination Inability to stand or hop on one foot, poor performance on heel-knee test.

Line walk. Inability to walk 90cm (3ft) in a straight line with tandem gait.

Incomplete handedness. Lack of definite preference for right or left hand in performing five simple tasks, such as drawing and throwing.

Crossed laterality. Difference in foot and hand preference in performing three simple tasks to show the former and five to show the latter.

Cortical sensory interpretation. Defective visual,

auditory, tactile or kinaesthetic perception, and knowledge of body parts.

Right-left discrimination. Inability to perform at least two of the following tasks: indicate own right hand, put right hand to own left ear, indicate own left leg.

Finger localization. At least two errors on one hand while identifying on diagram which hidden finger has been touched (finger agnosia).

Language ability. Inability to achieve at least two of the following: name penny, nickel and dime, count nine objects, name four colours.

Drawing ability. Inability to copy a triangle or simpler figures.

Hearing ability. Doubtful or impaired hearing in at least one ear.

EEG. Borderline or abnormal EEG.

Bender Gestalt Test. A standardized error score (Koppitz) exceeding 2 on the Visual-Motor test.

WISC Verbal/Performance difference. At least a 20-point disparity between Performance and Verbal scores.

Full-scale WISC/Goodenough difference. WISC Full-scale IQ at least 20 points greater than the average score for the Goodenough-Harris Draw-a-Man and Draw-a-Woman tests.

History of diseases possibly affecting the central nervous system. At least one of a wide range of diseases, including meningitis, brain tumour, measles with delirium, chronic ear-infection, convulsive disorders, encephalitis, emotional deprivation, psychosis.

8
Ophthalmic Disorders

Andrew Q. McCormick, Enid M. Tredger, Henry G. Dunn and Ruth V. E. Grunau

Several follow-up studies of low-birthweight children have noted the relatively high frequency of ophthalmic disorders, particularly oxygen-induced ocular disease and defects of ocular motility. Drillien (1961*b*) reported such disorders in 27 (37 per cent) of 72 school-age children with birthweights ≤1361g born between 1948 and 1960. In 13 cases the child was blind or had a significant visual handicap. Lubchenco *et al.* (1963*b*) followed 63 children with birthweights ≤1500g born between 1947 and 1950. At the age of 10 years, ophthalmological examination demonstrated permanent visual impairment due to retinopathy of prematurity (ROP)* in 16 and due to other eye disorders in three, and myopia and strabismus in 19 more, *i.e.* an over-all visual morbidity of 60 per cent (38 of 63 children). Similarly, Dann and colleagues (1964) examined 100 children, mostly between the ages of four and 18 years, who had been born prematurely weighing ≤1000g, or whose weight fell within that range in the postnatal period. The frequency of serious eye-defects was 59 per cent. McDonald (1967) recorded ophthalmological findings for 1081 children at the ages of six to eight years who had been born between 1951 and 1953 weighing ≤1814g: 3.7 per cent had cicatricial ROP and a further 2.2 per cent had myopia of −3D or more, most of which was thought to be the result of ROP. The incidence of squints, apart from those occurring in children with cerebral palsy, mental retardation, ROP or cataracts, was 7.1 per cent, compared to 2.8 per cent among normal school-entrants in England.

Wright *et al.* (1972) analyzed the findings for 65 children with birthweights ≤1500g born between 1952 and 1956, and for matched fullterm controls. On ophthalmological examination at 10 years about 11 per cent of the low-birthweight group had ROP, but none of the controls had. Strabismus was found about three times more frequently in the LBW group. None of these studies divided the LBW children into preterm AGA and SGA, and term SGA, as we have done.

Material and method

Eye examinations in the present study were carried out in the nursery and again after the general assessments at four and 6½ years. LBW infants were not examined until they were able to leave the incubator, *i.e.* at about one month. Control infants of full birthweight (FBW) were all examined in the first four days of life. Usually 1 per cent homatropine was used as a mydriatic, supplemented by 10 per cent phenylephrine if necessary. Lid retractors were used and the fundus was examined by direct ophthalmoscopy.

*The term 'retinopathy of prematurity' (Heath 1950) is now considered preferable to retrolental fibroplasia, although neither is ideal.

A staff ophthalmologist examined 259 LBW infants. 136 of these also had retinoscopy, but refractions were recorded for only 62. 190 FBW control babies were also examined in the nursery, and refraction was recorded for 158 of these.

For the older children, examination included muscle-balance studies and assessment of visual acuity. 260 LBW children were seen at four years, and 263 after their final assessment at 6½ years. 17 in the latter group were more than nine years of age and have been analyzed separately, in addition to 19 others who were re-examined at nine to 12 years. 119 FBW control children were examined at four years of age and 133 at 6½ years.

Most examinations after infancy were performed in the Outpatient Eye Clinic of the Vancouver General Hospital. Up to 1967, various staff ophthalmologists participated in the study; subsequently one ophthalmologist (A.Q.M.) took over the examination of all further follow-up cases. A few children were seen in private offices by ophthalmologists who filled in the standard forms for the study.

After 1967 the following routine was used in the Eye Clinic. Visual acuity was recorded, stereoscopic acuity was assessed with the Titmus stereo test (see Parks 1975), and colour vision was tested by American Optical Hardy-Rand-Rittler pseudo-isochromatic plates. A complete muscle-balance study was then carried out by an orthoptist, after which one drop of cyclopentolate 1 per cent was instilled into each conjunctival sac, followed by a second drop 10 minutes later, and cycloplegic refraction was performed 30 minutes after the first instillation. Following refraction, the ocular fundus was examined by direct ophthalmoscopy, the posterior pole and each of the four quadrants being checked. If anything suspicious was detected, binocular indirect ophthalmoscopy was carried out.

Of the 335 LBW children followed to school-age, 263 had an eye examination at 6½ years or later, while 44 were last examined at four years. 17 were seen only in the nursery, and 11 failed to have any examination by an eye specialist. Of the 139 FBW control children followed to school, only seven were not examined at or after 6½ years. Two of the seven were last examined at four years and the other five had been seen only in the nursery. (In addition, the 335 LBW and 139 FBW control children had their eyes examined in the general neuropaediatric assessment at 6 years.)

Results

Of the 335 LBW children followed to school-age, 60 had the ophthalmological defects shown in Table 8-I. One child who died in the nursery at six weeks had congenital bilateral cataracts and colobomata of the iris. No other cases of congenital cataract were encountered in our study.

In addition to these children with ophthalmological defects, two other boys had the diagnosis of *cortical blindness*. They are listed in the category of visual defects in Chapter 5. One of these has been re-examined at the age of 20 years. His eye-movements are random and purposeless, but the globes themselves, pupil response to light and blink response to light are all quite normal, suggesting a cerebral defect in a young man with a significantly small head, epilepsy and profound mental retardation. A similar child, whose mother attempted abortion at

TABLE 8-I

Ophthalmological defects in 335 LBW children

Congenital optic atrophy (OA)	1*
Congenital glaucoma	1
ROP† (retrolental fibroplasia)	12
Strabismus (excluding ROP and OA)	47
Total defects	61‡

*This girl had an extensive bilateral chorioretinopathy, with widespread pigment disturbance and optic atrophy. There was an unusual configuration of the nerve-head suggesting relatively early onset of intra-uterine inflammatory disease of non-specific aetiology. Serum tests for toxoplasmosis were negative.
†Retinopathy of prematurity.
‡N = 60 children; one child had both ROP and strabismus.

10 weeks, was born after 29 weeks gestation weighing 1474g. He had a stormy course in the nursery, with severe respiratory distress, pneumonia and hepatitis. Subsequently he had a significantly small head-circumference, length and weight, and at four months was noted to have continuous, purposeless eye-movements and a 'setting sun' sign. The globes themselves were normal. He was also severely mentally retarded and had febrile seizures. He died in an institution at 5 years 10 months.

The 139 FBW control children followed to school-age exhibited no ophthalmological abnormalities, except strabismus in five cases (3.6 per cent).

Retinopathy of prematurity (retrolental fibroplasia) and 'myopia of prematurity'

It is now 200 years since Scheele and Priestley independently discovered oxygen and described some of its biologically toxic effects. A period of intense medical interest in the element developed in the late 1940s and early 1950s when the administration of excessive oxygen to prematurely born infants was incriminated in the production of retinopathy of prematurity (ROP). The relationship between oxygen therapy and ROP was suspected by some clinicians and was proved statistically in the co-operative study organized by Kinsey (1956). It was also demonstrated in experimental work with kittens (Ashton *et al.* 1953, Patz 1957). The frequency of the disease duly declined when precautions were taken to avoid hyperoxia.

An editorial in the *American Journal of Ophthalmology* in 1955 stated: 'Retrolental fibroplasia is a unique disease in the annals of medicine. About 1942 it bowed into the ophthalmologic firmament, supposedly as a new and unheralded problem, caused blindness in approximately 8000 infants, and has now bowed out. All within a span of about 13 years . . .'. Unfortunately the promise of that editorial has not been kept. Although the incidence of ROP dropped sharply when the rôle of oxygen had been documented, there continued to be reports of the disease. Majima *et al.* (1972) analyzed cases of ROP in one Japanese hospital in the five-year period from 1967 to 1971. They found that as many as six of every seven

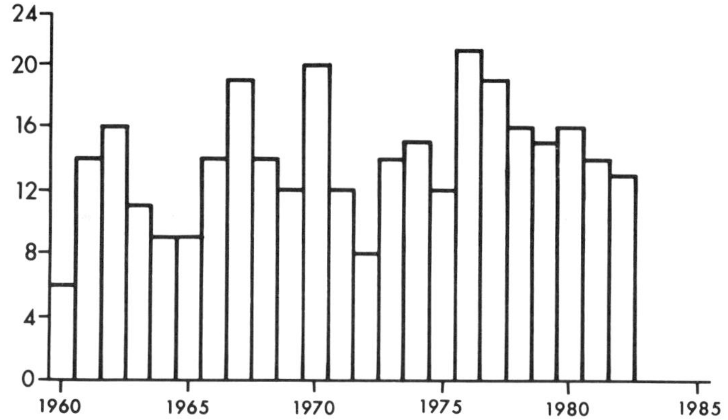

Fig. 8-1. Number of children legally blind as a result of retinopathy of prematurity notified to Canadian National Institute for the Blind from 1960 to the end of 1982.

infants (86 per cent) with birthweights <1250g had retinopathy, compared to only two of 62 infants (3.1 per cent) with birthweights between 2001 and 2250g. Retinopathy occurred in 80 per cent of infants with gestations of less than 30 weeks, in contrast to only 6.7 per cent of babies with gestations of 35 to 38 weeks. Cases also have been reported among LBW infants who have not had oxygen therapy, and even in term infants (Bruckner 1968, Kalina *et al.* 1972, Majima *et al.* 1972, Kraushar *et al.* 1975, Adamkin *et al.* 1977). In isolated instances the condition has been present at birth (Karlsberg *et al.* 1973).

It has been suggested that the prevalence of the disease was increasing again as more very small infants were being preserved with intensive perinatal care (Mushin 1974, McCormick 1977, Gunn *et al.* 1978). However, better examination techniques have made it possible to detect very mild cases, and the majority of recent cases have been mild. Phelps (1981) summarized reports from various centres in the 1970s by stating that active proliferative retinal disease was common among preterm survivors, but cicatricial sequelae generally were limited to infants with birthweights <1500g. The incidence of *blindness* among VLBW infants in different series ranged from 1.8 to 4.0 per cent and was skewed heavily towards those weighing <1000g at birth. Among these smallest survivors, cicatricial disease occurred in 22 to 42 per cent and blindness in 5 to 11 per cent. Phelps calculated that at these rates in the United States, 2100 infants would be affected annually by cicatricial ROP, and 546 had been blinded in 1979. Statistics compiled by the Canadian National Institute for the Blind indicate a lower frequency of blindness (Fig. 8-1), as only about 15 (range six to 21) children have been registered as blind each year in the Canadian population, which is about one-tenth that of the United States. Pomerance *et al.* (1982) found that of 51 survivors with birthweights ≤1000g, 12 (24 per cent) developed ROP, but only one of 19 infants was at stage IV or V. In another series the annual incidence of ROP among VLBW survivors was 35 to 36 per cent, but none was blinded (Shohat *et al.* 1983).

The concept of the pathogenesis of ROP has also changed in the past few years. Lubchenco *et al.* (1972*a*), in a follow-up study of LBW children at 10 years, found little difference in the frequency of visual disorders between children who had had a high environmental oxygen concentration in the nursery and those who had had 40 per cent or less. However, ROP was less severe for those with low oxygen-levels. According to Phelps (1981), 'this disorder is caused first by prematurity and only secondarily by oxygen'. A co-operative study by Kinsey *et al.* (1977) showed that the association between ROP and the duration of oxygen exposure was significant only for infants weighing >1500g, and the condition was not significantly associated with the number of episodes of arterial PO_2 greater than 70mmHg. However, there was an association between ROP and apnoea requiring bag and mask ventilation.

Low birthweight and repeated or prolonged exposure to high levels of oxygen are still considered important in this condition, but other contributing factors have been shown to play a significant rôle, *e.g.* low gestational age, apnoeic spells, septicaemia, degree of illness, blood transfusion and mechanical ventilation (Gunn *et al.* 1980). Thus ROP is now considered a multifactorial disease. The frequent association between ROP and intraventricular haemorrhage has also been pointed out (Procianoy *et al.* 1981). Whether exchange and simple transfusions represent a risk factor for ROP (Cornet *et al.* 1976, Clark *et al.* 1981), when duration and intensity of oxygen therapy have been considered, is still controversial (Sacks *et al.* 1981). Similarly, the protective effect of vitamin E has to be weighed against its possible risks (Phelps 1982). Shohat and colleagues (1983) report that the factors significantly associated with the disease are apnoea with mask and bag ventilation, prolonged parenteral nutrition, number of blood transfusions, episodes of hypoxaemia and hypercarbia, and particularly hypocarbia.

Baum (1971) described the prevalence of tortuosity of retinal vessels in a group of LBW children examined in their late teens, and suggested that this represented a 'forme fruste' of retrolental fibroplasia. ROP often leads on to myopia (Fletcher and Brandon 1955, Gunn *et al.* 1980), and it is controversial whether 'myopia of prematurity' exists as a separate entity.

Results

Of the 12 children in our study identified as having ROP, three are blind, and two of these have total bilateral retinal detachment. Of the remaining nine, one did not have visual acuity recorded; two read 6/6 with their better eye, five read 6/9 with their better eye and one was restricted to 6/12, so none of these represent a significant visual handicap. (These visual acuities are measured with the best spectacle correction.)

Severe ocular damage was noted in the three blind children when they were still in the nursery. Six others were classified as being highly myopic at four years (one also had a posterior staphyloma), and it was not until the 6½-year examination that the changes were interpreted as being due to ROP.

Eight of these 12 children weighed ≤1500g at birth (VLBW), and five of these were preterm AGA, while the remaining three were of uncertain gestational age. Of the remaining four, two were preterm AGA, one was SGA, and one was of uncertain gestational age. Eight are singletons and four are twins (belonging to three pairs). All but one had supplemental oxygen therapy in the incubator, generally at a concentration of less than 40 per cent, but ranging up to 85 per cent in cases of severe respiratory distress. The three who are blind had had the highest concentrations for the longest periods. They were all preterm AGA infants weighing ≤1500g. One of them is otherwise normal neurologically, one has cerebral palsy and the third is mentally retarded. Of the remaining nine children who are less severely visually handicapped, only two are neurologically normal. It is interesting that two cases are twins of similar birthweight who both had respiratory distress; one required environmental oxygen in higher concentration for a somewhat longer period and subsequently had more impaired eyesight. The minor manifestations of retinal disease in his twin sister probably would have been missed if she had not been examined with such care, in view of his serious retinopathy. It is also noteworthy that the one SGA case received no supplemental oxygen and was born at 38 weeks gestation weighing 1928g. He was the heaviest of the 12.

Strabismus

Estimates of the prevalence of strabismus in normal children have varied from about 2 to 7 per cent in different surveys. In a large-scale Danish study, Frandsen (1960) found that it rose from about 1 per cent in the first year to a maximum of about 7 per cent at six to seven years and then fell gradually to 0.8 per cent in the late teens. The frequency of squint averaged about 4.5 per cent in children attending normal schools, without sex variation. It was also noted that there was a marked predominance of *convergent* squints in the early years of life, and there was a suggestion of an inverse relationship between intelligence and the frequency of strabismus. In the survey of 1000 families in Newcastle upon Tyne (Miller *et al.* 1960), about 4.7 per cent of children were found to have a persisting squint during the first five years. Children receiving deficient physical care had squints twice as frequently as the remainder, and at three years of age children with squints were significantly below average in height. In the British National Child Development Study, 492 of 14,110 children (3.5 per cent) aged seven years had strabismus in 1965 (Alberman *et al.* 1971). This is close to the frequency of 2.8 per cent among school entrants aged five to six years estimated by the British Ministry of Education in 1964.

Many previous investigators have found an increased frequency of strabismus among LBW children. As early as 1934, Hess and co-authors reported that 14.4 per cent of 250 prematurely born children had a squint, compared to 1.3 per cent of 156 children born at term. Studies by Castrén (1955) had similar results. Conversely, Scobee (1951) reviewed a personal series of 230 cases of strabismus among children of all ages and found that 31 (13.5 per cent) had been 'premature' at birth, whereas the incidence of prematurity among the general population in that area was only 3 per cent. Drillien (1964) noted that 7.4 per cent of LBW children with birthweights <2500g had strabismus during the first five years of life. Among these, the prevalence was only 5.2 per cent in the group weighing >2041g, whereas it was 11 per cent in the birthweight group 1588 to 2041g, and no less than 16.3 per cent among those weighing ≤1588g. McDonald (1967) found a frequency of 10 per cent in children with a birthweight ≤1814g when those with cerebral palsy and mental retardation were included, and 7.5 per cent when children with these defects and

TABLE 8-II
Details of 47 LBW children with strabismus

		N		*N*
Sex: female		31	EEG at 6½ yrs:	
male		16	Normal	17
			Abnormal	16
Original type of strabismus:			Borderline	6
Esotropia		35	Not recorded	8
Exotropia		12	Strabismus surgery:	
			Performed	18
Gestational age category:			Not performed	29
Preterm AGA		22		
SGA		22	Outcome:†	
Uncertain		3	Residual esotropia	29
			Residual exotropia	14
Neurological status at 6½ yrs:			Exophoria	1
Normal		15	Esophoria	1
Abnormal		32	Monofixational phoria	1
Minimal brain dysfunctions	16*		Uncertain	1
Cerebral palsy	11		Visual acuity:	
Mental retardation	5		6/6 and 6/6	15
More than minimal brain dysfunctions	3		6/6 and 6/12 or better	9
			6/6 and less than 6/12	2
Epilepsy	1		Less than 6/6 in each eye	17
Aphasia	1		Unknown	4

*Some children had more than one abnormality.
†Dissociated vertical divergence recognized in four cases.

those with ROP, myopia, cataract and nystagmus were excluded. Wright *et al.* (1972) reported nine cases of strabismus among 65 VLBW children, whereas there were only three among an equal number of FBW controls.

The association of squints with various types of brain dysfunction is well established. Frandsen (1960) found that the frequency of strabismus in schools for retarded children ranged from 10 to 30 per cent, compared to 4.5 per cent in normal schools. With regard to cerebral palsy, Freud (1893) considered that convergent squint occurred in 30 per cent of cases of cerebral diplegia, and was particularly common when this was associated with prematurity. Douglas (1961) found a manifest squint in 37 per cent of 168 patients with cerebral palsy. He also pointed out that the ratio of convergent to divergent squint was 2.7:1 in that series, and thus distinctly lower than that of 10:1 for the general population in Dundee, Scotland. The problems of strabismus in cerebral palsy were reviewed by Smith (1963), who also commented on the early onset of squints in this condition, the problem of determining unequivocally which are paralytic or concomitant, and the difficulties of treatment. Douglas (1963) examined 104 children whose squint had been detected in the first year and found a high frequency of low birthweight (18.2 per cent), malformations recognizable at birth (14.5 per cent) and spastic types of cerebral palsy (6.7 per cent). Alberman *et al.* (1971) found that the frequency of cerebral palsy, mental subnormality or clumsiness among children with squints was twice that of a control group, and the proportion with poor speech, left or mixed

TABLE 8-III
Analysis of LBW children with and without strabismus

	Strabismus *(N = 47)*		*No strabismus* *(N = 196)*		*Significance*
Sex: female	31	(66%)	89	(45%)	$\chi^2 = 5.61$
male	16	(34%)	107	(55%)	$p < 0.02$
Plurality:					
Singletons	37	(79%)	144	(73%)	$\chi^2 = 0.55$
Twins	10	(21%)	52	(27%)	NS
Birthweight (g):					
Mean ± SD	1688	290	1738	283	$t = -1.06$ NS
Gestational age category:					
Preterm AGA	22	(47%)	115	(59%)	
SGA	22	(47%)	73	(37%)	$\chi^2 = 3.44$
Uncertain	3	(6%)	6	(3%)	NS
LGA	—		2	(1%)	
WISC Full-scale IQ:					
Mean ± SD	89.9	18.1	98.4	14.1	$t = -2.93$ $p < 0.005$
Social class I-III	12	(25%)	47	(24%)	
IV	15	(32%)	80	(41%)	$\chi^2 = 1.365$
V	20	(43%)	69	(35%)	NS
Neurological status:					
Normal	15	(32%)	127	(65%)	$\chi^2 = 15.55$
Abnormal	32	(68%)	69	(35%)	$p < 0.0001$

handedness and signs of maladjustment was also significantly raised. Children with squints but no other evident neurological or mental defects still included an unduly high proportion of poor readers, and they also scored badly on a test of copying a design. Hence they may be assumed to have had an abnormally high prevalence of MBD, although they performed as well as controls in tests involving intellectual rather than visual ability. Also, Levinson *et al.* (1951) and Stillerman *et al.* (1952) and their colleagues found an unusually high frequency of abnormal EEGs in children with strabismus, particularly occipital foci.

Results

In the present study, among 335 LBW children who were followed to 6½ years there were 47 (14 per cent) with some form of strabismus not attributable to retrolental fibroplasia or other defect resulting in diminished visual acuity, whereas there were only five cases (3.6 per cent) among the 139 FBW control children examined at the same age. If children with severe cerebral palsy or mental retardation are excluded, the figures are 12 per cent for the LBW group and 2.9 per cent for the FBW controls.

There was no uniformity of care for these children with strabismus, as they were treated by various ophthalmologists in the community. Evaluation of the final outcome and visual acuity in 27 of the 47 LBW children and five FBW controls with strabismus was carried out by one of us (A.Q.M.), with the assistance of the

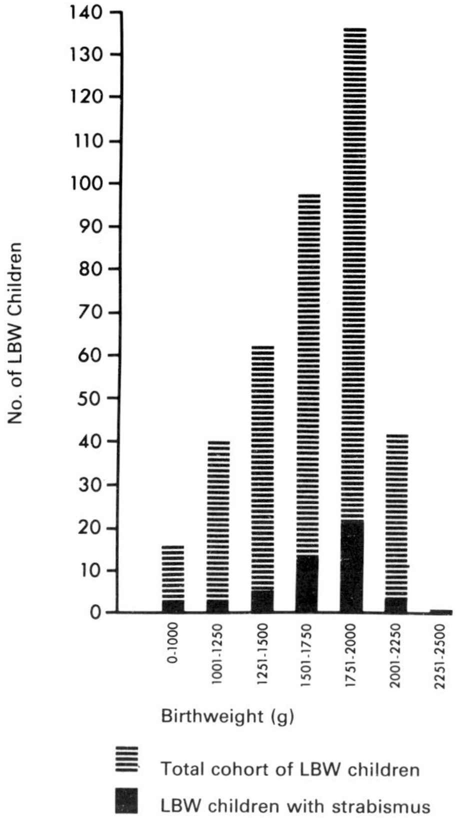

Fig. 8-2. Birthweight distribution of LBW children with strabismus and of total LBW cohort. No notable difference is evident.

orthoptists. Relevant information for the remaining 20 LBW children was supplied by their ophthalmologists. Care was taken to obtain information about the original deviation before corrective surgery. The data for the 47 LBW children are summarized in Table 8-II. An analysis of these children and the LBW children without strabismus is shown in Table 8-III.

Whereas ROP occurs chiefly in infants with birthweights <1500g, the distribution of birthweights among the LBW children with strabismus resembles that for the total cohort (Fig. 8-2).

Types of strabismus

Of these 47 children, 35 had esotropic and 12 exotropic deviations before surgery. Thus the ratio is about 2.9:1, distinctly lower than that reported in the general population with strabismus, and not greatly different from that reported in association with cerebral palsy. None of the five FBW control children with strabismus had exotropic deviation.

Stereo acuity could be measured in 25 of the 47 LBW children by the Titmus stereo test. Six (24 per cent) had 40 seconds of arc stereo acuity, and all originally

TABLE 8-IV

Type of strabismus *vs.* neurological status and EEG findings for LBW children at 6½ years

	Esotropia	*Exotropia*	
	(N = 35)	(N = 12)	
Neurological status:			
normal	10	5	
abnormal	25 (71%)	7 (58%)	$\chi^2 = 0.7052$ NS
	(N = 27)	(N = 12)	
EEG: normal	10	7	
borderline	4 } (63%)	2 } (42%)	
abnormal	13 }	3 }	$\chi^2 = 1.968$ NS

TABLE 8-V

Neurological status *vs.* visual acuity of 43 LBW children with strabismus

Neurological status	*6/6 6/6*	*6/6 ≥6/12*	*6/6 <6/12*	*Neither eye 6/6 but >6/9>6/12*	*Neither eye 6/6 but ≤6/9≤6/12*
Normal	7	1	2	4	—
Minimal brain dysfunctions	7	6	—	—	3
Cerebral palsy	1	2	—	3	2
Mental retardation	—	—	—	1	—
Cerebral palsy + mental retardation	—	—	—	1	1
More than minimal brain dysfunctions	—	—	—	—	2

TABLE 8-VI

Analysis of matched pairs of neurologically normal children with and without strabismus

		N	*Strabismus*			*No strabismus*			*Significance*
Placement* at yr 3 in school		14	1	2	3	1	2	3	
			12	2	—	12	2	—	
Reading level at yr 5	Mean	12		18.50			18.58		t = −0.27
	SD			3.38			2.53		NS
Arithmetic level at yr 5	Mean	12		17.75			17.42		t = 0.12
	SD			1.83			1.66		NS
Spelling level at yr 5	Mean	12		17.92			18.50		t = −0.79
	SD			2.72			1.66		NS
Writing level at yr 5	Mean	11		17.73			18.18		t = −0.97
	SD			2.93			1.40		NS
Bender Gestalt score at 6½ yrs	Mean	15		0.39			0.17		t = −0.89
	SD			0.94			1.09		NS
Crawford Dexterity score									
Part I	Mean	12		5.67			7.67		t = −1.59
	SD			3.14			2.46		NS
Part II	Mean	12		9.41			11.17		t = −1.66
	SD			2.87			1.72		NS

*1 = at grade level or above; 2 = below grade level; 3 = special class or special school.

had exotropic deviations. 15 children (60 per cent) had peripheral fusion only. Four were alternators and had no binocularity at all. No child with esotropic deviations achieved better than peripheral fusion.

When the type of strabismus was analyzed in relation to neurological status and EEG findings, the correlations shown in Table 8-IV were obtained. The children with exotropia appear to have a higher proportion with normal neurological status and EEG findings, but the differences are not significant.

The five cases of strabismus among the FBW controls had the following diagnoses (one case each): accommodative esotropia; monofixation syndrome; Duane's retraction syndrome; intermittent esotropia; and variable esotropia with hypertropia suggestive of dissociated vertical divergence.

Vision

Reliable measurements of visual acuity in each eye were obtained for 43 of the 47 LBW children at the age of 6½ years. 15 of these (35 per cent) had 6/6 vision in each eye; nine (21 per cent) had 6/6 in one eye and 6/12 or better in the other; two (5 per cent) had 6/6 in one eye and less than 6/12 in the other. The remaining 17 of the 43 (39 per cent) had less than 6/6 vision in each eye. Of the 15 children with 6/6 vision in both eyes, seven are neurologically normal and eight are abnormal, mostly mildly so. On the other hand, the eight children with at most 6/9 and 6/12 vision are all neurologically abnormal (Table 8-V).

Other features

To determine the composition of the segment of LBW children with strabismus, comparisons were made with the remainder of the LBW group who had an eye examination at six to nine years. Again, ROP and OA cases were excluded. There were no significant differences between the LBW children with and without strabismus in plurality, mean birthweight, category of weight for gestational age at birth, or social-class distribution. However, differences that did occur in the group with strabismus were that it contained significantly more girls ($p<0.02$), the mean WISC Full-scale IQ was significantly lower ($p<0.005$), and it contained a highly significantly greater proportion with abnormal neurological status ($p<0.0001$).

The various types of neurological abnormality appeared to be similar in each group, except that 11 of 32 (34.4 per cent) neurologically abnormal children with strabismus had cerebral palsy, compared to only nine of 69 (13 per cent) of those with neurological abnormality but no squint. The proportion of abnormal and borderline EEGs was also significantly higher in the strabismus group (see Table 13-XII). It was noted that of the 16 LBW and two FBW children with strabismus and abnormal EEGs in our series, only two had occipital spike foci in their records.

There were statistically significant differences in the school placement of children with and without strabismus in the third and seventh years in school. In the third year, 29 per cent of those with and 12 per cent of those without strabismus were in either a special class or special school ($\chi^2 = 8.67$, $p<0.01$). By the seventh year the proportions were 47 per cent and 15 per cent ($\chi^2 = 15.16$, $p<0.0005$).

The two groups were also compared on scores derived from the teacher's rating of the child's level of reading, arithmetic, spelling and writing at the end of the fifth year in school. There were no statistically significant differences, but there was a consistent trend in favour of the children without strabismus.

The question arose as to whether poor learning by children with squints was due to disturbed brain function or was secondary to poor vision or stereopsis in association with the squint itself. Therefore the 15 children with normal neurological status in the LBW group with squints were matched with 15 children with normal status in the non-squinting LBW group (Table 8-VI). The children were matched for sex, birthweight (within 250g, except in one case where the difference was 340g), maturity and social class (grouping I to III, IV and V). Placement information for the third year in school was available for 14 of the 15 pairs, and the distribution was identical for the two groups. Neither did teachers' ratings for reading, arithmetic, spelling or writing in the fifth year in school show any significant difference. Similarly, there was no marked difference in the Bender Gestalt scores at 6½ years. A trend of possible interest occurred in the Crawford Dexterity Test, in which the children without strabismus obtained distinctly but not significantly better scores, which might be attributable to their better stereoscopic visual acuity.

It may be concluded that strabismus in itself is not a serious handicap to learning. The associated disturbance of brain function appears to be much more important as a cause of learning disability.

In seven of the 47 cases the strabismus had already been noted in the first year (cases secondary to ROP and congenital optic atrophy being excluded). Four of these seven had cerebral palsy and another had minimal cerebral dysfunction; the other two were otherwise neurologically normal at 6½ years. Although these are small numbers, they suggest a high rate of cerebral palsy among cases of strabismus with early onset.

Table 8-II also shows the eventual outcome for eye-muscle balance in these children. While some defect in balance always remained, the results in terms of visual acuity are quite gratifying. Even for those with cerebral palsy, for whom the results of surgery for strabismus are usually less satisfactory than for those with normal neurological status (Edwards and Moran 1974), only three of the 10 children with known visual acuity have 6/9 or worse in the better and 6/12 or worse in the poorer eye (see Table 8-V).

Refraction

The final word on the refractive state of newborns' eyes has not yet been written. Duke-Elder (1970) stated that all eyes are hypermetropic at birth, and that 'it is an extraordinary fact that an approximation to emmetropia is maintained throughout infancy and childhood in spite of great alterations in the constituents of the refractive system'. Graham and Gray (1963) also found general hypermetropia of moderate degree in 98 fullterm infants. However, Mehra and Vaithilingam (1965) reported hypermetropia in only 79 per cent of 100 fullterm newborns, astigmatism greater than two dioptres in 12 per cent and myopia in 9 per cent. Goldschmidt (1969) reviewed the literature and examined 356 neonates with birthweights

>2500g: he concluded that 24.2 per cent were myopic. He considered that the lack of conformity in the results of various studies was due to the technical difficulties of the examination, differences in the genetic composition of the groups, and the varying degrees of maturity of the babies, for which birthweight was only one criterion. He stated that 'in the last months of pregnancy and the first months of life the eyes develop considerably, and there is reason to believe that the refraction also changes'. That no entirely satisfactory method is available for refractive measurement of the eye of the newborn, and particularly of LBW infants, is also suggested by the scarcity of comment on details of technique in textbooks of refraction and of paediatric ophthalmology.

For newborn LBW infants, the only large survey of refraction was recorded by Fletcher and Brandon (1955). They studied 462 'premature' infants and followed them for six months. They found a high and fluctuating degree of myopia during the neonatal period, more marked in the smaller infants. Unfortunately, it appears that only 45 of this group were seen with dilated pupils and only 10 were examined by means of retinoscopy; the remainder were assessed only with the ophthalmoscope. The authors failed to mention any difficulty in viewing the fundus because of the slightly cloudy cornea found in many LBW newborns or because of remnants of the pupillary membrane (Gans 1959), or of the hyaloid vascular system. Finally, while many of the infants had active ROP, with some clouding of the vitreous, the authors made no mention of any difficulties in examining them. It is well-established that ROP is associated with myopia in later infancy and childhood, but it has not been demonstrated that these changes are manifest in the acute early stages of the disorder.

In 1952, Gleiss and Pau performed serial refractions in 23 'premature' infants without ROP and found that there was a distinct tendency for hypermetropia to increase and myopia to decrease during the last two months before term. Graham and Gray (1963) compared 150 'prematures' with 98 fullterm infants: the former showed a tendency to low myopia and emmetropia, in contrast to the hypermetropia of the fullterm babies. Honegger (1969) also commented on the diminishing myopia of the prematurely born, as judged by the ophthalmoscope. Lomičkova (1972) followed 160 LBW newborns prospectively: below 1600g the frequency of myopia exceeded that of hypermetropia, but above 2200g hypermetropia became more frequent. Refraction studies also showed the exclusive presence of myopia until the 31st weeks after conception. In all the term SGA children hypermetropia was present at delivery.

Sorsby and colleagues (1961) have documented the evolution of normal refractive changes after the age of three years, *i.e.* a gradual reduction of hyperopia after infancy. Castrén (1955) found hypermetropia in 90 per cent and myopia in 3.3 per cent of a group of ex-premature older children, whereas hypermetropia was encountered in 94 per cent and myopia in only 2.3 per cent of fullterm control children at school-age. Wright and associates (1972) examined 65 LBW children and matched controls at 10 years and found no statistical difference in the prevalence of hypermetropia and myopia when the eyes were otherwise normal.

In our study the refractions in the nursery were carried out by four staff

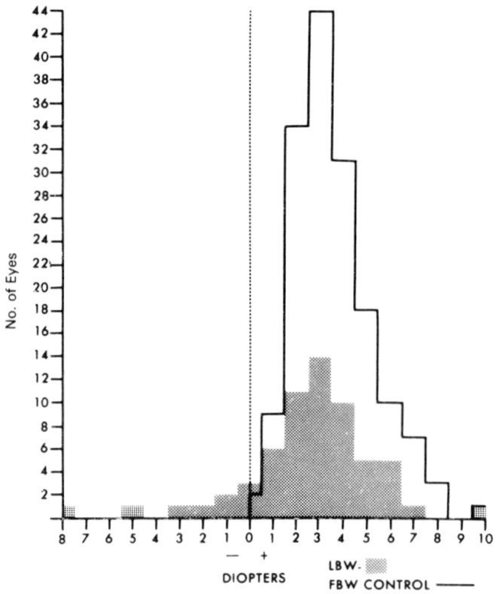

Fig. 8-3. Refraction (right eye) for LBW infants at a mean chronological age of one month shows a tendency towards less hyperopia than among FBW infants at one week of age. Myopic refractive errors were encountered only in LBW infants.

ophthalmologists who had somewhat different criteria for the diagnosis of the refractive state of the eye, and slight differences in the technique of examination. Nevertheless, their results tend to confirm the change from myopia to hyperopia before term.

Results

While refractions were actually recorded in only 62 of the LBW nursery examinations, the refractive state was noted in 63 others. Myopia was reported in 12 (9 per cent) of these 125 LBW infants. No myopia was present in 182 similar examinations of FBW control infants. 10 of the 12 were preterm AGA and the other two were SGA. Only one of these myopic children had myopia at a later examination (−0.5 at 6½ years), when 10 of them were seen again, and none had any signs of ROP.

It should be remembered that the LBW infants were not examined until they were able to leave the incubator (average age about one month), whereas the control infants were all examined within the first four days of life.

The eyes of the infants with recorded refraction tended to become more hyperopic as term approached. Figure 8-3 shows the distribution of recorded refractions, and Table 8-VII the mean values for refractions for preterm AGA, SGA and control infants. It can be seen that the differences between the mean refractive errors of the LBW and FBW infants are significant, and the difference between preterm AGA and SGA mean values just reaches significance. However, the conceptional-age difference should be noted, and it is of interest that the mean refractive error of SGA infants at term was identical to that of the FBW controls.

As the children became older the refractive states of the eyes of preterm AGA and SGA babies appeared to become similar. Table 8-VIII gives the mean refractive values at ages four and about 6½ (extending up to nine) years, and also for a small group of LBW children who are now more than nine years old. The values for

TABLE 8-VII

Mean refractive values in various birthweight groups in newborn nursery

	N	*Concept. age at eye exam. (wks) (mean)*	*Refractive value*† *(mean)*	*Significance*
LBW AGA	39	37.5	+2.04	t = −1.989
LBW SGA	20	40.6	+3.50	p = 0.05
Total	62*	38.4	+2.60	t = −2.875
FBW controls	158	40.6	+3.50	p <0.005

*Total includes those with uncertain length of gestation.
†Spherical equivalents.

TABLE 8-VIII

Mean refractive values in various birthweight groups at various ages

	Mean refraction right eye					
	N	*4 yrs*	*N*	*6½–9 yrs*	*N*	*>9 yrs*
LBW AGA	79	+0.95D	119	+0.80D	13	+0.70D
LBW SGA	58	+0.94D	79	+0.80D	19	+0.80D
Total	144	+0.92D } *	206	+0.79D } **	34	+0.74D
FBW controls	119	+1.12D	130	+1.08D		

*t = −1.73, NS; **t = −2.93, p <0.005.

TABLE 8-IX

Refractive values at about 6½ years

	N	*Plano to +2.00 sph.*	*>+2.00 sph.*	*Myopic sph. error*	*Hyperopic astigmatism <1D*	*Hyperopic astigmatism ≥1D*	*Myopic astigmatism <1D*	*Myopic astigmatism ≥1D*
LBW	206	148 (71.8%)	5 (2.4%)	6 (2.9%)	11 (5.3%)	7 (3.4%)	19 (9.2%)	10 (4.9%)
FBW controls	130	92 (70.8%)	4 (3.1%)	2 (1.5%)	6 (4.6%)	4 (3.1%)	16 (12.3%)	6 (4.6%)

TABLE 8-X

Corrected visual acuity at 6½ to 7 years

	N	*6/6*	*6/7.5*	*6/9*	*6/12*	*6/18*	*6/21*	*6/24*	*6/30*	*6/60*
LBW	205	159 (77.6%)	26 (12.7%)	8 (3.9%)	7 (3.4%)	—	1	1	2	1
FBW controls	132	121 (91.6%)	5 (3.8%)	3 (2.3%)	2 (1.5%)	1	—	—	—	—

preterm AGA and SGA show no significant difference at the three age-levels. The FBW control children still appear to be slightly more hyperopic at four and 6½ years. The difference between the mean refractive values of the total LBW and FBW groups is not significant at four years but reaches significance at 6½ to nine years.

However, if the types of refractive error are analyzed in detail, as evaluated by one examiner (A.Q.M.) at about 6½ years, the results shown in Table 8-IX are obtained for the older LBW children with major eye-defects (*i.e.* excluding ROP and OA) and for the FBW control children. It can be seen that when the cases of simple myopia and myopic astigmatism are added together there is little difference in the relative frequency of myopia between the two groups.

Table 8-X compares the corrected visual acuity in either eye or, if different, in the poorer eye at 6½ to seven years, again determined by the same examiner. There is little apparent difference between the corrected visual acuities of LBW children without major visual handicap and the FBW controls: 97.6 per cent of the former and 99.2 per cent of the latter have visual acuity of 6/12 or better in the poorer eye. (This arbitrary value was chosen because it appears to represent a limit permitting normal and adequate visual function.) However, only about three-quarters of LBW children actually achieved 6/6 vision in both eyes, compared to nine-tenths of the controls, and visual acuities below 6/12 in the poorer eye evidently are more liable to occur in the LBW category.

Discussion

Retinopathy of prematurity (ROP) occurred in up to 25 per cent of LBW children studied by earlier workers, depending on birthweight and intensity of oxygen therapy (Drillien 1961*b*, 1964; Lubchenco *et al.* 1963*b*). McDonald (1967) analyzed the outcome for children born between 1951 and 1953 weighing ≤1814g and found that ROP had affected 7.7 per cent of the infants, but had regressed in about half the cases. On follow-up at six to eight years, 3.7 per cent had residual disease of sufficient severity to cause blindness in one-half of the children and severely impaired visual acuity in the rest. In addition, 2.2 per cent were reported to have a refractive error of −3D or more in one or both eyes, often non-progressive and without evidence of cicatricial ROP.

Our study was concerned with a similar birthweight category (mostly ≤2041g), but with children born between 1959 and 1965. As the risk of oxygen therapy was recognized, care was taken to avoid excess, but 12 of 335 children (3.6 per cent) followed to the age of 6½ years still had residual ROP, sufficient to cause blindness in three. However, this group of 12 children includes eight in whom the disorder caused no visual loss, or a loss so small as to result in near-normal vision in at least one eye. Seven of these were classified as highly myopic and/or astigmatic at four years and were recognized as representing mild residual ROP at 6½ years. We believe that nearly all cases of severe 'myopia of prematurity' diagnosed by previous authors were similar to these. In the examination of ex-LBW children with possible minor manifestations of ROP it is essential that the eyes be inspected with the pupils dilated and that an indirect ophthalmoscope be used so that the whole of the peripheral retina and vitreous can be thoroughly visualized.

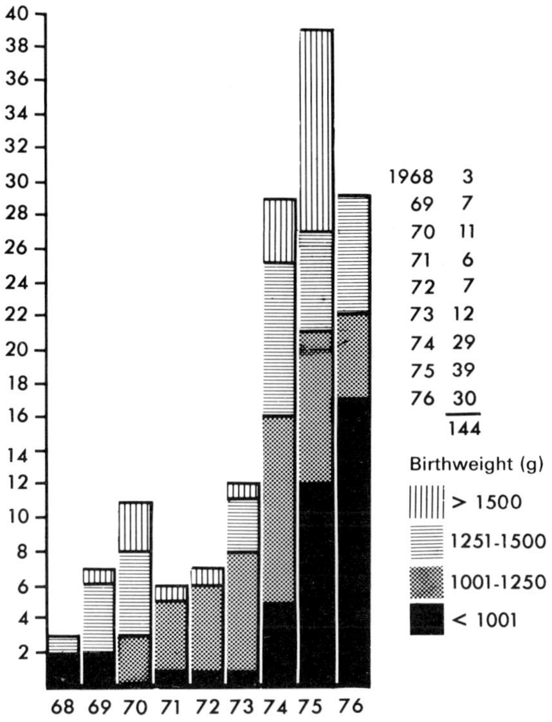

Fig. 8-4. The increasing frequency of retinopathy among LBW infants at the Vancouver General Hospital between 1968 and 1976 is only partly accounted for by the increased survival of babies with very low birthweights.

Fortunately the frequency of serious ROP appears to be falling further as a result of careful analysis of blood gases in intensive care of the newborn. Stewart and Reynolds (1974) reported no case of blindness and only one of partial sightedness among 95 infants at follow-up, and in the one affected case the visual impairment was due to congenital cataracts. Similarly, Davies and Tizard (1975) found impaired vision in only 2.4 per cent of 165 VLBW infants. On the other hand, as more careful ophthalmological examinations are made in the nursery, it is clear that mild degrees of retinopathy are still common, especially among infants with birthweights ≤1250g (Mushin 1974, McCormick 1977, Phelps 1981). These mild cases may show only abnormal development of retinal vessels, without any evidence of fibrous tissue behind the lens (Mushin 1974), so the term 'retinopathy of prematurity' is preferable to 'retrolental fibroplasia'. However, one of our cases illustrates that affected infants are not necessarily premature. When the condition occurs at term or in infants who had not been exposed to oxygen, the question arises as to whether they may have some form of retinal dysplasia which is clinically indistinguishable from ROP and may occur particularly in SGA infants (Svedbergh 1975, McCormick 1977).

Our own recent experience confirms the great frequency of the minor forms of the disease. Among 114 cases of ROP in the years 1968 to 1975, only seven are legally blind (visual acuity of 6/60 or less in the better eye with correction). Figure 8-4 shows the increased frequency of the condition as observed by a single examiner

(A.Q.M.) in the Intensive Care Nursery of the Vancouver General Hospital. It also illustrates that the infants with the lowest birthweight, who are now surviving in increasing numbers, are only partially responsible for this increase. We do not think that more careful ophthalmoscopic examinations account for any of the increase, but the greater numbers of newborns transferred from other hospitals recently may play a significant part (Pomerance *et al.* 1982).

It has also been suggested that the infant's fundi should be inspected repeatedly during oxygen therapy, since the early changes in the retinal vasculature may serve as a warning sign of the disease (Lomičkova and Melichar 1968, Patz 1968). However, it is still controversial whether an early stage of vasospasm is observable in the human infant, and once abnormal proliferative vascular changes are visible in the peripheral retina the damage has already been done. It is also technically difficult to visualize the retina of small preterm infants clearly, partly because of the immaturity of the eye itself and partly because the infant is in an incubator and frequently attached to a respirator. Thus the ophthalmologist hardly plays a rôle in the prevention of the condition, but even minor degrees of damage should be identified, as they may be associated with subsequent myopia.

The prevention of ROP appears to be dependent on continuous monitoring of arterial oxygen tensions, on a search for pharmacological agents to prevent the obliterative vascular changes in the presence of high ambient oxygen concentration, and on methods to control the onset of premature labour (James and Lanman 1976). With respect to oxygen therapy, the dilemma is that too-liberal use may cause blindness, whereas excessive restriction may cause more LBW babies to die, particularly during the first day of life (Avery and Oppenheimer 1960, Cross 1973, Bolton and Cross 1974). The American Academy of Pediatrics has made recommendations how to deal with this dilemma (see James and Lanman 1976). At present it appears that vitamin E may prove to be useful in the prevention of retinopathy (Phelps 1982): the full effect of appropriate doses on the newborn remains to be evaluated, but its use for premature babies might have the dual advantage of also protecting them against intraventricular haemorrhage, as suggested by recent studies (Chiswick *et al.* 1983, Speer *et al.* 1984).

With respect to strabismus in LBW children, it is clear that this has a significant association with abnormal neurological status and EEG, and thus presumably is often 'neurogenic'. Of the 47 cases in our series, 22 were preterm AGA and an equal number were SGA, while the length of gestation was uncertain for three. As in the cases of McDonald (1967) and Lomičkova (1971), there was no marked tendency for squints to occur in the lighter children, as happens in ROP (see Table 8-II). The neurological and intellectual implications of strabismus require more emphasis among paediatricians and ophthalmologists; the frequent association between strabismus of early onset and cerebral palsy should also be noted. The relatively high frequency of *divergent* squints in our children confirms the findings by Lomičkova (1972) in a similar group at 10 years and is analogous to the situation with cerebral palsy (Douglas 1961). It should be added that we have only analyzed our cases of strabismus and not the phorias which were noted by the ophthalmologist in the majority of the children. We have also refrained from trying to specify how many cases had a paralytic component or evidence of eye-muscle fibrosis (as in Duane's retraction syndrome).

Congenital bilateral cataracts were found in 10 (1.3 per cent) of 759 singletons with birthweights <1800g by McDonald (1967) and in only one of our 480 patients weighing less than 2041g. McDonald noted that these patients tended to be relatively mature but unduly small, and that mental retardation and a history of seizures were more common. We can only explain the discrepancy between McDonald's finding and our own by assuming that her survey may have occurred at the time of some viral epidemic, but she stated that there were no indications of rubella.

Like Castrén (1955), we found that the mean refractive error of LBW children at a later age is less hyperopic than that of FBW controls. The reason for this is not clear, but one may wonder whether oxygen therapy and subclinical retinopathy play a rôle in causing the difference. In two recent studies it was shown that the prognosis for 'myopia of prematurity' is quite good, as refraction changes towards emmetropia by seven years (Scharf *et al.* 1978), but at 18 years myopia was still slightly more frequent among the LBW subjects than the FBW controls (Fledelius 1980).

Thus, apart from major visual handicaps caused by congenital eye-defects or ROP, the visual acuity of LBW children does not appear to be greatly impaired. However, it is evident that less than perfect vision is somewhat more common in LBW than in FBW children.

Summary

Totals of 259 LBW and 190 FBW control infants were examined by a staff ophthalmologist in the nursery. At four years 260 LBW and 119 FBW children had an ophthalmological assessment, and again at 6½ years 263 LBW and 133 FBW children had a further eye examination. The eyes of the 335 LBW and 139 FBW children followed to school-age also were examined repeatedly during neuropaediatric assessments up to the age of 6½ years.

Of the 335 LBW children followed to 6½ years, 60 (17.9 per cent) had ophthalmological defects: congenital optic atrophy (one), congenital glaucoma unilaterally (one), retinopathy of prematurity (ROP) (12) and strabismus, excluding ROP and optic atrophy (47*).

Only one child who died in the nursery had congenital cataracts (and colobomata of the irides). Two boys were cortically blind, with normal eyes. They had significantly small head circumferences and one was profoundly and the other severely mentally retarded. These two are considered to have cerebral rather than ocular defects.

There were no ophthalmological abnormalities among the 139 FBW children followed to school-age, apart from strabismus in five cases (3.6 per cent).

Of the 12 children with ROP, three are blind and seven have myopia of more than −3D in at least one eye. Seven were preterm AGA, length of gestation was

*One child had both retinopathy and strabismus not attributable to poor vision.

unknown for four and only one was SGA. Eight were singletons and four were twins. Eight had birthweights <1500g.

The 47 cases of strabismus not attributable to ROP or other primary eye-defect represent 14 per cent of the LBW children, in contrast to only 3.6 per cent (five of 139) of the FBW controls at 6½ years. Of the 47, about one-half were preterm AGA and the others were SGA. 33 had esotropic and 14 exotropic deviations, a ratio of 2.9:1, contrasting with a reported comparative ratio of about 10:1 in the general population. Strabismic children with visual acuity of 6/9 in one eye and 6/12 or worse in the other were always neurologically abnormal in this series. In general, the group with strabismus contained a significantly greater proportion with abnormal neurological status, had a significantly lower mean WISC Full-scale IQ, and a higher proportion of abnormal or borderline EEGS. Their mean grade-placement, reading and arithmetic skills at school also were lower than those of children without strabismus. Among seven children whose strabismus had been noted in the first year of life (and was not due to ROP or other eye-defect), four had cerebral palsy. No significant difference in school performance was demonstrable when 15 strabismic LBW children with *normal* neurological status were compared to 15 matched non-squinting LBW children who were also neurologically intact. It was concluded that strabismus tends to be associated with various forms of cerebral dysfunction, but in itself causes little scholastic handicap.

Refractions in the nursery showed a tendency for the eyes of SGA and FBW control infants to be more hyperopic in comparison with AGA preterm infants. Mild myopia was found in 12 (9 per cent) of 125 LBW infants without retinopathy, and in none of 182 FBW controls. 10 of the 12 with myopia were AGA preterm and two were SGA. When 10 of these children were re-examined at 6½ years, only one had mild myopia. The findings are consistent with the view that the eyes of normal infants are myopic at the beginning of the last trimester of pregnancy and become hyperopic as term approaches.

By the age of six years the refractive states of the eyes of AGA preterm and SGA children had become similar, but LBW children had a significantly lower mean hyperopic refractive error than the FBW controls.

Apart from cases of ROP, refractive errors were no more common among LBW than FBW control children, but only 78 per cent of LBW children actually achieved 6/6 vision in both eyes, compared to 92 per cent of the FBW group.

Acknowledgement: The authors express their gratitude to Drs. A. Cohen, W. D. McKinlay, E. L. Smith and A. J. Stewart for participation in these studies; to many other ophthalmologists for permission to quote their findings; to Dr. A. J. Elliot and Dr. S. M. Drance for their advice and encouragement; and to the Department of Bio-Medical Communications, University of British Columbia, for help with the Figures.

9
Hearing Impairment and Associated Factors

Bryan R. Clarke, Robert F. Conry and Henry G. Dunn

Over the past 30 years a number of studies have examined the relationship between deafness and low birthweight. The results have been inconsistent, and one reason may be changes in classification and definition of LBW children referred to in the first two chapters.

One of the earliest studies was conducted by Johnsen (1952). Excluding cases with recognized hereditary conditions or haemolytic disease of the newborn, he retrospectively examined the possible causes of deafness in 39 children with sensorineural hearing-loss and found that 23 per cent had birthweights of ≤2500g, compared with only 7 per cent in the general population. Somewhat similarly, Cubert (quoted by Campanelli *et al.* 1958) analyzed the clinic records for 145 consecutive children with sensorineural hearing-loss and found that 15.1 per cent had such a low birthweight. Barton *et al.* (1962), in a retrospective study of 270 severely deaf children born in Northumberland and Durham, England, between 1945 and 1954, reported a 'prematurity' rate of 12.5 per cent in the whole cohort, and of 21 per cent among the 121 unexplained cases. Danish and Levitan (1967) showed that the proportion of LBW children among pupils at the Pennsylvania School for the Deaf rose from 21.4 per cent of the cases with congenital non-hereditary deafness in 1960-61 to 36.2 per cent of such cases in 1964-65. This represented an increase from 3.7 per cent of the total number of deaf students in the earlier period to 11.3 per cent in the later period. Vernon (1967) reviewed the pre-admission evaluations of 1468 children at the California School for the Deaf (Riverside) between 1953 and 1965 and determined that 17.4 per cent had birthweights below 2500g. Thus it appears to be well established that children with congenital deafness are two to three times more likely than the general population to have a low birthweight. However, it needs to be clarified whether these deaf children are light because of poor intra-uterine development or because of short gestation.

Sensorineural deafness among LBW children

There has been much difference of opinion on the question of whether there is an increased frequency of sensorineural deafness among LBW children. Perhaps this depends to some extent on the degree of care with which hearing defects have been investigated.

Alm (1953) presented a tabular survey of 49 research studies from 1913 to 1952, in which abnormalities of 'premature' children were examined, but there was no reference to hearing loss. Campanelli *et al.* (1958) reported that seven (16 per cent) of a sample of 44 LBW children had bilateral sensorineural hearing impairment, extending from moderate to severe, at six to seven years, whereas a control group of 44 FBW children all yielded results within normal limits for both pure-tone and speech stimuli.

Other investigators, however, have found a lower frequency of sensorineural hearing-loss among LBW children. Harper and Wiener (1965) reported a frequency of 3.6 per cent, compared to less than 1 per cent in a control group of full term children. Robinson and Robinson (1965) encountered only one case of bilateral congenital deafness among 135 LBW children, and that appeared to be hereditary deafness since two siblings also were born deaf.

In studies of LBW children with birthweights ≤1800g, McDonald (1962, 1967) found only 19 (1.7 per cent) of 1128 children with moderate or severe sensorineural deafness. However, since that survey was based on questionnaires completed by public-health nurses, detailed audiological examination may not have been performed for each child. McDonald (1967) also noted that hearing loss was significantly rarer in twins than in singletons (0.3 *vs.* 2.4 per cent). 16 (4.1 per cent) of 387 single children with a gestation period of less than 33 weeks had hearing loss, compared to only two (0.6 per cent) of 339 single children with a gestation period of 33 weeks or longer. There was no association with low birthweight other than that attributable to gestational age.

Corner (1960), in a follow-up study of 174 infants with birthweights <1500g identified eight (4.6 per cent) with hearing loss, of whom three had cerebral palsy with a history of kernicterus. Drillien (1961*b*) found six (12 per cent) of 49 children with birthweights <1360g to have definite hearing defects. Similarly, Lubchenco *et al.* (1972*a*) encountered sensorineural hearing-loss in 10.5 per cent of 63 VLBW children (≤1500g) who survived to 20 to 25 years of age. Wright *et al.* (1972) found three children with bilateral deafness and two with a unilateral defect among 65 VLBW children who survived to the age of 10 years, but in only one of 65 matched FBW controls. Depending on whether a further 'premature' with 'auditory aphasia' was included, the incidence of hearing deficits among VLBW children thus was 7 or 9 per cent. On the other hand, Dann *et al.* (1964) found only two children with sensorineural deafness among 100 who had weighed ≤1000g in the neonatal period. Davey (1962) also reported only one such patient, and another with conductive and possibly superadded sensorineural defect, among 93 testable children with birthweights <1360g. In contrast, Davey found 25 children with conductive losses, and she concluded that the incidence of sensorineural problems in LBW children had been over-emphasized.

Neonatal mortality and morbidity have declined since the introduction of more intensive perinatal care since about 1965, as discussed in Chapter 1. The frequency of hearing loss among survivors often was determined after relatively brief follow-up. In one series of 88 VLBW survivors who were re-examined at a mean age of four years, only one (1.1 per cent) had a hearing defect (Mercer *et al.* 1978). Similarly, Bjerre (1975*b*) noted that only 1.4 per cent of LBW children had hearing loss at a mean age of five years. However, Winkel *et al.* (1978) investigated 91 four- to six-year-old children with birthweights <2000g born in Copenhagen between

1967 and 1969: 19 per cent had a sensorineural hearing-loss, regardless of whether or not they had been treated with kanamycin. Another careful study also reported sensorineural loss in 9 per cent of VLBW children at a mean age of 6.5 years (Abramovich *et al.* 1979), and this is close to the 9.7 per cent found by Bergman *et al.* (1985). Also, among infants with birthweights ≤1000g, who now survive in increasing numbers, the reported rate of hearing loss has still ranged from 3.7 per cent (Stewart *et al.* 1977) to 9.3 per cent (Pape *et al.* 1978).

It is hard to compare these figures with those for the general population, since estimates of the latter vary greatly, according to the criteria used. For instance, Harper and Wiener (1965) stated that about 0.5 to 1 per cent of American schoolchildren had hearing defects. More accurately, Fraser (1976*a*) considered that severe degrees of hearing loss in childhood could affect 0.1 per cent of the population in economically advanced countries, and a greater proportion in less privileged regions. Less severe hearing-loss is more common, and if relatively mild hearing-loss and unilateral deafness are included the proportion may be as much as 5 per cent.

In any event, the present consensus appears to be that indeed there is an increased frequency of sensorineural deafness among LBW children. It is still poorly documented whether this happens predominantly among preterm or among SGA children. As noted above, Drillien (1961*b*) found hearing defects particularly among children with birthweights <1360g, and McDonald (1967) concluded that the correlation was between deafness and short gestation, rather than birthweight. Fitzhardinge and Steven (1972*b*) tested the hearing of 87 SGA infants born at term and found only one with unilateral nerve deafness and three with mild conductive loss, but they did not have a control group of preterm AGA children. Drillien (1972) encountered five deaf children among 27 with severe handicap when 283 LBW children with birthweights <2000g were examined at one to three years: four of these were SGA and only one was AGA and preterm.

Pathogenesis of deafness in LBW children

There is still considerable disagreement about the pathogenesis and the following mechanisms have been proposed, which may occur in conjunction.

Haemorrhage into the inner ear

This was postulated many years ago (Voss 1923, Albrecht 1930). Keleman (1963) also suggested that the damage to the organ of Corti was due to a toxic and irreversible effect of extravasated blood. LBW infants tend to have immature blood-vessels and can have clotting defects (Gray *et al.* 1968), particularly when there has been severe asphyxia at birth (Chessells and Wigglesworth 1971). Buch (1966) demonstrated that haemorrhage into the temporal bones of newborn infants occurred almost exclusively in the 'premature', and suggested that traumatic obstetric procedures played an important rôle in its causation. Spector *et al.* (1978) demonstrated the extension of cerebral and ventricular haemorrhages into the inner ear of infants who died after receiving ventilatory support for respiratory distress.

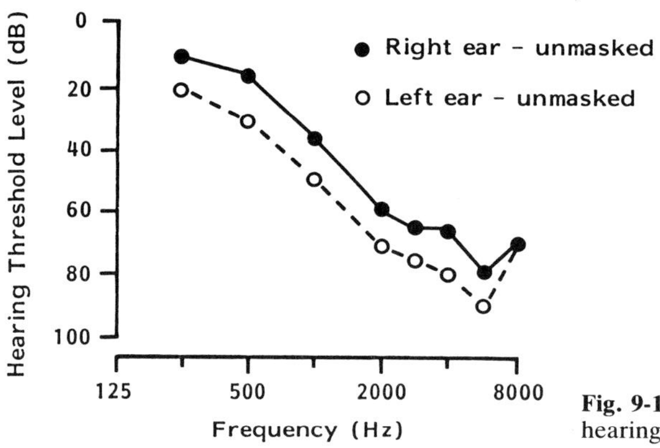

Fig. 9-1. Audiogram of child with sensorineural hearing-loss.

Jaundice

Kernicterus is well documented as a cause of sensorineural deafness, particularly in haemolytic disease of the newborn due to Rh incompatibility (Lande 1948, Crabtree and Gerrard 1950, Fisch and Osborn 1954, Johnston *et al.* 1967). In these cases of congenital deafness the lesion is usually in the cochlear nuclei, and principally in the dorsal nuclei, where the fibres which carry the high-frequency sound impulses are concentrated. In an important study, Fisch (1955) found that the audiograms of deaf children who had had neonatal jaundice, haemolytic disease, 'prematurity' or anoxia tended to be gently or sharply sloping, thus indicating effective loss of hearing for high frequencies (Fig. 9-1). This could be explained by particular damage to the dorsal cochlear nuclei, which are among the areas richest in capillary vessels and thus perhaps particularly vulnerable to hyperbilirubinaemia. However, Blakeley (1959) noted that all 20 patients with perceptive hearing-loss after erythroblastosis had recruitment and aural-harmonic thresholds suggestive of damage to the cochlea.

In 1961, Fisch and Norman reported that six of 50 children who were jaundiced at birth later had high-tone sensorineural hearing-loss. Corner (1960) also found a correlation between neonatal jaundice and subsequent deafness, but McDonald (1967) concluded that deafness was not significantly related to neonatal jaundice in 19 of the LBW children with perceptive hearing-loss. Barton *et al.* reported in 1962 that only 18 per cent of the 'premature' infants among the unexplained cases of deafness in her survey had a history of severe jaundice. However, Barton subsequently reviewed the birth records of all 'premature' infants at one hospital between 1949 and 1954 and found that among 191 children with neonatal jaundice 11 proved to have sensorineural hearing-loss at follow-up, whereas no high-frequency deafness was detected among 78 'premature' controls with birthweights ≤1815g (4lbs) who had not been jaundiced (Barton 1964). Keaster *et al.* (1969) followed 405 children who had haemolytic disease or hyperbilirubinaemia as newborns and found that 17 (4.2 per cent) had sensorineural hearing-loss. While this incidence was similar to that among unselected children, the frequency of educationally handicapping hearing-problems was greater.

Anoxia

Fisch (1955) postulated that in perinatal anoxia, as in kernicterus, the cochlear nuclei in the brainstem were liable to be damaged, and particularly the dorsal cochlear nuclei, which would account for high-frequency hearing-loss. He pointed out that the dorsal cochlear nuclei, which are responsible for hearing sounds of higher frequency, were phylogenetically younger than the rest of the auditory apparatus and thus presumably more vulnerable; that they were more exposed than the ventral nuclei as they bulged into the fourth ventricle from the floor; that they were extremely vascular and thus probably had a high oxygen consumption; and that vascularity was bound up with an extremely complicated structure and rich synaptic connections, and therefore presumably with greater sensitivity to anoxia. This view was supported by Hall (1962), who found a definite loss of cells in the cochlear nuclei of fatally asphyxiated children. Histological investigation of these children demonstrated that the ventral cochlear nucleus had lost 41.8 per cent of its cells and the dorsal cochlear nucleus had lost up to 65 per cent. Norman (1964) mentioned that destruction of both medial geniculate bodies could also account for central deafness after birth injury.

Other parts of the auditory pathways are similarly vulnerable. Thus Windle (1961) found that the nuclei of the inferior colliculi of asphyxiated monkeys were damaged most commonly, and Hall (1963) confirmed such damage in some asphyxiated infants. Bosher (1972) pointed out that the human cochlea itself is uniquely vulnerable to perinatal anoxia, which may initiate degeneration in the presence of other deleterious factors. According to this hypothesis, multiple adverse perinatal factors may act synergistically to produce failures of homeostasis of the endolymphatic fluid, similar to those postulated to be responsible for the inner-ear degeneration of deaf white cats (Bosher and Hallpike 1966). The examination of the cochlea in the temporal bone presents technical difficulties, but Hall (1964) concluded from his histological studies that the massive loss of cells in the cochlear nuclei of asphyxiated infants lent support to Fisch's (1955) view pointing to central damage, whereas the finding of smaller and more dubious changes in the peripheral sense-organ indicated that the affection of the cochlea was probably of secondary significance. This particular problem may be clarified by studies of brainstem auditory evoked responses (*e.g.* Schulman-Galambos and Galambos 1975, Cox *et al.* 1984).

Ototoxic drugs

Marcus *et al.* (1963) studied 35 deaf 'premature' children and found that 29 had been treated wtih dihydrostreptomycin in excess of the standard recommended daily doses. This drug gradually fell into disfavour as its disastrous effects on hearing became generally known (Shambaugh *et al.* 1959). Streptomycin itself is probably more toxic to the vestibular than to the auditory system, and both McDonald (1967) and Lubchenco and colleagues (1972*a*) considered that treatment with this antibiotic could not be incriminated conclusively in the causation of hearing loss ascertained by prospective studies of LBW children. They concluded that neonatal anoxia was an important aetiological factor in deafness and that the association between the administration of oxygen or antibiotics (including streptomycin) and deafness was secondary, since such treatment tended to be given to children whose clinical condition was most serious. Nevertheless, there is continuing concern about the ototoxicity of maternal abortifacients like quinine, and about antibiotics given to the infant, such as kanamycin (Yow and Tengg 1961), though some studies demonstrated no ototoxic effect of kanamycin in a dosage of 10 to 15mg/kg per 24 hours for five to 10 days (Eichenwald 1966, Sanders *et al.* 1967, Winkel *et al.* 1978). Certain preparations of vitamin K have been implicated in the past in indirectly causing jaundice when given in excessive doses (Fisch and Norman 1961).

Other factors

Fraser (1964) studied the causes of deafness amongst 2355 children at special residential schools throughout Great Britain and the Irish Republic. He was able to assign a definite cause for 1509 of these cases, including perinatal events such as 'jaundice of prematurity', haemolytic disease of the newborn, birth injury and the use of streptomycin. The remaining group of 846 contained a large excess of LBW children (103), suggesting that apart from the risk of jaundice, birth injury and streptomycin, 'prematurity' was associated with subsequent deafness in some nonspecific manner. On the other hand, Fisch (1964) considered that 'uncomplicated prematurity' was not the cause of hearing impairment and that only the complications of low birthweight, such as anoxia and kernicterus, were responsible. Fraser (1976*b*) concluded from his own studies that the relationship between perinatal problems and subsequent deafness was complicated and that multiple genetic and environmental variables were liable to interact in causing impaired hearing. This view is supported by the findings of Schulte and Stennert (1978), who applied audiometric tests to preterm infants and found no relationship of hearing loss with gestational age, hyperbilirubinaemia, drugs or length of stay in an incubator, but a strong correlation between hearing loss and 'perinatal non-optimal score', *i.e.* the sum of perinatal risk-factors (Prechtl 1967). Bergman *et al.* (1985) noted the highest frequency of hearing loss (28.6 per cent) in LBW survivors of neonatal seizures.

It should be mentioned that often there is only scant information in the literature concerning the audiological status of the individuals examined. Frequently references are made to a mild or moderate hearing-loss in one or both ears, with little or no quantitative data to document the extent of the loss. It is the purpose of the present study to re-examine the questions of whether hearing loss is one of the serious risks arising from low birthweight and whether it is more liable to occur in preterm AGA or SGA children.

Material and method

Between March 1968 and March 1974, audiometric data were collected on the available LBW children and FBW controls in this study. The children were approximately 6½ years of age at the time of testing. Of those examined, 205 were

LBW* and 123 were FBW controls (see Chapter 2). By design, birth status was not made known to the examiner at the time of testing.

A Maico 24 audiometer was used to test hearing of pure tone by air conduction (and bone conduction where necessary) at 250, 500, 1000, 2000, 3000, 4000, 6000 and 8000HZ in each ear (see Newby 1979 for procedural details). The Wepman Auditory Discrimination Test (1958) and standard speech-hearing tests (Newby 1979) were administered only to children with average thresholds greater than 25dB through the speech range.

Testing was conducted individually in a custom-built sound-treated booth which meets the ASA standard for background noise level. The TDH 39 earphones were replaced by Maico aural domes (calibrated audiometric headset noise barriers)†. Equal amounts of practice were given to the children before they entered the booth, to ensure that they understood the task of taking a peg from a pegboard each time a tone was heard. The same equipment was used on all occasions, and all but a few children were tested by the senior author.

Results

The criterion for hearing impairment was a threshold greater than 45dB above audiometric zero for any frequency in the speech range (500 to 4000HZ). The audiograms were then classified according to site of lesion. A *sensorineural* loss was diagnosed when bone-conduction patterns closely resembled those of air conduction. On the other hand, *conductive* losses were diagnosed when bone conduction was normal and air-conduction levels were lower than normal. In these cases an abnormality of the external and/or middle ear usually could be demonstrated. There were no cases of a sensorineural loss with superadded conductive defect at the time of testing.

A further unusual response was observed and classified as minimal high-frequency loss. This was defined as a loss of 30dB or more at 4000HZ and 35dB or more at 6000 and 8000HZ, where responses to lower frequencies were normal and responses to speech-hearing tests were adequate.

The Committee on Conservation of Hearing of the American Academy of Ophthalmology and Otolaryngology (1959) recommended a classification of hearing handicap based on the average threshold level for 500, 1000 and 2000HZ in the better ear. However, Davis and Silverman (1970) warned that 'deviations above or below those that enter into the average may be of medical significance', and further, that 'this summarizing constant cannot legitimately be used to classify individuals for educational purposes'. It has been criticized, for example, for having its lower limit too high and for not including higher frequencies in the average of the speech range (Kryter 1973). Since this averaging classification has to be

*Although a detailed audiological examination was performed on only 205 of the 335 LBW children followed to the age of 6½ years, pains were taken to include all those suspected clinically of having any hearing defect. It is possible, but unlikely, that there were one or two further cases among the other 130 children.

†The authors acknowledge the Western Institute for the Deaf, Vancouver, for the use of their facilities and some testing services.

TABLE 9-I

Pure-tone air conduction thresholds for LBW children with sensorineural loss

		Hearing thresholds in dB (ISO)								
		250	*500*	*1000*	*2000*	*3000*	*4000*	*6000*	*8000*	*Hz*
Bilateral										
Case	*Ear*									
24	R	10	15	10	10	30	45	60	80	
	L	10	10	10	30	50	65	70	60	
68	R	—	—	—	—	—	—	—	—	
	L	—	—	—	—	—	—	—	—	
73	R	0	0	5	15	50	55	80	75	
	L	0	0	10	15	60	70	80	75	
136	R	30	25	40	60	*	70	*	*	
	L	35	30	50	75	*	80	*	*	
313	R	35	35	35	55	60	60	60	65	
	L	40	50	65	70	70	80	80	80	
380	R	30	55	65	70	*	70	*	80	
	L	55	70	65	70	*	70	*	80	
421	R	10	15	35	60	65	65	80	70	
	L	20	30	50	70	75	80	90	70	
487	R	55	80	90	95	—	—	—	—	
	L	50	80	90	95	—	—	—	—	
Unilateral										
33	L	40	50	65	70	70	80	80	80	
120	R	5	10	20	40	45	45	60	60	
465	L	10	5	5	15	50	55	50	40	
466	L	10	5	0	15	45	55	45	40	

—No response at limits of audiometer.
*Not obtained.

TABLE 9-II

Frequency of hearing defects

	LBW		*Controls*	
	N	*%*	*N*	*%*
Sensorineural				
Bilateral	8	3.9	0	0
Unilateral	4	2.0	0	0
Conductive	13	6.3	3	2.4
Minimal high-frequency loss				
Bilateral	7	3.4	3	2.4
Unilateral	2	1.0	2	1.6
Normal hearing	171	83.4	115	93.5
Total	205		123	

modified by other pertinent considerations, it was not applied to the present data. The results of audiograms are presented in full in Table 9-I. All cases of sensorineural loss were characterized by an increasing drop at high frequencies (see Fig. 9-1).

The results summarized in Table 9-II show a higher frequency of hearing defects among LBW children than among the FBW controls. There were eight bilateral and four unilateral cases of sensorineural loss among the LBW children, and none in the control group. The corresponding percentages of conductive losses were 6.3 per cent, compared to 2.4 per cent. Some clinical details of the 12 LBW children with sensorineural hearing-loss may be noted:

(1) Nine of the 12 children are boys, as are all but one of the eight with bilateral hearing-loss.
(2) Ten of the 12 children were preterm AGA, only one was SGA and the length of gestation for the remaining girl was uncertain.
(3) Half the affected children were twins.
(4) Some abnormality of delivery had occurred in nine of the 12 children.
(5) Neonatal jaundice had been noted in all but one. However, it had only been sufficiently marked to make the attending physician check serum bilirubin levels in eight of the 12, and for seven of these the maximum level had been 15mg/100ml (255μmol/l) or more. Only one child had been given a replacement transfusion.
(6) Neurological abnormalities were found after birth in 11 of these 12 infants, but subsided during the stay in the nursery in seven of them. All the children with bilateral sensorineural loss had other neurological sequelae, and all four whose neurological findings were still abnormal at the time of discharge from the nursery had more severe defects than minimal cerebral dysfunction.
(7) Respiratory problems were encountered in all the children who had bilateral hearing-loss, but there was considerable variation in the time oxygen had been administered, ranging from only the first day to as long as 31 days.
(8) Systemic antibiotics were administered to seven of the eight infants with bilateral hearing-loss, but only four of the seven had aminoglycosides.
(9) Two of the eight children with bilateral sensorineural loss were noted to have neonatal hypoglycaemia.

Goodman and Kruskal's gamma correlation coefficients (Freeman 1965) were computed to determine the significance of the relationships between sensorineural loss and each of a number of potential causative factors and associated outcomes. The variables examined included: sex, social class, birthweight, preterm AGA *vs.* SGA, serum bilirubin level, antibiotics and other medication in the newborn period, and neurological status and EEG at approximately 6½ years.

Statistically significant coefficients were obtained for the relationships between sensorineural loss and: neonatal serum bilirubin level ($p = 0.007$); neurological status at about 6½ years ($p = 0.013$); use of antibiotics in the newborn nursery ($p = 0.016$); and incubator time ($p = 0.048$). No other gamma coefficient was significant at the 5 per cent level.

We thought it desirable to estimate the degree of *unique* contribution of each of these predictors to variation in the dependent variable, sensorineural hearing-

TABLE 9-III

Prediction of sensorineural hearing-loss from selected variables

Predictor	*Eta squared*	*Beta squared*	*df*	*F*	*p*
Incubator time	0.317	0.188	4, 31	3.62	<0.025
Bilirubin level	0.293	0.135	4, 31	3.09	<0.05
Antibiotics	0.082	0.025	1, 34	2.33	NS
Multiple R	0.508		27		<0.01

loss. We also wished to obtain an estimate of the multiple correlation between the set of significant predictors and the dependent variable. For these purposes the technique of Multiple Classification Analysis was selected (Andrews *et al.* 1967).

A computer program was obtained from the OSIRIS data analysis system developed at the University of Michigan by the Inter-University Consortium for Political Research (Le 1972). This technique examines the relationship between several predictor variables and a dependent variable. It assumes that the effects of the predictors are additive, and determines a coefficient for each predictor variable, while the effects of the other predictors are not allowed to vary. The dependent variable should be a dichotomy, and the predictors may be on nominal or ordinal scales.

Two analyses were performed: one for determining the predictability of sensorineural hearing-loss from incubator time, bilirubin level and use of antibiotics; the other for determining the predictability of ultimate neurological status from the same three predictors. Thus both hearing loss and neurological status were treated as dependent variables. Hearing loss was entered into the analysis as a dichotomous measure and neurological status was entered as an ordinal measure, with four levels ranging from normal to major abnormality. The three predictors were entered as ordinal measures in both analyses.

Since Multiple Classification Analysis is invalid when the dependent variable is markedly skewed, not all the non-hearing loss (NHL) cases could be included*. Thus the NHL cases were randomly sampled with the ratio of 1:8. This yielded a sample of 36 for this analysis: the 12 sensorineural loss cases and 24 NHL cases.

The results of the analysis for the outcome of hearing loss are summarized in Table 9-III. In this table the term 'eta squared' is the sum of squared unadjusted deviations between a predictor and the dependent variable, and 'beta squared' is the corresponding squared adjusted, *i.e.* partial, correlation. Thus beta squared is the proportion of variance in the dependent variable which is uniquely associated with the corresponding predictor. As indicated in the table, incubator time and neonatal serum bilirubin level are both systematically associated with unique variations in sensorineural hearing-loss, while the use of antibiotics is not.

*The proportion of hearing-impaired cases was 12/205, equal to 0.059; the greatest deviation from 0.50 considered allowable for the dependent variable was 0.25 to avoid intolerable skewness in the dependent variable.

TABLE 9-IV

Prediction of neurological status from selected variables

Predictor	*Eta squared*	*Beta squared*	*df*	*F*	*p*
Incubator time	0.182	0.200	4, 31	1.68	NS
Bilirubin level	0.111	0.212	4, 31	<1	NS
Antibiotics	0.007	0.041	1, 34	<1	NS
Multiple R	0.191		27		NS

The results for the analysis of subsequent neurological status are given in Table 9-IV. A similar pattern of outcomes is noted, though the multiple correlation coefficient is much smaller than in the case of hearing loss, and relationships between predictors and the dependent variable are not statistically significant.

To investigate further the extent of the association between these predictor variables and sensorineural hearing-loss, graphs were prepared to illustrate the relationships between the two significant predictors, *i.e.* bilirubin level and incubator time, and the dependent variable.

Figures 9-2 and 3 give the probability of hearing loss as a function of (1) serum bilirubin level, and (2) incubator time. Although the number of cases is small, it is clear from Figure 9-2 that the probability of hearing loss in general is an increasing function of neonatal maximal serum bilirubin level. In Figure 9-3 it is apparent that the probability of hearing loss generally is an increasing function of incubator time in this study, and that a high probability of sensorineural hearing-loss is a risk associated with an incubator time greater than four weeks.

Discussion

Sensorineural hearing-loss

Although auditory screening tests had been carried out during infancy in the present sample, the LBW children were not examined audiologically until they were about six years of age and, as in other studies, the assumption that these children were born with a sensorineural loss or that they acquired it in the early postnatal period may be questionable. On the other hand, the zero frequency in the FBW control group and the high frequency in the LBW group tend to support this assumption.

As mentioned in the introduction, estimates of the frequency of sensorineural hearing-loss among LBW children have ranged widely in different studies. However, the frequency of 3.9 per cent with bilateral and 2.0 per cent with unilateral sensorineural loss among the 205 LBW children in the present series is close to the prevalence of 3.6 per cent reported by Harper and Wiener (1965). It is also close to the proportion of 4.6 per cent found by Corner (1960) in VLBW infants. Barton *et al.* (1962) calculated that *severe* deafness was present in 1.7 out of every 1000 'premature' infants who survived, and that the incidence was higher for infants with birthweights ≤1815g. Depending on the definition of severity, it might be

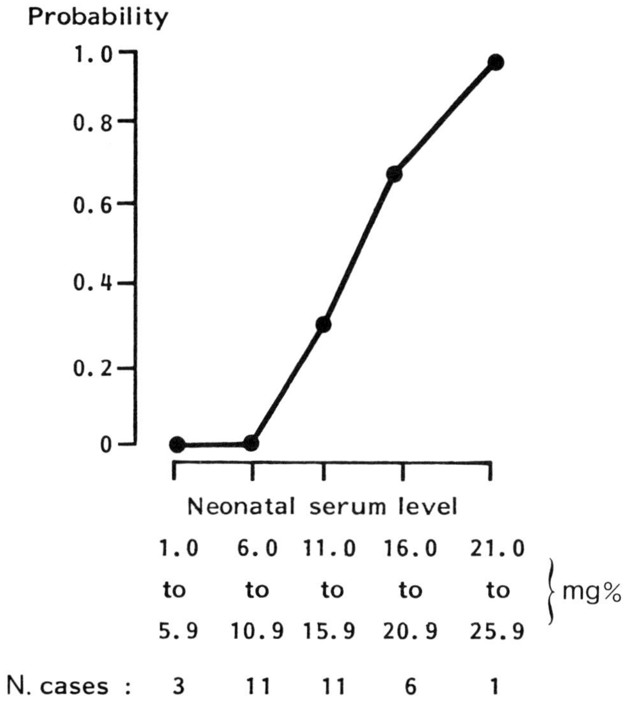

Fig. 9-2. Probability of sensorineural hearing-loss as a function of neonatal serum bilirubin level.

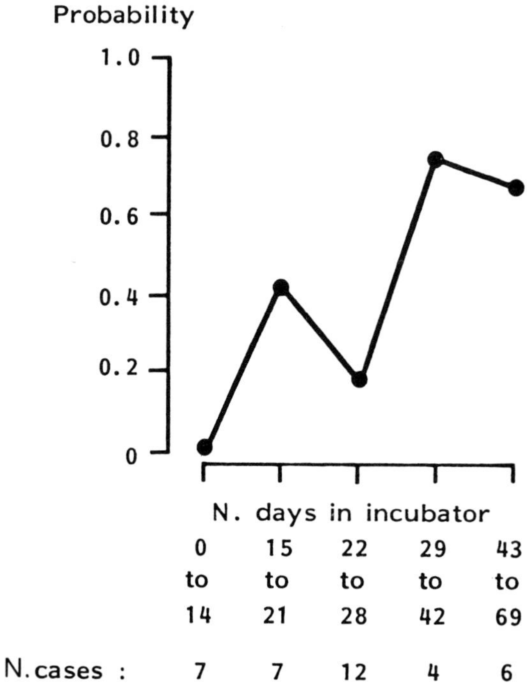

Fig. 9-3. Probability of sensorineural hearing-loss as a function of time spent in incubator.

postulated that two of our patients (1 per cent) were affected to this extent, and it should be recalled that most of the patients in our study had birthweights <2041g. Presumably the frequency of sensorineural deafness in LBW survivors has fallen along with that of other neurological sequelae with the advent of intensive perinatal care. It is noteworthy that in our series sensorineural hearing-loss (like ROP) occurred predominantly among preterm infants and was no less common in twins than in singletons.

Hyperbilirubinaemia

The relationship of hearing loss to serum bilirubin level has been demonstrated to be significant (see Table 9-III, Fig. 9-2). This is consistent with the findings by previous investigators of LBW children (Corner 1960, Barton 1964, Fisch 1964).

From our own case material, Crichton *et al.* (1972*a*) selected 30 LBW children who had maximum neonatal serum bilirubin levels above 20mg/100ml (340μmol/l) and compared them with two groups of 30 matched controls each, for whom the levels were, respectively, 11 to 19.9mg (187 to 338μmol/l) and below 11mg/100ml (187μmol/l). It was found that cerebral palsy, hearing defects and minimal cerebral dysfunction occurred in all three groups, without significant differences. However, there were trends towards lower mean global IQ scores and more abnormal and borderline EEGs in the children who had had higher neonatal serum bilirubin levels. Of the two cases with marked deafness in those 90 children, one occurred in the group with the highest and the other in the group with intermediate bilirubin concentration. It was clear that larger numbers of children would need to be analyzed to obtain statistically significant results.

Anoxia

Respiratory problems occurred in all the infants who subsequently had bilateral hearing-loss and in two of the four with unilateral hearing-loss. This frequency of 10 out of 12 infants with subsequent hearing-loss contrasts with the occurrence of respiratory abnormalities in 138 (42.9 per cent) among the other 322 LBW children followed to school in our series ($\chi^2 = 6.128$ with Yates' correction, $p<0.02$). In the absence of blood-gas measurements the degree of anoxia is hard to quantitate, but oxygen was administered in the incubator to 11 of the 12 infants; also at least three required oxygen to establish respiration and two others needed respiratory assistance. Whereas eight of the 12 infants required oxygen for more than 48 hours, only 108 (34.4 per cent) of the remaining 314 LBW infants did so ($\chi^2 = 3.938$ with Yates' correction, $p<0.05$).

While it was not possible to demonstrate any significant correlation between oxygen concentration in the incubator and subsequent deafness, our data support the assumption of previous authors that anoxia plays a part in damaging the auditory pathways and may aggravate the effect of hyperbilirubinaemia.

Incubator time

The number of days spent in an incubator was significantly greater for the hearing-impaired group than for a random sample of LBW children with normal hearing in our cohort. As shown in Figure 9-3, it also seems that a high probability of sensorineural hearing-loss is associated with an incubator time greater than four weeks.

There has been some disagreement between previous workers as to whether deafness in such babies merely reflects the severity of their initial clinical state, which necessitated long-term incubator-care, or whether the noise in the incubator could itself have a harmful effect on hearing. Seleny and Streczyn (1969) examined 17 incubators and found that the linear sound pressure-levels caused by the motor and fan fell in the range of 68 to 82dB at 125Hz. External noise source had an additive effect of 4 to 7dB for each octave band. They regarded this to be not only above the recommended acceptance level but also to be very close to the danger area in view of the prolonged exposure time. Dayal and co-authors (1971) found that hair-cell damage in guinea pigs following exposure to noise and simultaneous administration of ototoxic antibiotics was greater than the additive effect of each one. Falk and Farmer (1973) also analyzed noise from infant incubators and detected a 74.5dB noise level, with a frequency distribution mainly below 500Hz. Blennow and associates (1974) recorded similar findings and pointed out the possible risks. Douek and colleagues (1976) showed that adult guinea pigs subjected to incubator noise had no significant loss of outer hair-cells, but infant guinea pigs subjected to similar sound intensities had considerable loss of outer hair-cells. Further animal experiments demonstrated that noise trauma may aggravate the effects of anoxia and antibiotics on hearing. Accordingly, these authors also considered that incubator noise could damage the hearing of LBW babies. The problem was discussed in detail by Falk, in consultation with the Committee on Environmental Hazards of the American Academy of Pediatrics (1974), and it was suggested that manufacturers of incubators should reduce the noise from motors as much as possible, that physicians should limit the use of aminoglycoside antibiotics and other potential ototoxic drugs, and that hospital personnel should eliminate unnecessary noise in the premature nursery. It was also recommended that the effects of noise, with or without ototoxic drugs, on subsequent hearing, speech and language development should be studied further. Stennert *et al.* (1977) then found in a retrospective study of high-risk LBW children that hearing defects were correlated with the duration of incubator care, but only insofar as the association was correlated with a non-optimal perinatal risk-score (Prechtl 1967), *i.e.* an eventful neonatal period. In contrast to our own findings, the authors noted that infants raised in an incubator for longer than 20 days (up to 62 days) showed no correlation between hearing defects and duration of incubator stay. The same group of authors (Schulte *et al.* 1977) also studied the effect of preterm delivery and a three-week period of incubator care on the development of auditory evoked responses (AER) by comparing infants of the same conceptional age but with different extra-uterine life spans. The maturation of the AER was nearly identical inside and outside the uterus in otherwise normal low-risk newborns.

Schulte and Stennert (1978) concluded that the duration of exposure to incubator noise was not responsible for substantial hearing loss in preterm infants, though possibly it might play an additional rôle along with other factors. The same conclusion was reached by Stewart and Abramovich (1979), who examined the hearing of 111 VLBW infants at a mean age of 6½ years. They found that 10 (9 per cent) had a sensorineural hearing-loss. None of the audiograms of these 10 children showed notches at 4000Hz, which are characteristic of damage to the cochlea from long-term exposure to noise. Also, the mean duration of incubator stay did not differ between children with sensorineural hearing-loss and those without, whereas perinatal illnesses, particularly those likely to have caused hypoxia, were significantly associated with sensorineural hearing-loss, and jaundice appeared to have an additive effect. Table 9-I demonstrates that the audiograms of the children in our study also failed to show notches at 4000Hz. Winkel *et al.* (1978) did find such 'noise dips' in 52 per cent of 56 incubator-treated children with normal hearing, and in only one of 18 who had not been in an incubator, but noted that it did not cause any clinical symptoms. One may conclude that the noise in commercially available incubators in current use is not a major cause of sensorineural hearing-loss, and at most may be a contributory factor.

Antibiotics

A variety of antibiotics was used for our patients. Only three of the 12 children with sensorineural hearing-loss received streptomycin, two had kanamycin, and none were given dihydrostreptomycin. Falk and Farmer (1973) implied that the use of potentially ototoxic antibiotics in noisy incubators exposed the newborn to a further risk. In our study there was a significant correlation between sensorineural loss and the use of antibiotics, but their use did not have any predictive value by itself, and it was not independent of incubator time, as it should be to estimate unambiguously the interactive effects of two variables.

Neurological status

Only two of the 12 children were considered to be neurologically normal in other respects; both had only unilateral hearing-loss. Of the remaining 10, two had cerebral palsy (right spastic hemiparesis, asymmetrical spastic quadriparesis) and both these children and one other were also mentally retarded (global IQ below 70); the remaining seven had other evidence of cerebral dysfunction (minimal in two, more than minimal in five). None of the children had the choreo-athetoid type of cerebral palsy which has long been considered a common after-effect of kernicterus (Yannet and Lieberman 1946, Lande 1948, Gerrard 1952, Perlstein 1960), and this may again emphasize the complex interaction of jaundice with anoxia and other factors in LBW children. Although serum bilirubin levels and incubator times are not significant predictors of neurological status, it is apparent that neurological impairment is generally part of a syndrome in which low birthweight, neonatal hyperbilirubinaemia and anoxia, length of incubator time, and bilateral or unilateral hearing-loss are associated.

Conductive hearing-loss

Robinson *et al.* (1967) found conductive hearing-loss in 3.5 per cent of Vancouver schoolchildren. A similar percentage (2.4) was obtained for the FBW controls in the present study, but for the low-birthweight sample the frequency was more than twice as high (6.3 per cent).

McLellan *et al.* (1962) examined 49 petrous temporal bones, including the ear-drum, from 28 unselected LBW infants. Microscopic examination of histological sections revealed pus in the middle ear in 19 of the 28 cases. Those authors suggested that otitis media may play an important rôle in the morbidity and mortality of 'prematures'. Davey (1962) found that 25 out of 93 children with birthweights <1360g had conductive losses; and McLellan and Struck (1965), studying babies whose mothers had premature rupture of the amniotic membranes, found a rate as high as 36 per cent. Since the children in the present study did not have detailed audiometric testing until the approximate age of 6¾ years, it might be speculated that improved paediatric care, and especially the use of antibiotics, had reduced the frequency of conductive loss in LBW children, but not to the same degree as in the controls. It would seem that the susceptibility of LBW children to respiratory infections still puts them at risk with respect to conductive hearing-loss.

Minimal high-frequency hearing loss

As shown in Table 9-II, the prevalence of minimal high-frequency loss was about 4 per cent, with little difference between the LBW and FBW children. This proportion with minimal high-frequency disorders is greater than that for high-frequency *deafness* noted by Anderson (1967) and Sheridan (1972). Other studies have shown that various factors may attenuate the reliability of measuring high-frequency losses. Goetz (1972) showed that the audiometric configurations of normal children differ significantly between first and subsequent tests. Her results provide support for the hypothesis that test anxiety affects the results of the first examination, especially at higher frequencies. There is also evidence (Newby 1979) that subjects may not respond reliably to test tones of high frequency because of the standing wave phenomenon caused by occlusion of the external canal. Further, it is known that audiometer earphones are least stable at very high frequencies. The minimal high-frequency losses reported in this and other studies therefore may be artefacts, with little clinical importance.

Summary

Audiometric evaluations were carried out on a population of 205 LBW children and 123 FBW controls at a mean age of about 6¾ years.

Eight LBW children (3.9 per cent) had a bilateral and four (2.0 per cent) a unilateral sensorineural high-frequency loss. No case of sensorineural hearing-loss was found among the controls. There were 13 (6.3 per cent) cases of conductive loss among the LBW sample, compared with three (2.4 per cent) among the FBW controls.

Nine of the 12 children with sensorineural hearing-loss were boys, as were all but one of those with bilateral loss. 10 of the 12 were preterm AGA children and only one was SGA. For the remaining girl the length of gestation was uncertain. Half the affected children were twins.

Some abnormality of delivery had occurred in nine of the 12 infants. Neonatal jaundice had been noted in all but one; the serum bilirubin level had been checked in eight of these 12, and for seven the maximum levels had been 15mg per cent (255μmol/l) or more.

Respiratory problems had been encountered in all eight children with bilateral hearing-loss, and in two of the four with unilateral loss. This contrasts with 42.9 per cent with neonatal respiratory problems among the other 322 LBW children followed to school ($p<0.02$). All but one of the 12 children with sensorineural hearing-loss had received oxygen as newborns—seven of the eight with bilateral loss and one of the four with unilateral loss, *i.e.* a total of two-thirds, had required oxygen for more than 48 hours, whereas only 34.4 per cent among the other 314 LBW children in the total cohort had needed it for this length of time ($p<0.05$).

Two of the eight children with bilateral sensorineural loss also had neonatal hypoglycaemia. Systemic antibiotics were administered to seven of the eight infants with bilateral loss.

Neurological abnormalities were found after birth in 11 of the 12 infants, but in seven cases subsided during the stay in the nursery. All the children with bilateral loss and two of the four with unilateral loss had neurological sequelae; two had spastic forms of cerebral palsy with mental retardation, one was mentally retarded, and seven had various degrees of other cerebral dysfunction.

Correlation coefficients showed significant relationships between sensorineural hearing-loss and maximal neonatal serum bilirubin level, use of antibiotics and incubator time, and neurological outcome. Subsequent multiple classification analyses showed that while neonatal serum bilirubin level and incubator time were each significant predictors of sensorineural loss, this was not the case with the use of antibiotics.

Neurological sequelae appeared to be closely associated with the syndrome of low birthweight, neonatal hyperbilirubinaemia and hypoxia, extended incubator-time and sensorineural hearing-loss.

ADDENDUM

Vestibular Function

*R. Patrick Gannon**

Only a few investigators have studied vestibular function in LBW children. Fisch and Osborn (1954), reporting on 891 children with congenital sensorineural hearing-loss, included a subgroup of 68 'premature' children and stated that vestibular function in this group was normal in all cases. Fisch (1964) has also pointed out that the vestibular system, developmentally and phylogenetically, is older than the hearing system; accordingly, if the vestibular apparatus is intact in cases with severe congenital deafness, we can deduce that the developmental fault occurred at a later

*The writer is indebted to Margaret Roberts, M.Sc., for technical assistance.

TABLE 9-V

Proportions of children with normal findings on audiological and vestibular tests

Group	*N*	*Mean age (yrs)*	*Pure-tone test N*	*%*	*Speech test N*	*%*	*Impedance N*	*%*	*ENG N*	*%*
Normal birthweight with normal hearing	10	7.3	9	90	10	100	8	80	8	80
Low birthweight with normal hearing	10	10.9	7	70	10	100	2	20	8	80
Low birthweight with sensorineural loss	8	11.6	0	0	4	50	4	50	6	75

stage of embyronic development than if both systems were involved together. Although it might seem reasonable for perinatal anoxia or neonatal hyperbilirubinaemia to affect chiefly the auditory system, the proportion of deaf children who also have abnormal vestibular function has varied in different studies. Arnvig (1955), like Fisch and Osborn, found no notable changes in vestibular function among LBW children. Marcus *et al.* (1963) examined 35 deaf children who had been born prematurely and found that 26 had no vestibular function. It was markedly reduced in eight and only one had normal function. The authors noted that dihydrostreptomycin had been administered in excess of the standard recommended daily dose to 29 of these children, and thus appeared to be largely responsible for the impairment of cochleovestibular function. Nonetheless, vestibular function also was absent or markedly reduced in four children who had not received this drug; they had had only procaine penicillin and 7.5mg of vitamin K. Winkel and colleagues (1978) performed caloric testing on 91 four- to six-year-old children with birthweights <2000g and found only one to be abnormal, but obtained inconclusive results in several others.

For children of any birthweight who had been jaundiced because of haemolytic disease of the newborn, the proportion reported with impaired vestibular function has ranged from 2 per cent (Schneeweiss *et al.* 1970) to 11.8 per cent (Weber and Ströder 1973). Among 20 children who were considered deaf as a result of haemolytic disease, six were found to have some evidence of vestibular damage on caloric testing, but the extent of the impairment appeared to be unrelated to the degree of hearing-loss (Blakeley 1959). Hervei *et al.* (1977) investigated both cochlear and vestibular function by unsophisticated techniques in 72 children aged four to seven years who had had neonatal hyperbilirubinaemia and had not received any ototoxic drugs. Contrary to previous reports, they found increasingly serious impairment of vestibular function among patients who had had prolonged jaundice and concluded that the vestibular apparatus was more sensitive to bilirubin than the cochlea. The degree of damage to the two systems was not parallel.

As part of the present study, it was considered desirable to perform complete audio-vestibular investigations of the children with sensorineural deafness, using electronystagmography in addition to other techniques.

Material and method

Eight of the 12 LBW children with some degree of sensorineural loss (five bilateral, three unilateral) were compared with 10 LBW and 10 FBW children, all with normal hearing and selected randomly from the study population (Table 9-V). The mean age of the two LBW groups was 10.9 years for those with normal hearing and 11.6 for those with sensorineural loss. The mean age of the FBW control group with normal hearing was more than three years younger.

The audiometric testing procedures carried out on all children were pure-tone air and bone conduction audiogram, speech-reception threshold and discrimination, and impedance audiometry and stapedius reflex thresholds. Pure-tone testing was performed with a Madsen OB-70 audiometer in a soundproof room of custom construction. Impedance audiometry was carried out with a Madsen ZO-70 in a quiet but not soundproof room. All equipment was calibrated to ANSI 1969 standards. Vestibular function was examined according to a modified Fitzgerald and Hallpike (1942) method, using electonystagmographic recording. Surface electrodes positioned around the eyes to record horizontal and vertical nystagmus were connected to an Elema-Schonander Mingograph 81 recorder. Calibration of the equipment was performed using voluntary 10° eye-movements in horizontal and vertical planes. Recordings were made of spontaneous, positional and gaze nystagmus. Caloric responses to 30°C and 44°C irrigations of 30 seconds duration were recorded for right and left ears. The results were calculated according to the following formula*:

$$\mathrm{CP} = \frac{\mathrm{RC} + \mathrm{RH} \sim \mathrm{LC} + \mathrm{LH}}{\mathrm{RH} + \mathrm{RC} + \mathrm{LH} + \mathrm{LC}} \times 100\% \qquad \mathrm{DP} = \frac{\mathrm{RC} + \mathrm{LH} \sim \mathrm{LH} + \mathrm{RH}}{\mathrm{RH} + \mathrm{RC} + \mathrm{LH} + \mathrm{LC}} \times 100\%$$

Canal paresis less than 15 per cent was considered to be within normal limits, 15 to 20 per cent was considered borderline, and greater than 20 per cent was considered a significant impairment of the labyrinth giving poorer response.

Results

Audiology

Pure tone. Hearing was considered to be normal if the thresholds at all frequencies were 25dB or better. Of the 10 FBW normal-hearing controls, nine had completely normal hearing, and one had a mild conductive loss in both ears, but only the left was significantly abnormal. (This child had a cold on the day of the test.)

Among the 10 in the LBW normal-hearing control group, seven had normal results and three had a mild conductive impairment. One of the three had a cold on the day of the test, one had had a fractured skull and one had a scarred left drum and a history of ear infection.

All eight in the LBW sensorineural-loss group had some degree of sensorineural hearing-loss. This confirmed previous test results for these children.

*CP = canal paresis; DP = directional preponderance; RH = right-ear 44°C irrigation; RC = right-ear 30°C irrigation; LC = left-ear 30°C irrigation; LH = left-ear 44°C irrigation.

Speech tests. Speech testing consisted of speech-reception thresholds and discrimination scores. The FBW and LBW normal-hearing controls all had normal results.

In the LBW sensorineural-loss group, four had entirely normal speech-discrimination scores, three showed mild impairment, such as would be consistent with their pure-tone audiograms, and one had no response to speech stimuli, which was also consistent with the degree of hearing loss.

Impedance audiometry. In the FBW normal-hearing control group eight had entirely normal impedance results, one had elevated reflex thresholds as a result of a mild conductive loss caused by a cold, and one who had had a skull fracture had elevated reflexes in one ear.

In the LBW normal-hearing control group only two had normal results; eight had abnormal results associated with either Eustachian-tube dysfunction or a history of a middle-ear disease.

Four in the LBW sensorineural-loss group had normal results and four showed elevation of stapedius reflex thresholds.

Vestibular function

Of the 10 FBW normal-hearing controls, eight had normal results, one showed a mild positional nystagmus of questionable significance but with normal calorics, and one showed a 36 per cent right labyrinthine impairment. This child had had mumps and chickenpox, with febrile convulsions, and on one occasion had drunk paint thinner.

The 10 LBW normal-hearing control children included eight with normal vestibular function; one had a questionable spontaneous nystagmus and one had definite spontaneous nystagmus with a high directional preponderance, for which there was no obvious cause. One of the group had impaired caloric responses.

Of the eight children with LBW sensorineural hearing-loss, six had entirely normal vestibular function, one showed a questionable positional nystagmus but normal caloric responses, and one had a mild but significant asymmetry of caloric responses, without other evidence of vestibular abnormality. These results are summarized in Table 9-V.

Discussion

The purpose of this investigation was to document the occurrence of vestibular abnormalities among LBW children with sensorineural hearing-loss. Without the use of statistics, it is clear that the frequency of vestibular abnormality among these children is not significantly greater than in the LBW or FBW normal-hearing groups. Therefore, although there is an increased frequency of sensorineural hearing-loss in LBW children, in this small series there is no obvious association between sensorineural hearing-loss and vestibular abnormalities in LBW children.

Table 9-V suggests that there may be significant differences in the findings on impedance audiometry. χ^2 tests showed that the difference between the FBW and LBW normal-hearing groups was significant beyond the 0.05 level. Further, the difference on impedance testing between the FBW group and the two LBW groups combined also was significant beyond the 0.05 level. This suggests that abnormal middle-ear function, as determined by impedance audiometry, is more prevalent among LBW children than the FBW controls (see pp. 161-2).

Summary

Audio-vestibular investigations, including impedance audiometry, estimation of stapedius reflex thresholds and electronystagmography, were performed on eight of the 12 LBW children with sensorineural deafness described in the main section of this chapter and also in 10 LBW children with normal hearing at a mean age of 11.6 and 10.9 years, respectively. The same studies were performed on 10 random FBW control children with normal hearing from the prospective study at a mean age of 7.3 years.

Of the 10 FBW normal-hearing control children, nine were found to have completely normal hearing and one had a mild conductive loss on pure-tone testing. On speech tests all 10 had normal results. On impedance audiometry eight had entirely normal results, one had elevated reflex thresholds owing to a mild conductive loss, and one had elevated reflexes in one ear after a skull fracture. Vestibular function was normal in eight, while one showed a mild positional nystagmus of questionable significance and one showed a 36 per cent right labyrinthine impairment, possibly acquired.

Of the 10 in the LBW normal-hearing group, seven had normal results on pure-tone audiometry, while three a had mild conductive loss. All had normal results on speech testing. However, only two had normal findings on impedance audiometry; eight had abnormal results associated either with Eustachian-tube dysfunction or a history of middle-ear disease. Vestibular function was normal in eight, while one had a questionable spontaneous nystagmus and one had definite spontaneous nystgamus, without obvious cause.

All eight LBW children with sensorineural loss had abnormal findings on pure-tone testing. On speech tests, four had normal discrimination scores, three showed mild impairment and one had no response to speech stimuli, consistent with the degree of hearing loss. On impedance audiometry, four had normal results and four showed elevation of stapedius reflex thresholds. On electronystagmography, six had normal vestibular function, one showed a questionable positional nystagmus, and one had a mild but significant asymmetry of caloric responses, without other evidence of vestibular abnormality.

The frequency of vestibular abnormality among LBW children with hearing loss is not significantly greater than in LBW and FBW control children with normal hearing. The finding in the main section of this chapter that LBW children are significantly more subject to abnormal middle-ear function than FBW controls is confirmed by the results of impedance audiometry.

10
Communication Skills

Dorothy M. Washington, Annetta K. McBurney and Ruth V. E. Grunau

The literature contains a number of studies dealing with the developmental patterns of LBW children (Centano *et al.* 1956; Dann *et al.* 1958, 1964; Drillien 1961*a*; Wiener *et al.* 1968; Beargie *et al.* 1970; Neligan *et al.* 1976; Caputo *et al.* 1979; Friedman and Sigman 1981). However, only a limited number have been concerned specifically with communication skills. Kastein and Fowler (1959) investigated 'premature' children within two weeks of their second birthday. In the four categories used in their final assessment (severely retarded, retarded, adequate and superior), only 25 of the 60 children had adequate or superior language development.

Rabinowitch *et al.* (1961) discussed psychological test findings for 50 children who had been 'premature' and for 50 controls. They also collected data from parents concerning the children's early language development and found that, on average, 'premature' children had mastered sentences at the age of 27 months, compared to 23 months for the controls. Drillien (1961*a*), in a longitudinal investigation of the mental development of 540 prematurely born children, used a selection of tests based on the Gesell Scale and Terman-Merrill L Form to study the ability to name, to describe pictures and to state the use of common objects at three and four years. (The development of speech and language was not discussed as a separate cognitive area.) Fitzhardinge and Steven (1972*b*) noted delayed onset of speech in SGA children: speech defects featuring immaturity of reception and expression were found in 33 per cent of the boys and 26 per cent of the girls.

Rubin *et al.* (1973) showed that measures of language development, school readiness and academic achievement discriminated LBW children from controls at four to seven years. Neligan and co-authors (1976) also reported a greater frequency of language difficulties among their LBW children compared to FBW children, but suggested a strong environmental influence on language competence at five to seven years of age.

The most comprehensive study of the speech and language development of 'premature' and control children, by de Hirsch *et al.* (1964), considered 15 dimensions of the oral language of children between five and six years of age. This formed part of a larger longitudinal investigation aimed at predicting children's reading, writing and spelling performance at the end of Grades 2 and 3 by means of a battery of 46 maturational tests administered in kindergarten. The findings were that 'in seven of the 15 areas tested, namely tapped patterns, language comprehension, word finding, number of words used, mean of five longest sentences, sentence elaboration and definitions, the premature children's performance was indeed inferior to that of children born at term. It is suggested that these findings result from the premature children's lingering neurophysiological immaturity'.

Method

The present study used data from repeated neurological and psychological examinations from birth to 6½ years, and school progress up to Grade 3. For specific speech and language skills the children were seen individually at the age of about four years in a clinical setting, and were tested in a single session lasting approximately one hour. Children whose language development might differ somewhat from the norm were excluded, namely twins, children with a bilingual background and those with an IQ <80, with marked neuromotor involvement (chiefly more than minimal cerebral palsy), with hearing difficulties and with gross emotional disturbance. The sample then consisted of 357 boys and girls, of whom 243 were LBW and 114 were FBW controls.

Assessment

The speech and language pathologist examined the children at four years of age. At 6½ years the psychologist added further data. The areas assessed were speech mechanisms (tongue elevation and protrusion, movement of soft palate, articulation and phonation) and language (vocabulary, receptive and expressive language, auditory memory, ability to receive and process auditory information in a temporal sequence and psychometric assessment of functional language skills). The psychometric measures at 6½ years were the Wechsler Intelligence Scale for Children (WISC) Verbal Subtests, the Benton Sentence Repetition Test and the Illinois Test of Psycholinguistic Abilities (ITPA) Vocal Encoding Subtest. The following sources also were used:

(1) Griffiths Mental Development Scale (Division C) for hearing and speech at ages three, six, 12 and 18 months, giving data on comprehension, expressive language and communication skills. According to Griffiths, a high score suggests a 'verbal child'.

(2) Medical records concerning language development at the four-year and 6½-year examinations.

(3) Psychological tests at 6½ years: WISC Verbal Subtests, Benton Sentence Repetition Test and ITPA Vocal Encoding.

(4) Reading: Stanford Achievement Test in Grade 1; word meaning, paragraph meaning.

(5) Speech and language examination by a speech and language pathologist (see next section).

Speech and language test at four years

The speech pathologist's evaluation at four years included the physical speech mechanisms of lips, tongue and soft palate, as well as a screening test for hearing deficiencies. In a play session at the beginning of the test period the child's ability to recognize common objects, to name them and respond to questions about them was evaluated. Maturity of sentence development was judged by the number of words, length of utterance, use of compound and complex sentences, and correct use of syntax. This was evaluated according to the over-all response throughout the test period. Assessment of articulation included two considerations: first, words from the Hejna (1955) Articulation Test were introduced to evaluate the articulation of vowels and diphthongs, and of initial and final consonants; and second, connected speech and over-all intelligibility. De Hirsch *et al.* (1964), and others, have indicated that there is a significant number of children whose articulation of isolated words and short phrases is entirely acceptable, but whose speech tends to disintegrate under the stress of having to organize complex thought-units into verbal form. Therefore the frequency of articulatory errors when using single words was compared to the number of errors made during story-telling, in response to questions and in conversational speech to produce an over-all intelligibility score.

Procedure

The mother (or accompanying adult) and the child were introduced to the examiner in the waiting-room. If the child was reluctant to accompany the examiner to the testing-room the mother remained with the child, but she was encouraged to be strictly non-participatory. The child was given time to become familiar with the surroundings—to wander about the clinic, examine the one-way mirror and ask questions—before being invited to sit on a small chair at the kindergarten table, with the examiner seated opposite at the same level.

Screening for hearing was done on portable apparatus. After a brief explanation and demonstration of 'whistles', and the use of marbles to signal that a 'whistle' had been heard, a sweep test of each ear at 10 or 15dB (depending on the level of background noise) was performed over 500 to 4000Hz to determine whether hearing was within the normal range or whether referral for a complete hearing examination was needed.

Before removing the apparatus, the child was asked to help put the marbles back into the container, counting as each one was put back. Frequently the child also named the colours of the marbles.

To test naming familiar objects, small toys representing animals and well-known objects were presented one at a time for the child to handle and comment on. These included a horse, cat, dog, rabbit, lion, cars of different sizes and colours, baby doll, doll's bottle and shoes, a cup, spoon, comb and scissors.

The child and the examiner carried on a conversation about the colours of the cars, the name and kind of pet(s) in the child's own home, and about brothers and sisters (older, younger, bigger, smaller). The examiner gathered much information during this informal period about the child's ability to comprehend language, to make simple statements, the use of syntax and the variety of sentence types.

The child was then ready to accept a more formal type of articulation test, which was presented as a game. Items from three-year to six-year levels of the Hejna Test were used, but most four-year-olds completed the entire test. The child's responses were entered on a scoring sheet, with appropriate comments indicating verbal behaviour and attitude toward testing.

Sentence development was further evaluated from the child's response to coloured pictures of the everyday activities of small children. The child was invited to comment on what they showed, and free and spontaneous use of speech and language reflected the child's ability to use expressive language effectively.

A penny sucker was used to examine oral structures (instead of a tongue-depressor), to assess the condition of the teeth, palate, lips, and mobility of the tongue.

The examination ended with a brief session between the parent (or accompanying adult) and the examiner.

All these procedures were scored, and responses were evaluated and recorded in terms of specific responses. An over-all classification was made of the child's speech and language, and the ability to communicate at the four-year level. A reasonably accurate over-all classification can be made, at least in the three categories of average, below average and markedly deficient. The categories of above average and superior were also used in this study.

Analysis of data

The data were analyzed to identify measures indicating differing patterns of language development of *(a)* LBW SGA, preterm AGA and FBW children, and *(b)* boys and girls. Neurological status at four and 6½ years and EEGS at 6½ years were also evaluated in relation to language scores for the same groups.

Results

Comparison of language scores (chronological listing)

As a group, FBW children were significantly better than the combined groups of LBW SGA and preterm AGA children at three, six, 12 and 18 months on the Griffiths Speech and Hearing Subtest, in several areas of the speech and language assessment at four years, and in over-all ratings of speech assessment in the medical examination at four years ($\chi^2 = 7.34$, $p<0.025$). The areas examined at four years are given below, together with the areas of superior performance by the FBW children.

Speech mechanisms (lip retraction, *etc.*): differences were slight but tended to favour the FBW group.

Phonation: similar results were obtained for both groups.

Articulation: vowels and diphthongs ($\chi^2 = 7.18$, $p<0.05$); initial consonants ($\chi^2 = 6.49$, $p<0.05$); final consonants ($\chi^2 = 8.24$, $p<0.05$); connected speech (slight but non-significant trend favouring the controls); intelligibility of speech (similar results obtained by both groups).

Receptive language: points to named objects (similar results for both groups); follows oral serial directions ($\chi^2 = 7.70$, $p<0.05$).

Expressive language: spontaneous verbalization and naming of objects (for both, slight but non-significant trends favoured the controls).

Vocabulary: nouns and verbs (slight but non-significant trend favoured controls); adjectives (similar results for both groups); prepositions ($\chi^2 = 7.99$, $p<0.05$); conjunctives ($\chi^2 = 10.69$, $p<0.005$); articles (slight but non-significant trend favoured controls); sentence length ($\chi^2 = 20.71$, $p<0.001$).

TABLE 10-I

Communication skills: areas of significant differences† between LBW-SGA and FBW control children

	SGA (N = 93–105)		*FBW (N = 91–114)*			
Test	*Mean*	*SD*	*Mean*	*SD*	*t*	*p*
Griffiths: speech and hearing: 3 mths	94.5	18.5	101.9	12.4	2.34	<0.05
6 mths	96.9	17.6	102.3	11.5	2.11	<0.05
12 mths	95.7	16.2	104.5	10.3	4.54	<0.001
18 mths	88.8	15.1	96.4	11.5	4.02	<0.001
Speech assessment (4 yrs)*					χ^2	*p*
Articulation: initial consonants					8.33	<0.025
final consonants					9.60	<0.01
Receptive language: follows oral serial directions					4.66	<0.025
Expressive language: prepositions					8.03	<0.025
conjunctives					9.46	<0.01
sentence length					21.6	<0.001
Echolalia					6.31	<0.05
Over-all classification					9.09	<0.025
Medical examination						
articulation: 6½ yrs (normal *vs.* all other)					6.40	<0.05
WISC (6½ yrs)					*t*	*p*
Digit Span	8.8	3.3	11.0	2.8	4.38	<0.001
Verbal IQ	96.8	13.4	110.1	11.4	6.45	<0.001
Sentence repetition	9.8	2.3	11.5	2.3	4.41	<0.001

*20 items or categories.

TABLE 10-II

Communication skills: significant differences† between LBW preterm AGA and FBW control children

	Preterm AGA (N = 129–138)		*FBW (N = 91–114)*			
Test	*Mean*	*SD*	*Mean*	*SD*	*t*	*p*
Griffiths: speech and hearing: 3 mths	85.0	19.3	101.9	12.4	5.53	<0.001
6 mths	85.7	16.9	102.3	11.5	6.94	<0.001
12 mths	89.0	17.0	104.5	10.3	8.89	<0.001
18 mths	87.7	15.1	96.4	11.5	5.24	<0.001
Grade 1 Stanford Achievement:						
Word meaning	17.5	10.1	23.9	7.9	2.89	<0.005
Paragraph meaning	14.5	9.4	19.9	9.4	2.10	<0.05
Speech assessment (4 yrs)*					χ^2	*p*
Receptive language: follows oral serial directions					5.97	<0.025
Expressive language: prepositions					6.18	<0.05
conjunctives					9.48	<0.01
sentence length					13.01	<0.025
Over-all classification					7.07	<0.05
WISC (6½ yrs)					*t*	*p*
Vocabulary	10.2	2.4	11.0	2.2	1.98	<0.05
Digit Span	9.7	2.8	11.0	2.8	2.70	<0.01
Verbal IQ	100.9	11.6	110.1	11.4	4.84	<0.001

*20 items or categories. † All differences favour FBW groups.

TABLE 10-III

Communication skills: significant differences between preterm AGA and SGA children

Test	*Preterm AGA (N = 129–138) Mean*	*SD*	*SGA (N = 93–105) Mean*	*SD*	*t*	*p*
In favour of SGA						
Griffiths: speech and hearing: 3 mths	85.0	19.3	94.5	18.5	2.22	<0.05
6 mths	85.7	16.9	96.9	17.6	3.22	<0.005
12 mths	89.0	17.0	95.7	16.2	3.01	<0.005
In favour of preterm AGA						
Sentence repetition (6½ yrs)	11.1	2.5	9.8	2.3	2.93	<0.005
Speech assessment (4 yrs)* Phonation: quality (adequate *vs.* all other)					χ^2 4.73	<0.05

*20 items or categories.

Echolalia: a non-significant trend favoured the controls.
Over-all classification: outstanding plus above average/average/below average plus deficient (χ^2 = 19.42, p<0.001); and at 6½ years more problems with articulation were evident among the LBW children (χ^2 = 16.11, p<0.025).

At 6½ years, significant differences in favour of the FBW group were found in all tests given at that age: WISC Verbal IQ (t = −6.07, p<0.001); Sentence Repetition (t = −2.85, p<0.01); Stanford Achievement (word meaning) test in Grade 1 (t = −3.00, p<0.01); and Stanford Achievement (paragraph meaning) test in Grade 1 (t = −2.16, p<0.05).

When the results for LBW SGA and preterm AGA children were compared separately with those for the FBW controls, 16 and 14 areas, respectively, of significant difference were found (Tables 10-I and II).

In a few of the areas examined the SGA and preterm AGA groups differed significantly from each other, the differences being in favour of the SGA group in the Griffiths Speech and Hearing Subtest at three, six and 12 months, but thereafter (*i.e.* at four and 6½ years) in favour of the preterm AGA children (Table 10-III).

Comparison of boys' and girls' language scores

Sex differences were examined within the LBW SGA, preterm AGA and FBW groups. Few differences in language function between boys and girls were noted in the medical and psychological evaluations. However, the FBW girls performed better than the boys on the Griffiths Division C Test at 18 months and on two sections of the Grade 1 Stanford Achievement Test. The speech pathologist's analysis at four years also yielded two areas of significant difference between the FBW boys and girls. In the LBW SGA and preterm AGA groups, five and eight tests, respectively, distinguished boys from girls. Sentence length was the only item that distinguished boys from girls within each of the three groups. In the over-all assessment of speech and language at four years, placement of the LBW girls was significantly higher than

TABLE 10-IV

Communication skills: significant differences[†] between males and females

SGA (males N = 41–44, females N = 52–61)		
Speech and language (4 yrs)*	χ^2	*p*
Articulation: connected speech	7.15	<0.05
Expressive language		
Spontaneous verbalization	14.14	<0.01
Names objects	13.88	<0.005
adjectives	7.72	<0.05
prepositions	7.61	<0.05
conjunctives	7.09	<0.05
articles	9.58	<0.01
Sentence length	10.33	<0.05
Over-all assessment		
Outstanding + above average/ average/below average + deficient	10.51	<0.01
Pre-term AGA (males N = 67–73, females N = 62–65)		
Speech and language (4 yrs)*		
Articulation: initial consonants	7.13	<0.05
Receptive language: follows oral serial directions	8.69	<0.005
Expressive language:		
Names objects	10.65	<0.05
sentence length	11.02	<0.05
Over-all classification	8.07	<0.05

FBW (males N = 45, females N = 45–47)	*Male*		*Female*			
	Mean	*SD*	*Mean*	*SD*	*t*	*p*
Griffiths speech and hearing (18 mths)	92.1	9.3	100.3	12.1	4.04	<0.001
Grade 1 Stanford Achievement:						
Word meaning	20.0	7.6	26.5	6.6	3.56	<0.001
Paragraph meaning	13.7	7.1	23.8	9.1	4.74	<0.001
Speech Assessment (4 yrs)*:		χ^2	*p*			
Vocabulary: adjectives		7.12	<0.05			
sentence length		10.77	<0.005			

*20 items or categories. [†] All differences favour females.

that of the LBW boys (χ^2 = 10.51, p<0.01) (Table 10-IV).

Thus in all tests in which differences were found the girls performed better than the boys, and generally speaking these differences were in the areas of vocabulary and expressive language.

Neurological status in relation to language scores

Abnormal neurological status at four years was significantly associated with poorer performance language scores in each of the three groups, particularly in the case of the FBW children's responses in the speech and language examination at that age (Table 10-V). At 6½ years abnormal neurological status also was associated with poor language scores in the majority of language measures (Table 10-V).

TABLE 10-V

Neurological status at four and at 6½ years *vs.* language scores: correlation of abnormalities

		LBW SGA (N = 93–105)				Preterm AGA (N = 129–138)				FBW (N = 91–114)			
		Mean	*SD*	χ^2	*p*	*Mean*	*SD*	χ^2	*p*	*Mean*	*SD*	χ^2	*p*
Four years													
Speech and language													
Over-all assessment								16.22	<0.005			27.54	<0.001
Vowels and diphthongs												10.18	<0.005
Initial consonants												16.67	<0.001
Final consonants												16.67	<0.001
Connected speech				6.27	<0.025			6.03	<0.025			12.84	<0.001
Intelligibility of speech								6.03	<0.025				
Follows oral serial												10.35	<0.005
directions								7.27	<0.01			10.35	<0.005
Spontaneous verbalization								8.31	<0.005				
Names objects				10.63	<0.005			12.34	<0.025			19.00	<0.001
Names animals				13.20	<0.005			12.34	<0.01			25.72	<0.001
Names pictures				13.20	<0.005			12.34	<0.01			19.00	<0.001
Nouns								6.70	<0.01			17.26	<0.001
Verbs								6.70	<0.01			24.13	<0.001
Prepositions				6.27	<0.025			3.89	<0.05			22.57	<0.001
Conjunctives				6.27	<0.025							26.80	<0.001
Articles												26.80	<0.001
Approx. length of sentence												6.01	<0.025
Medical examination													
Language												62.45	<0.001
Articulation				10.48	<0.05			10.01	<0.05			19.63	<0.001
6½ years				*t*				*t*				*t*	
Sentence repetition	1*	10.89	2.30	4.32	<0.001								
	2	8.45	2.13										
Vocal encoding	1									−0.43	0.69		
	2									−0.89	0.55	2.56	<0.01
WISC vocabulary subtest	1	10.74	3.47	1.72	<0.05	10.92	2.51	2.38	<0.01				
	2	9.37	3.05			9.60	2.34						
WISC verbal IQ	1	102.96	11.40	4.08	<0.001	102.05	10.72	1.77	<0.05	110.65	10.73	2.90	<0.005
	2	89.50	14.10			96.96	12.64			97.08	15.73		
WISC Full-scale IQ	1	105.00	11.10	5.02	<0.001	104.23	9.35	2.52	<0.01	111.29	9.57	2.97	<0.005
	2	90.62	11.72			98.12	10.51			96.92	17.10		

*1 = normal, 2 = abnormal status.

EEGs in relation to language scores

Very few significant associations were found between abnormal *vs.* normal EEGS at 6½ years and language measures at four years. At 6½ years the psychometric tests did show significant differences in WISC Verbal IQ scores as a function of EEG rating for the LBW SGA and FBW groups, but not for preterm AGA.

Discussion

The finding of delayed development in many aspects of speech and language in our LBW cohort is consistent with earlier reports of group differences in communication skills between LBW and FBW children (de Hirsch *et al.* 1964, Rubin *et al.* 1973, Neligan *et al.* 1976). As advised by Dr. Ruth Griffiths, we did not apply any 'correction for prematurity' by adjusting for conceptional age, and this explains why the LBW SGA infants, who largely were born at term, obtained higher mean Griffiths Speech and Hearing scores in the first year than preterm AGA infants, whose brains were more immature at birth (see Table 10-III). This difference was also demonstrated with respect to over-all Griffiths GQ scores in Chapter 4.

Recent studies have continued to show delayed language development in LBW infants: however, conclusions about the persistence of language difficulties beyond early childhood have varied somewhat, depending on whether the language scores were adjusted for prematurity. Siegel *et al.* (1982) found that LBW children had poorer comprehension and expression on the Reynell Language Scale at two, three and four years compared to FBW children. As might be expected, these differences were more significant when scores were *not* adjusted for gestational age at birth. On the other hand, Ungerer and Sigman (1983), also using the Reynell Scale, reported that LBW children had significant delays in language ability at 22 months, but that these problems mostly were overcome by three years if corrections for gestational age were made. In contrast, Siegel (1983) argued that it is inappropriate to correct for prematurity beyond the first few months of life.

Studies of the intellectual development of LBW children provide indirect indications of their functional competence with language. Caputo *et al.* (1981) found that visuomotor aspects of cognitive functioning were relatively more impaired than verbal abilities in a sample of LBW children followed to middle childhood. However, they pointed out that their LBW sample had relatively high birthweights and fewer neurological and intellectual defects than had emerged in other studies (Wiener *et al.* 1968, Wright *et al.* 1972). Rubin and colleagues (1973) did not report Verbal and Performance IQs separately, but WISC Full-scale IQs were lower than those of the controls. The present study found a lower mean Verbal IQ score in the LBW group, indicating long-term differences in language-based intellectual competence (see Chapter 4).

Respiratory distress syndrome (RDS) and intracranial haemorrhage are common complications among immature LBW infants. Survivors of severe RDS have a greater frequency of developmental deficits, particularly those with very low birthweights (≤1500g) (Bacola *et al.* 1966, Roberton and Tizard 1975), and the same applies to survivors of intraventricular haemorrhage (Palmer *et al.* 1982). Earlier studies of infants with milder RDS who received respiratory assistance had suggested that they may have early developmental delays (Fisch *et al.* 1968), but by the age of four years have no significant lowering of IQ scores (Robertson and Crichton 1969, Ambrus *et al.* 1970, Fisch *et al.* 1975). However, more recent studies have tended to show an increased prevalence of hyperactivity and delayed production of language among such children. Field *et al.* (1979) consider a broadly normal IQ (≥85) to be a crude estimate of intellectual functioning, as children with learning disabilities or minimal brain dysfunctions will not be identified. They compared RDS survivors with fullterm control children and found more hyperactivity and slower language development at two and four years among the former, despite normal IQ scores. In a later study the same authors again demonstrated delayed language skills at two years (Field *et al.* 1981). Interestingly, language development was evaluated by systematic analysis of a taped sample, recorded during play involving mother and child, not unlike the semi-structured play with the speech pathologist in the present study. Preterm infants who had had RDS used fewer words, and had a smaller vocabulary and a shorter mean length of utterance than term infants. The home environments of the preterm and control infants did not differ. In both these studies scores were adjusted for gestational age at birth.

While our findings are consistent with those in the recent literature, it must be repeated that our data were obtained mostly in the years 1963 to 1970, and since then a number of new ways have been developed to test the various parameters of vocal language. Following the work of Roger Brown (1973), a mechanism (Mean Length of Utterance) has been developed by which to assess a child's syntactic level. Similarly, phonological assessment has extended our understanding of the child's use of language, and while traditional segmental analysis has not been entirely replaced, phonological analysis provides greater understanding of children's speech patterns (Ingram 1978). Sophisticated language-based tests, using data from psycholinguistic and neurolinguistic studies, have also been developed to provide a clearer definition of the subgroups of language users and of the abnormalities of language development (see Rapin 1982).

Even so, the linguistic development of LBW infants has hardly begun to be evaluated in depth. To our knowledge no attempts have been made to distinguish children exhibiting delays in language development from those with *disorders* of communication (Rutter and Martin 1972). Rocissano and Yatchmink (1983) point out the limitations of assessment tools such as the Peabody Picture Vocabulary Test and the Reynell Scale, which provide information on relative performance in comparison to a set of norms but do not assess the child's ability to control and utilize structural and semantic features of language.

Parmelee (1981) reviewed studies concerned with possible effects of prolonged exposure of the infant's immature nervous system to noise in the incubator and nursery environment (see Chapter 9). He concluded that the potential long-term influence of the unusual auditory environment on the preterm infant is unclear, although studies have found no significant correlation between length of stay in the incubator and auditory discrimination at four months (O'Connor 1980) or neurosensory hearing-loss in childhood (Schulte and Stennert 1978).

Increasing attention is being paid to the importance of demographic variables and parent-infant interactions in the cognitive development of high-risk infants (Beckwith *et al.* 1976, Parmelee 1981). Caregiver-infant interactions have been shown to have a marked effect on receptive language skills. Rocissano and Yatchmink (1983) stressed the highly variable outcome among LBW infants: they attempted to identify adult-infant interactions which facilitated language development and which might explain the heterogeneity of linguistic competence. They proposed that the caregiver should monitor the infant's focus of attention and use it as a source for interchange to make the most of the high-risk child's limited resources for the learning of language (see also Bloom *et al.* 1974, Hoff-Ginsberg and Shatz 1982).

We conclude that there is fairly consistent evidence for low birthweight being related to delays in the acquisition of language and speech. The appropriateness of applying corrections for prematurity in the evaluation of language beyond the first few months of life needs careful consideration, as such adjustments of scores may mask important long-term differences between LBW and FBW children. Environmental features may contribute significantly to differential development; some important transactional relationships between vulnerable infants and their caregivers have been delineated (Sameroff and Chandler 1975, Rocissano and Yatchmink 1983). Estimates of the prevalence of neurodevelopmental communication disorders, as opposed to delays in language development, of LBW children are not yet available. Ultimately the course of language development may be more helpful than global IQ scores in predicting cognitive capabilities and 'minimal brain dysfunctions'.

Summary

Longitudinal follow-up of the language and speech development of LBW and FBW control children showed differences continuing up to 6½ years of age. There were significant differences favouring the FBW controls on the Griffiths Speech and Hearing Subscale at three, six, 12 and 18 months; with respect to articulation, following oral serial directions, length of sentences, use of prepositions and conjunctions, and over-all ratings of speech and language development at four years; and in verbal intelligence, short-term auditory memory and reading comprehension at 6½ years.

During the first year of life (at three, six and 12 months) mean language development in the LBW SGA group was ahead of that in the AGA preterm group. At 18 months there was no significant difference, but by the ages of four and 6½ years differences favoured the AGA preterm group.

Some sex differences emerged; girls scored higher than boys in vocabulary and expressive language. Abnormal neurological status (including MBD) was associated with poorer performance on speech and language measures.

Acknowledgement: The authors are indebted to Dr. John Gilbert and Dr. Henry Dunn for reviewing their manuscript and for helpful comments.

11
Educational Achievement

Ruth V. E. Grunau

A number of studies have been concerned with the school performance of low-birthweight children, and the literature has been reviewed by Benton (1940), Alm (1953), Dunham (1955), Wiener (1962), Harper and Wiener (1965), Caputo and Mandell (1970), Balow *et al.* (1975/76) and Friedman and Sigman (1981). In general, very low birthweight has been found to be associated with relatively poor progress at school.

Drillien (1961*b*) found that high proportions of children with birthweights ≤1360g required special educational placements. Of the 69 children in her sample, one-half were ineducable in regular school because of mental and/or physical handicaps; one-quarter were 'dull' children being educated in regular schools; and the remaining quarter attended regular schools and performed appropriately for age, but all except two were in the lower levels of their classes. Wiener (1968) reported that at 12 to 13 years grade placement varied significantly with birthweight: 45 per cent of the lighter LBW, 57 per cent of the larger LBW and 72 per cent of FBW children were in the appropriate grade at school. Wiener noted that birthweight contributed to reading and arithmetic scores, independently of social class and neurological impairment, which supported the view that low birthweight may result in relatively poor school performance into early adolescence. On the other hand, Robinson and Robinson (1965) showed that poor reading in their LBW as compared to their FBW samples was probably related to social class rather than birthweight. At eight years of age their group with the lowest birthweights (≤1500g) scored considerably lower than the larger LBW group on a reading test, but the smallest babies tended to be from the lowest social-classes, so birthweight and social class were confounded, making it difficult to interpret the results.

In view of the established relationship between low social-class and low birthweight (Rider *et al.* 1955), and between low social-class and poor school performance, it is important that appropriate methods be employed so that birthweight can be considered independently from social class. The degree to which low birthweight itself affects school performance, independent of social class, is still unclear. Davie *et al.* (1972) found that 'educational backwardness' was nearly twice as frequent among preterm children as among those born at 37 to 42 weeks. Early delivery also led to low 'copying design' scores after allowing for social class and birth order. Balow *et al.* (1975/76) have summarized studies on perinatal events as precursors of reading disability; low birthweight was the most extensively studied variable. Those authors concluded that none of the studies they reviewed was free of methodological problems: however, the weight of evidence did suggest a correlation between low birthweight and reading disability.

The literature contains very little information comparing the school performance of preterm AGA and preterm and term SGA LBW infants. Rubin *et al.* (1973) compared LBW preterm and term children's abilities in reading, spelling and arithmetic and found that although the LBW children were significantly delayed compared to FBW controls, there was no significant difference between the two LBW groups. Drillien (1970) found that adverse effects of being SGA were demonstrable up to 12 years of age in children from average or poor working-class families, but not from superior homes.

In 1971 our team of investigators reported that preterm AGA children obtained significantly better class placements than SGA children, and that poorer school performance by the SGA group seemed to be related to a somewhat lower mean IQ and a greater frequency of neurological abnormalities (Dunn *et al.* 1971). Neligan *et al.* (1976) found no statistically significant difference on a reading test between random control, short-gestation, 'rather light-for-dates' and 'very light-for-dates' children. However, the mean birthweights of the groups were 3508g, 2415g, 2071g and 2397g, respectively. If lighter LBW children had been studied the outcome might have been different. Parkinson *et al.* (1981) found that SGA children had more difficulties at school compared to classroom controls, and that the children most likely to show poor school achievement and behaviour problems were boys whose head growth slowed before 34 weeks gestation.

In general, it appears that school performance is most impaired among VLBW children, and not as markedly among children at the upper end of the LBW distribution. However, there is considerable variation in the outcome within any given birthweight group. It has been unclear, as yet, to what extent there may be differences in school performance between preterm and SGA children.

In our prospective study of the neurological development of LBW children, educational data were collected annually as the children progressed through school. The aim of this aspect of the survey was to compare the school performance of: (1) LBW (≤2041g), FBW (>2500g) and classroom control children; (2) AGA preterm and SGA children; and (3) lighter (≤1750g) and heavier (1751 to 2041g) LBW children.

Method

Information on school progress was available for 320 of the 480 LBW children (≤2041g at birth) and for 153 of the 203 FBW children (>2500g at birth). The FBW infants were selected to reflect the social-class distribution of the LBW group (see Chapter 2 for a full description of the sample selection).

The LBW sample consisted of 170 AGA preterm, 128 SGA, two LGA and 20 infants with unknown lengths of gestation. An additional group of classroom control (CC) children was used. Public-health nurses selected two children of normal birthweight from the LBW child's classroom (almost always of the same sex as the LBW child). These CC children provided a good comparison group for the LBW children, since variables such as teachers and school districts were held constant. In addition, social-class differences were controlled insofar as the school draws from a particular neighbourhood.

Extensive medical, psychological, social and educational data were collected for the LBW and FBW children. Only educational data were collected for the CC

TABLE 11-I

Socio-economic status of SGA, AGA preterm, all LBW and FBW children at 6½ years of age*

Social class	*Unknown gestation and LGA*	*SGA*	*AGA preterm*		*All LBW*	*FBW*	
I	3	8(6%)	14(8%)		25(8%)	7(5%)	
II	—	10(8%)	7(4%)		17(5%)	7(5%)	
III	1	11(9%)	24(15%)	$\chi^2 = 5.49$ NS	36(12%)	12(9%)	$\chi^2 = 3.19$ NS
IV	5	46(37%)	64(38%)		115(37%)	61(43%)	
V	13	49(40%)	58(35%)		120(38%)	54(38%)	
Total	22	124	167		313	141	

*Social class unknown for 7 LBW and 12 FBW children.

group. Since data were not available for the whole sample for all measures, the numbers in the different comparisons varied. Year in school, rather than grade, was used so that all children were compared with peers of the same chronological age, regardless of grades failed in school.

The children's geographical location at year 1 in school was as follows: 76 per cent of the LBW, 75 per cent of the FBW and all of the CC children were living in the British Columbia (B.C.) Lower Mainland area; 18 per cent of the LBW and 20 per cent of the FBW were in the remainder of B.C.; and 6 per cent of LBW and 5 per cent of FBW children were in schools outside the province. CC children were not selected for study children outside the B.C. Lower Mainland area.

Socio-economic status (SES) was classified into five levels (Hollingshead 1957), with class I representing the highest and class V the lowest SES levels. The SES distributions of the LBW and FBW samples with school data showed no statistically significant differences (Table 11-I): 38 per cent of both the LBW and FBW children were in social-class V at 6½ years of age.

Standardized achievement testing

The Stanford Achievement Primary II Test Battery was administered during year 3 in school to children born in 1963 or later who lived in the B.C. Lower Mainland area at the time of testing.

Information from teachers

Report cards were requested for all the children up to the Spring of 1970. However, because of changes in the school system, report cards were found to be less informative than they had been before, so specific information was sought by means of a check-list. When this teachers' check-list was developed in 1970, report cards were requested only for children living outside B.C. On the check-list the teacher rated the child as below normal, normal or above normal on 16 items related to school achievement. The teacher also indicated the grade level at which the child was performing, on a scale, for reading, arithmetic, spelling and writing. The rating scale ran from early kindergarten to late Grade 7, with the choice of

TABLE 11-II

School placement of LBW and FBW children in school years 1 and 3

	At grade level	*Below grade level*	*Special class, school, institution*	χ^2	*p*
Year 1					
LBW (N = 313)	199(63%)	68(22%)	46(15%)	20.95	<0.000
FBW (N = 153)	119(78%)	32(21%)	2(1%)		
Year 3					
LBW (N = 303)	169(56%)	82(27%)	52(17%)	22.47	<0.000
FBW (N = 139)	105(75%)	30(22%)	4(3%)		

three levels for each grade. This information was converted to a score on a 25-point scale: a score of 25 indicated that the child's performance was above Grade 7.

School placement

Each LBW or FBW study child was rated as (1) in the regular stream at school, at the level to be expected or better; (2) in the regular stream but at least one grade-level below that expected for chronological age; or (3) in a special class, special school, or institution (other than private or parochial school). Over-all placement was determined from the teachers' information about performance in school: achievement on standardized tests was not considered. Information from report cards was part of the data used to determine over-all placement, but was not analyzed separately. Placement ratings were made for year 1 and year 3 in school for all LBW and FBW children for whom some form of educational data were available. These ratings were not appropriate for the CC group because of the method of their selection.

Results

Educational progress

The school placement of the LBW and FBW children was compared at year 1 and year 3 (Table 11-II). Data were available for 313 LBW children at year 1, of whom 63 per cent were at grade level, 22 per cent below grade level and 15 per cent in a special class, school or institution. Of the 153 FBW children, 78 per cent were at grade level, 21 per cent below and only 1 per cent in special educational settings. In school year 3, of the 303 LBW children only 56 per cent were at grade level, 27 per cent were below and 17 per cent were in a special setting. Of the 139 FBW children, 75 per cent were at grade level, 22 per cent were below and 3 per cent were in a special setting. The differences in school placement between the LBW and FBW groups at both these years were statistically highly significant (Table 11-II).

The LBW, FBW and CC groups were examined on the subtests of the Stanford test during year 3 in school*. LBW and FBW children with WISC Full-scale IQ scores

*No IQ measures were available for the CC children, but an IQ <80 should not occur in a regular classroom, from which this group was selected.

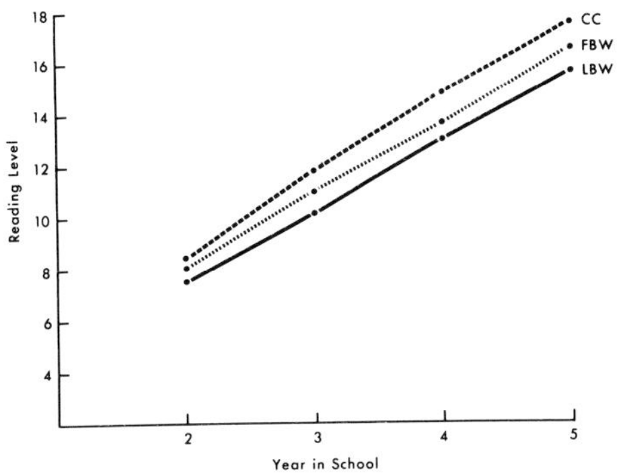

Fig. 11-1. Mean reading levels of LBW (N = 109-232), FBW (N = 106-134) and classroom control children (N = 107-165).

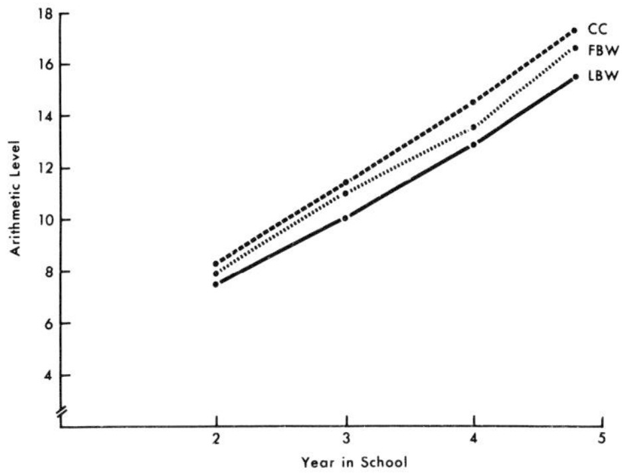

Fig. 11-2. Mean arithmetic levels of LBW (N = 109-234), FBW (N = 104-134) and classroom control children (N = 107-165).

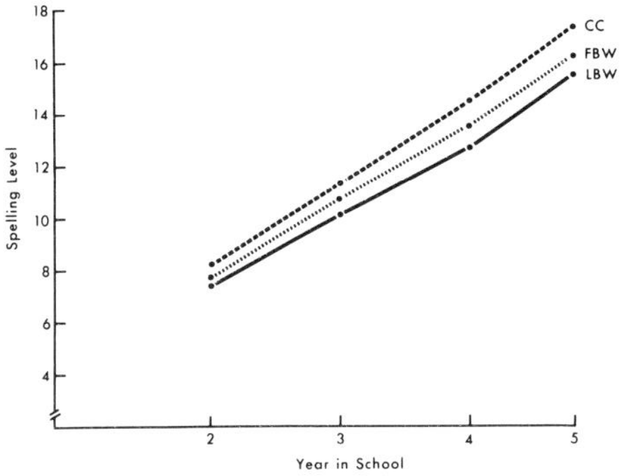

Fig. 11-3. Mean spelling levels of LBW (N = 106-233), FBW (N = 108-131) and classroom control children (N = 107-167).

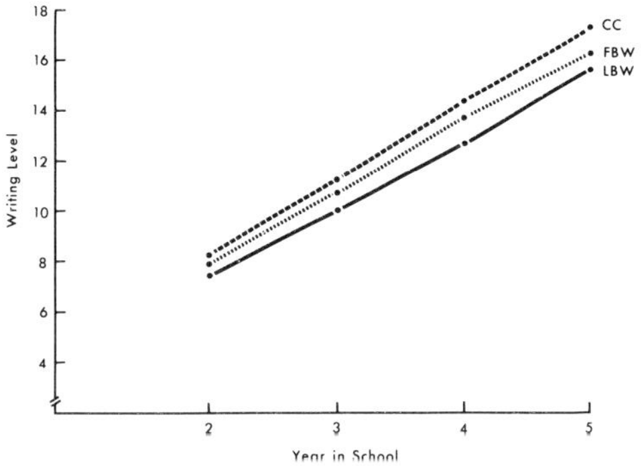

Fig. 11-4. Mean writing levels of LBW (N = 109-230), FBW (N = 106-134) and classroom control children (N = 107-165).

<80 at age 6½ were excluded from the analyses. Planned comparisons were carried out for statistical evaluation of the differences between the LBW *vs.* FBW and LBW *vs.* CC groups. As can be seen in Table 11-III, the means for the CC group were higher than those for the LBW and FBW groups for every subtest. There was a statistically significant difference between the means of the LBW and CC groups in each subtest. There were no statistically significant differences between the LBW and FBW groups, but in four of the six subtests the mean was higher for the FBW group.

The LBW, FBW and CC groups were compared on teacher ratings of level of achievement in reading, arithmetic, spelling and writing at each of years 2 to 5 in school to examine the differences between LBW *vs.* FBW and LBW *vs.* CC children (Table 11-IV, Figs. 11-1 to 4). The order of the mean scores was the same for each subject in each year: the LBW group had the lowest mean, the FBW group was somewhat higher and the CC group was highest. The difference between the LBW

TABLE 11-III

Comparisons of LBW*, FBW*, and classroom control (CC) children on Stanford Achievement Primary II Test Battery during year 3 in school

	LBW			*FBW*			*CC*			*Planned comparisons*			
										LBW vs. FBW		*LBW vs. CC*	
Stanford subtest	*N*	*Mean*	*SD*	*N*	*Mean*	*SD*	*N*	*Mean*	*SD*	*t*	*p*	*t*	*p*
Word Meaning	103	22.9	7.4	86	22.2	8.0	129	25.2	6.3	0.65	NS	−2.58	<0.01
Paragraph Meaning	103	34.5	12.7	86	36.0	13.5	129	41.4	10.0	−0.75	NS	−4.49	<0.000
Spelling	102	19.5	7.9	86	18.7	8.5	129	22.0	6.2	0.47	NS	−2.59	<0.01
Word Study Skills	101	41.3	12.4	86	43.4	13.1	128	46.4	9.6	−1.13	NS	−3.45	<0.001
Arithmetic Computations	103	26.8	11.2	86	30.0	12.6	128	32.6	11.4	−1.82	NS	−3.90	<0.000
Arithmetic Concepts	104	23.9	11.4	86	25.6	9.6	128	27.6	9.1	−1.05	NS	−2.63	<0.009

*LBW and FBW children with WISC IQ <80 at 6½ years excluded.

TABLE 11-IV

Comparisons of teacher's check-lists for reading, arithmetic, spelling and writing levels of LBW, FBW and classroom control (CC) children in school years 2 to 5

	LBW			*FBW*			*CC*			*Planned comparisons*			
										LBW vs. FBW		*LBW vs. CC*	
Teacher's check-list	*N*	*Mean*	*SD*	*N*	*Mean*	*SD*	*N*	*Mean*	*SD*	*t*	*p*	*t*	*p*
Year 2													
Reading	109	7.5	2.0	134	8.0	2.1	107	8.4	1.4	−1.98	<0.05	−4.12	<0.000
Arithmetic	109	7.5	1.8	134	8.0	1.6	107	8.3	1.4	−2.06	<0.04	−3.76	<0.000
Spelling	106	7.4	2.1	131	7.7	1.9	107	8.2	1.4	−1.47	NS	−3.44	<0.001
Writing	109	7.4	1.9	134	7.9	1.9	107	8.2	1.2	−2.20	<0.000	−3.80	<0.000
Year 3													
Reading	159	10.1	2.5	124	11.0	2.8	138	11.8	1.9	−2.81	<0.005	−6.62	<0.000
Arithmetic	160	10.0	2.4	124	11.0	1.9	138	11.4	1.4	−3.59	<0.000	−5.96	<0.000
Spelling	156	10.1	2.6	123	10.7	2.7	136	11.3	1.9	−1.95	<0.05	−4.95	<0.000
Writing	158	10.0	2.5	123	10.7	2.3	137	11.3	1.6	−2.45	<0.02	−5.53	<0.000
Year 4													
Reading	186	13.0	3.2	118	13.6	3.0	155	14.8	2.3	−1.66	NS	−6.05	<0.000
Arithmetic	183	12.9	3.0	115	13.5	2.2	155	14.5	1.8	−2.10	<0.04	−6.11	<0.000
Spelling	186	12.8	3.3	117	13.5	3.1	154	14.5	2.5	−2.01	<0.05	−5.93	<0.000
Writing	187	12.8	3.1	117	13.7	2.8	155	14.4	2.2	−2.80	<0.006	−5.76	<0.000
Year 5													
Reading	232	15.6	3.7	106	16.5	3.4	165	17.5	2.6	−2.09	<0.04	−6.07	<0.000
Arithmetic	234	15.5	3.4	104	16.6	2.8	165	17.3	1.9	−3.35	<0.001	−6.83	<0.000
Spelling	233	15.5	3.8	108	16.2	3.4	167	17.3	2.4	−1.83	<0.07	−5.92	<0.000
Writing	[illegible]	[illegible]	[illegible]	[illegible]	[illegible]	[illegible]	[illegible]	[illegible]	[illegible]	[illegible]	[illegible]	[illegible]	[illegible]

TABLE 11-V

School placement in year 3 of preterm and term SGA children

	At grade level	*Below grade level*	*Special class, school, institution*	χ^2	*p*
Preterm SGA (N = 60)	34(57%)	16(27%)	10(17%)	2.81	NS
Term SGA (N = 50)	23(46%)	12(24%)	15(30%)		

TABLE 11-VI

Comparisons of SGA *vs.* preterm AGA LBW children's school placement (years 1 and 3), Stanford Achievement Subtests (year 3) and teacher's check-list for reading, arithmetic, spelling and writing levels (years 2 to 5)

	SGA			*Preterm AGA*				
*School placement**	*1*	*2*	*3*	*1*	*2*	*3*	χ^2	*p*
Year 1 (N = 263)	72(62%)	23(20%)	20(18%)	95(64%)	36(24%)	18(12%)	1.81	NS
Year 3 (N = 257)	57(52%)	28(25%)	25(23%)	86(58%)	44(30%)	18(12%)	6.05	<0.05
Stanford (year 3)	*N*	*Mean*	*SD*	*N*	*Mean*	*SD*	*t*	*p*
Word Meaning	33	22.2	8.6	52	23.7	6.0	−0.85	NS
Paragraph Meaning	33	34.2	13.7	52	35.4	12.6	0.41	NS
Spelling	32	19.1	7.8	52	19.3	8.2	−0.07	NS
Word Study Skills	32	40.1	12.4	51	42.9	11.7	−1.03	NS
Arith. Computations	33	26.3	13.7	52	28.1	9.1	−0.64	NS
Arith. Concepts	33	22.9	11.1	52	24.5	7.4	−0.73	NS
Teacher's check-list	*N*	*Mean*	*SD*	*N*	*Mean*	*SD*	*t*	*p*
Year 2								
Reading	32	7.8	1.7	60	7.5	2.1	0.98	NS
Arithmetic	32	7.9	1.5	60	7.4	1.9	1.38	NS
Spelling	32	7.6	1.9	57	7.5	2.1	0.23	NS
Writing	31	7.7	2.1	61	7.3	1.8	0.95	NS
Year 3								
Reading	51	10.3	2.4	85	10.1	2.5	0.34	NS
Arithmetic	52	10.2	2.5	85	10.0	2.4	0.57	NS
Spelling	51	10.2	2.5	82	10.1	2.5	0.29	NS
Writing	52	10.0	2.4	83	10.0	2.3	−0.05	NS
Year 4								
Reading	66	12.7	3.3	97	13.2	3.1	−0.89	NS
Arithmetic	65	12.7	3.2	95	12.9	2.8	−0.54	NS
Spelling	66	12.6	3.6	97	12.7	3.0	−0.10	NS
Writing	66	12.6	3.4	98	12.7	2.9	−0.23	NS
Year 5								
Reading	82	15.9	3.8	113	15.5	3.7	0.79	NS
Arithmetic	82	15.4	3.4	115	15.5	3.4	−0.16	NS
Spelling	82	15.7	3.7	114	15.3	3.8	0.58	NS
Writing	80	15.6	3.5	113	15.6	3.3	−0.03	NS

*1 = at grade level, 2 = below grade level, 3 = special class, school, institution.

TABLE 11-VII

Comparisons of LBW boys *vs.* girls on school placement (years 1 and 3), Stanford Achievement Subtests (year 3) and teacher's check-list for reading, arithmetic, spelling and writing levels (years 2 to 5)

	Boys			*Girls*				
*School placement**	*1*	*2*	*3*	*1*	*2*	*3*	χ^2	*p*
Year 1 (N = 312)	83(55%)	36(24%)	31(21%)	115(71%)	32(20%)	15(9%)	10.53	<0.005
Year 3 (N = 316)	77(51%)	41(27%)	34(22%)	99(60%)	45(27%)	20(12%)	6.12	<0.047
Stanford (year 3)	*N*	*Mean*	*SD*	*N*	*Mean*	*SD*	*F*	*p*
Word Meaning	44	23.1	8.1	59	22.7	6.5	<1	NS
Paragraph Meaning	44	25.9	13.1	59	33.7	12.4	<1	NS
Spelling	44	18.2	8.9	58	20.4	7.0	2.29	NS
Word Study Skills	44	42.1	12.8	57	40.7	12.1	<1	NS
Arith. Computations	44	26.3	10.4	59	27.1	11.9	<1	NS
Arith. Concepts	44	24.1	9.6	59	22.7	9.1	<1	NS
Teacher's check-list	*N*	*Mean*	*SD*	*N*	*Mean*	*SD*	*F*	*p*
Year 2								
Reading	55	7.3	2.0	54	7.7	1.9	1.45	NS
Arithmetic	55	7.5	1.8	54	7.4	1.8	<1	NS
Spelling	53	7.3	2.1	53	7.5	2.1	1.16	NS
Writing	54	7.3	2.0	55	7.4	1.9	<1	NS
Year 3								
Reading	66	9.8	2.5	93	10.4	2.4	2.61	NS
Arithmetic	67	9.8	2.5	93	10.2	2.3	1.54	NS
Spelling	64	9.8	2.6	92	10.2	2.5	1.74	NS
Writing	66	9.5	2.5	92	10.3	2.4	4.89	<0.03
Year 4								
Reading	83	12.6	3.4	103	13.4	3.0	4.40	<0.04
Arithmetic	80	12.6	3.2	103	13.1	2.8	2.65	NS
Spelling	83	12.1	3.3	103	13.3	3.2	8.45	<0.004
Writing	83	12.2	3.3	104	13.2	2.9	7.13	<0.008
Year 5								
Reading	111	15.4	4.0	121	15.8	3.5	1.15	NS
Arithmetic	113	15.4	3.4	121	15.5	3.3	<1	NS
Spelling	113	15.0	4.0	120	15.9	3.6	3.58	NS
Writing	110	14.9	3.6	120	16.3	3.3	9.56	<0.002

*1 = at grade level, 2 = below grade level, 3 = special class, school, institution.

and CC groups was statistically significant for each subject in each year. There were also statistically significant differences between the LBW and FBW groups each year for all subjects, except spelling in year 2 and reading in year 4.

Comparisons within the LBW sample

A comparison was made between the SGA *vs.* preterm AGA groups and the term *vs.* preterm SGA groups. There was no statistically significant difference* between the preterm and fullterm SGA children in school placement at year 3 (Table 11-V), so for all further analyses those two groups have been combined.

Comparisons of the SGA and preterm AGA children in school placement, Stanford Achievement Test results and teacher ratings of reading, arithmetic, spelling and writing are presented in Table 11-VI. There were statistically significant differences in school placement between the SGA and preterm AGA children at year 3 (but not year 1), favouring the AGA preterm group. 23 per cent of

*Non-caucasians were excluded from the analyses which compared the school performance of SGA and preterm AGA LBW children. In cases of mixed percentage, mother's race determined that of the child.

TABLE 11-VIII

Comparisons of LBW children with birthweights ≤1750g *vs.* 1751 to 2041g in school placement (years 1 and 3), Stanford Achievement Subtests (year 3) and teacher's check-list for reading, arithmetic, spelling and writing levels (years 2 to 5)

	≤1750g			*1751 to 2041g*				
*School placement**	*1*	*2*	*3*	*1*	*2*	*3*	χ^2	*p*
Year 1 (N = 313)	36(58%)	37(25%)	25(17%)	113(69%)	31(19%)	21(13%)	3.63	NS
Year 3 (N = 303)	69(47%)	48(32%)	31(21%)	100(65%)	21(14%)	21(14%)	9.84	<0.007
Stanford (year 3)	*N*	*Mean*	*SD*	*N*	*Mean*	*SD*	*F*	*p*
Word Meaning	46	21.1	8.0	57	24.4	6.0	5.46	<0.02
Paragraph Meaning	46	31.0	12.7	57	37.3	12.1	6.21	<0.01
Spelling	45	18.4	8.3	57	20.6	7.5	3.04	NS
Word Study Skills	45	38.1	13.3	56	43.8	11.1	5.60	<0.02
Arith. Computations	46	23.6	12.1	57	29.3	9.9	7.24	<0.008
Arith. Concepts	46	20.4	9.8	57	25.6	8.3	8.36	<0.005
Teacher's check-list	*N*	*Mean*	*SD*	*N*	*Mean*	*SD*	*F*	*p*
Year 2								
Reading	47	7.1	2.73	62	7.8	1.6	3.91	<0.05
Arithmetic	47	7.0	1.9	62	7.8	1.6	6.01	<0.02
Spelling	47	6.9	2.3	59	7.8	1.8	4.79	<0.03
Writing	48	6.9	2.0	61	7.7	1.7	5.87	<0.02
Year 3								
Reading	79	9.9	2.7	80	10.4	2.3	2.29	NS
Arithmetic	79	9.7	2.5	81	10.4	2.3	4.75	<0.03
Spelling	78	9.7	2.7	78	10.4	2.3	2.82	NS
Writing	78	9.7	2.7	80	10.3	2.2	2.77	NS
Year 4								
Reading	90	12.5	3.2	96	13.5	3.2	6.54	<0.01
Arithmetic	89	12.3	2.9	94	13.5	2.9	8.87	<0.003
Spelling	90	12.2	3.3	96	13.3	3.2	7.77	<0.006
Writing	91	12.2	3.3	96	13.2	2.9	7.50	<0.007
Year 5								
Reading	108	15.0	3.9	124	16.1	3.5	5.94	<0.02
Arithmetic	108	14.9	3.7	126	16.0	2.9	5.90	<0.02
Spelling	107	15.0	4.1	126	15.9	3.5	4.24	<0.04
Writing	105	15.3	4.0	125	15.9	3.1	2.81	NS

*1 = at grade level, 2 = below grade level, 3 = special class, school, institution.

the SGA children were in a special class, school or institution, compared to only 12 per cent of the AGA preterm infants.

As mentioned earlier, children with a WISC Full-scale IQ <80 at 6½ years were excluded from analysis of the Stanford Achievement Test. None of the Stanford subtests showed a statistically significant difference between SGA and preterm AGA children. However, the mean was higher for the AGA preterm group on every subtest, indicating a consistent trend in their favour. There were no statistically significant differences between SGA and preterm AGA children in teacher ratings of reading, arithmetic, spelling or writing during school-years 2 to 5.

Sex differences and birthweight categories

A two-way analysis of variance* was carried out on each Stanford subtest and on all

*Univariate analysis of variance was used for statistical analysis of these and other variables, since data were available for varying numbers of children at each year in school. For multivariate analysis, only those children with data for each of years 2 to 5 and Stanford at year 3 would be used, which would greatly reduce the number of children in the analysis.

TABLE 11-IX

Comparisons of teacher's check-list for reading, arithmetic, spelling and writing levels of LBW children with birthweights ≤1750g *vs.* 1751 to 2041g, with social class and mother's education as covariates

	≤1750g			1751 to 2041g				
Teacher's check-list	*N*	*Mean*	*SD*	*N*	*Mean*	*SD*	*F*	*p*
Year 2								
Reading	41	7.2	2.2	56	7.8	1.7	3.61	<0.06
Arithmetic	41	7.2	1.7	56	7.9	1.6	7.94	<0.005
Spelling	41	7.1	2.2	54	7.8	1.9	4.25	<0.04
Writing	42	7.0	2.0	55	7.8	1.7	7.21	<0.008
Year 3								
Reading	67	10.0	2.6	75	10.4	2.3	1.33	<0.25
Arithmetic	67	9.8	2.5	76	10.4	2.3	3.33	<0.07
Spelling	66	9.8	2.7	73	10.4	2.4	1.68	<0.20
Writing	67	9.7	2.7	75	10.3	2.3	1.99	<0.16
Year 4								
Reading	78	12.4	3.0	89	13.4	3.2	7.54	<0.007
Arithmetic	77	12.4	2.9	87	13.4	2.9	6.51	<0.01
Spelling	78	12.2	3.3	89	13.1	3.1	6.15	<0.01
Writing	79	12.3	3.3	89	13.1	2.9	6.15	<0.01
Year 5								
Reading	93	15.1	3.9	114	16.2	3.5	5.12	<0.02
Arithmetic	93	15.1	3.7	116	16.1	2.9	4.72	<0.03
Spelling	105	15.2	4.0	103	16.0	3.4	3.67	<0.06
Writing	90	15.5	4.0	115	15.9	3.1	1.29	<0.26

teacher ratings of reading, arithmetic, spelling and writing for each year. The independent variables were two levels of birthweight (≤1750 *vs.* 1751 to 2041g) and sex. Table 11-VII shows the sex comparisons and Table 11-VIII the birthweight comparisons. The birthweight by sex interaction was not statistically significant in any of the analyses and therefore is not shown.

There were statistically significant differences between boys and girls in school placement in years 1 and 3. In year 1 only 55 per cent of the boys were at grade level or above, compared to 71 per cent of the girls. In the same year, 21 per cent of the boys and 9 per cent of the girls were in a special class, school or institution. The Stanford Achievement subtests showed no statistically significant differences between girls and boys. Analysis of variance of the reading, arithmetic, spelling and writing levels of LBW girls and boys showed statistically significant differences in favour of girls for reading and spelling in year 4, and for writing in years 3, 4 and 5 (Figs. 11-5 to 8).

The school placement of children with birthweights ≤1750g and those 1751 to 2041g showed no statistically significant difference in year 1. However, in year 3 school placement of the lighter LBW group was significantly poorer than that of heavier children (see Table 11-VIII). 47 per cent of the lighter LBW children were placed at grade level, compared to 65 per cent of the heavier LBW group. The latter performed significantly better than the lighter group on every Stanford subtest except spelling (which showed the same direction). There were statistically significant differences favouring the larger LBW children for arithmetic level in each of years 2 to 5, for reading and spelling in years 2, 4 and 5, and for writing in years 2 and 4 (Figs. 11-9 to 12).

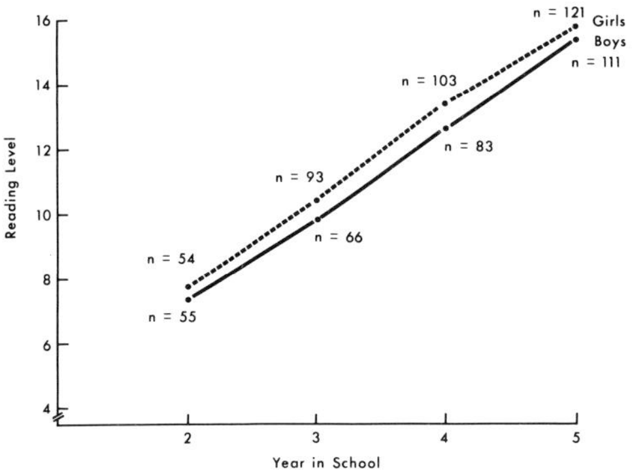

Fig. 11-5. Mean reading levels of LBW boys and girls.

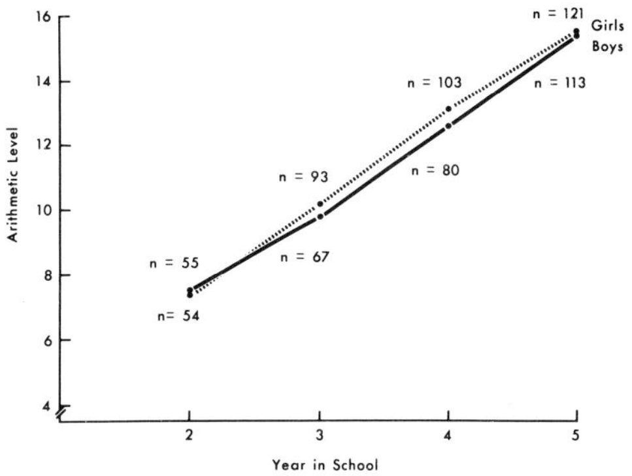

Fig. 11-6. Mean arithmetic levels of LBW boys and girls.

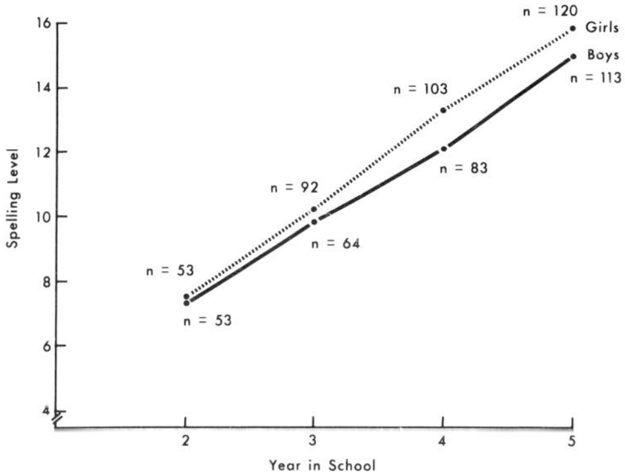

Fig. 11-7. Mean spelling levels of LBW boys and girls.

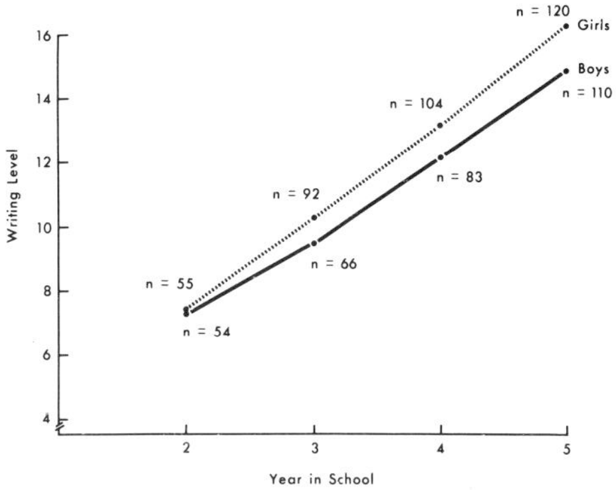

Fig. 11-8. Mean writing levels of LBW boys and girls.

The possibility was considered that some other hidden variable was responsible for these findings, rather than birthweight alone. In view of the known importance of socio-economic status in relation to both school performance and birthweight, the reading, arithmetic, spelling and writing performance of the birthweight groups were reassessed, using analysis of covariance to control for the effects of social class and mother's education (Table 11-IX). The means are higher for the children with birthweights 1751 to 2041g for every subject during school years 2 to 5. The analyses indicated statistically significant differences between the lighter and heavier LBW children for reading in years 4 and 5, arithmetic in years 2, 4 and 5, spelling in year 4 and writing in years 2 and 4. It was concluded, therefore, that these data reveal an effect of birthweight on school performance, independently of social class and mother's education.

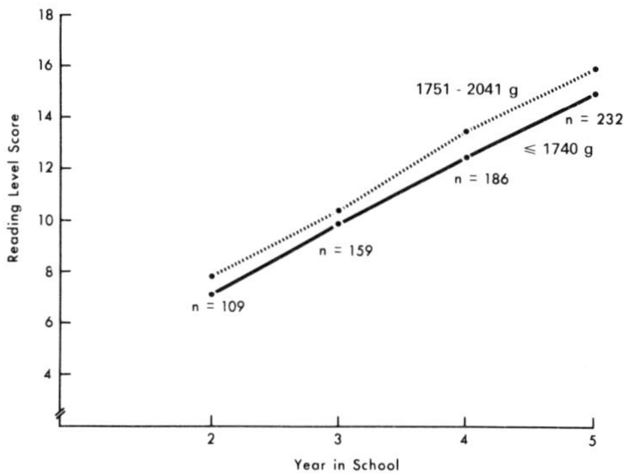

Fig. 11-9. Mean reading levels of LBW children with birthweights ≤1750g and 1751-2041g.

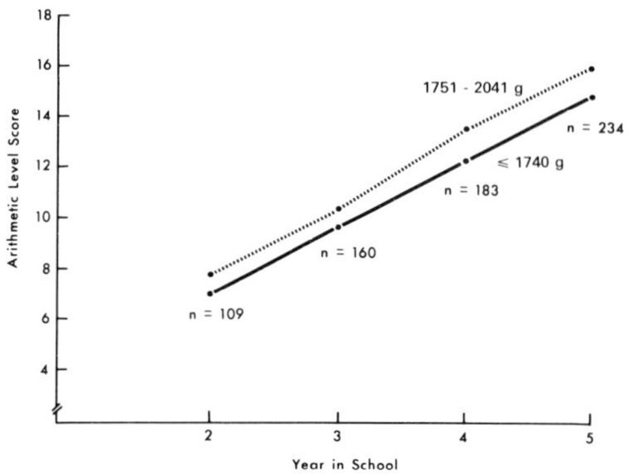

Fig. 11-10. Mean arithmetic levels of LBW children with birthweights ≤1750g and 1751-2041g.

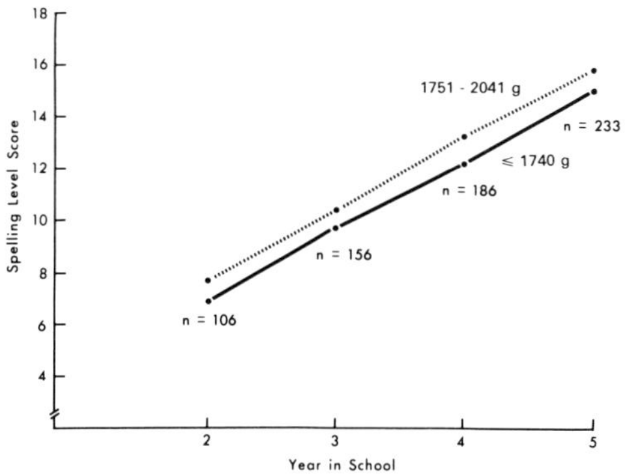

Fig. 11-11. Mean spelling levels of LBW children with birthweights ≤1750g and 1751-2041g.

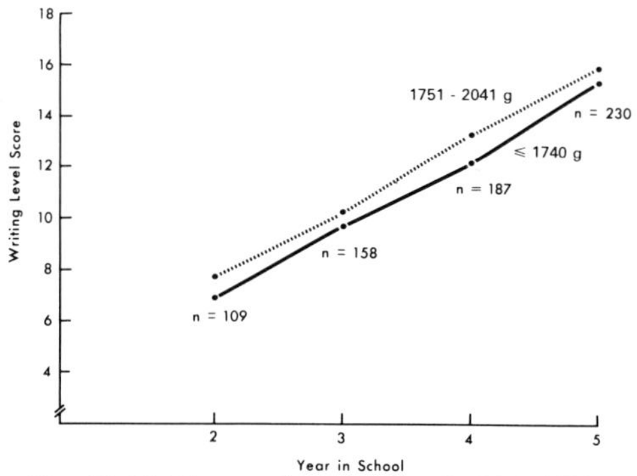

Fig. 11-12. Mean writing levels of LBW children with birthweights ≤1750g and 1751-2041g.

Socio-economic status (SES)

The LBW children's reading, arithmetic, spelling and writing levels during school years 2 to 5 were compared across three social-class groups—classes I to III combined, class IV and class V (Table 11-X). Newman-Keuls *post hoc* comparisons following each one-way analysis of variance indicated statistically significant differences between classes I to IV and V for every subject in years 2 to 4, and for arithmetic and writing in year 5. The differences between groups I to III, group IV and group V were statistically significant for reading and spelling in year 5 (Figs. 11-13 to 16).

SES within birthweight groups

School placement in year 3 of LBW children in social-classes I to IV was compared with social-class V (Table 11-XI). In the heavier LBW group, 74 per cent of children

TABLE 11-X

Comparisons of teacher's check-list for reading, arithmetic, spelling and writing levels of LBW children in social classes I-III, IV and V in school years 2 to 5

	Social class											
	(1) I, II, III			*(2) IV*			*(3) V*					
Teacher's check-list	*N*	*Mean*	*SD*	*N*	*Mean*	*SD*	*N*	*Mean*	*SD*	*F*	*p*	*Newman-Keuls Test Homogeneous subsets*
Year 2												
Reading	30	7.9	1.6	37	8.0	2.1	41	6.7	1.9	5.45	<0.006	(1,2)>(3)
Arithmetic	30	8.0	1.3	37	7.9	1.8	41	6.7	1.9	6.93	<0.001	(1,2)>(3)
Spelling	29	7.9	1.3	37	8.0	2.1	39	6.5	2.3	6.94	<0.001	(1,2)>(3)
Writing	31	7.8	1.6	37	7.8	1.8	40	6.5	2.0	6.25	<0.003	(1,2)>(3)
Year 3												
Reading	43	11.0	1.9	53	10.5	2.3	60	9.1	2.6	9.62	<0.000	(1,2)>(3)
Arithmetic	43	10.6	2.1	54	10.4	2.1	60	9.2	2.8	5.33	<0.006	(1,2)>(3)
Spelling	42	10.8	1.9	52	10.6	2.4	59	8.9	2.8	8.64	<0.000	(1,2)>(3)
Writing	42	10.7	2.2	53	10.5	2.2	60	9.1	2.6	7.59	<0.001	(1,2)>(3)
Year 4												
Reading	48	14.1	3.0	72	13.4	2.8	63	11.7	3.5	8.83	<0.000	(1,2)>(3)
Arithmetic	46	13.4	2.7	72	13.6	2.2	62	11.6	3.5	9.14	<0.000	(1,2)>(3)
Spelling	48	13.2	2.8	72	13.4	2.8	63	11.6	3.9	5.85	<0.003	(1,2)>(3)
Writing	48	13.0	2.5	72	13.5	2.7	64	11.7	3.7	6.26	<0.002	(1,2)>(3)
Year 5												
Reading	60	17.3	2.8	93	15.8	3.5	75	14.0	4.1	14.54	<0.000	(1)>(2)>(3)
Arithmetic	60	16.4	2.6	94	16.0	2.8	76	14.1	4.1	10.85	<0.000	(1,2)>(3)
Spelling	60	17.0	2.9	93	15.8	3.5	76	13.9	4.3	13.31	<0.000	(1)>(2)>(3)
Writing	58	16.5	2.6	93	16.2	2.9	75	14.2	4.4	10.48	<0.000	(1,2)>(3)

TABLE 11-XI

School placement in year 3 of LBW children in social classes I-IV versus V, within birthweight groups ≤1750g and 1751-2041g

	At grade level	*Below grade level*	*Special class, school or institution*	χ^2	*p*
≤1750g					
Social classes I-IV (N = 86)	47(55%)	31(36%)	8(9%)	19.58	<0.001
Social class V (N = 58)	18(31%)	17(29%)	23(40%)		
1751-2041g					
Social classes I-IV (N = 99)	73(74%)	18(18%)	8(8%)	12.68	<0.005
Social class V (N = 54)	25(46%)	16(30%)	13(24%)		

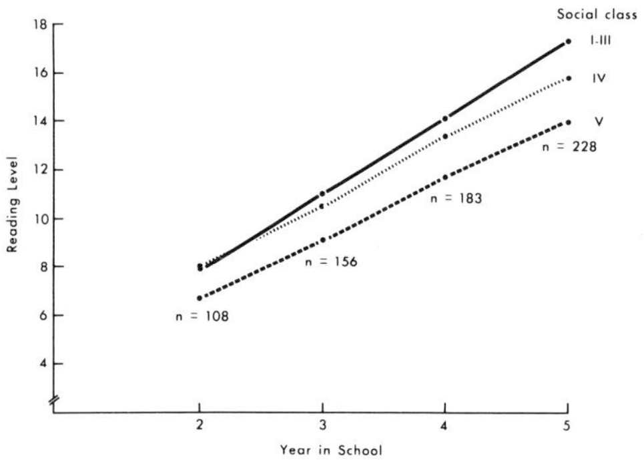

Fig. 11-13. Mean reading levels of LBW children in social classes I-III, IV and V.

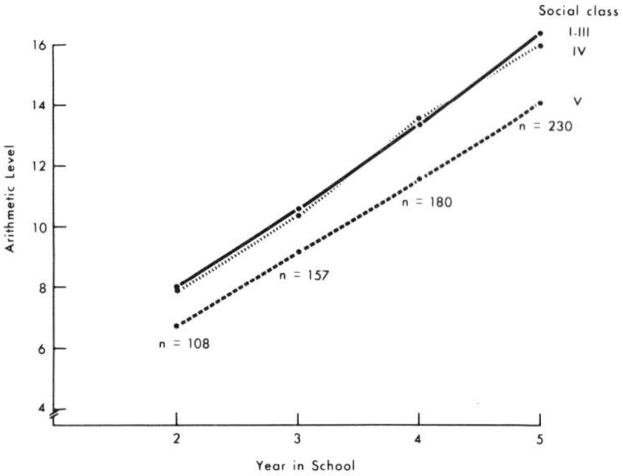

Fig. 11-14. Mean arithmetic levels of LBW children in social classes I-III, IV and V.

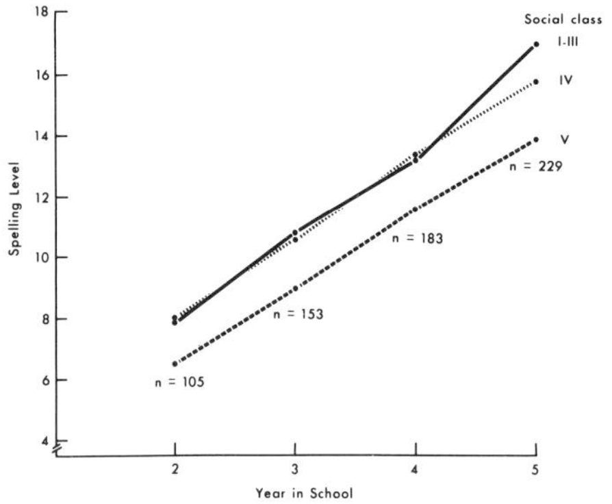

Fig. 11-15. Mean spelling levels of LBW children in social classes I-III, IV and V.

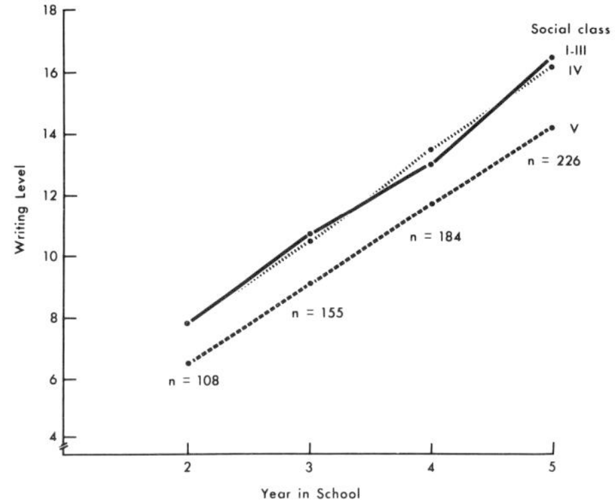

Fig. 11-16. Mean writing levels of LBW children in social classes I-III, IV and V.

in the higher social-classes (I to IV) were at grade level, whereas only 46 per cent of class V children were. Among the lighter LBW group, 40 per cent of social-class V children were in a special class, school or institution, compared to only 9 per cent of the higher SES group. These differences in school placement by social class were statistically significant.

Sex differences within birthweight group and SES

Comparison was made of school placement in year 3 of boys and girls within birthweight groups (<1750g *vs.* 1751 to 2041g) and social class (I to IV *vs.* V) (Table 11-XII). There were no significant differences between the placement of boys and girls within weight or social-class groups. It is noteworthy that within social-class V, boys and girls in the lighter LBW group and boys in the heavier LBW group had a high frequency (34 to 41 per cent) of special educational settings.

TABLE 11-XII

School placement of boys and girls within birthweight groups ≤1750g *vs.* 1751-2041g and social-class groups I-IV *vs.* V in year 3 in school

	*School placement**				
	1	*2*	*3*	χ^2	*p*
Social class I-IV					
≤1750g					
Boys (N = 33)	15(45%)	13(39%)	5(15%)	2.96	NS
Girls (N = 53)	32(60%)	18(34%)	3(6%)		
1751-2041g					
Boys (N = 52)	37(71%)	9(17%)	6(12%)	1.77	NS
Girls (N = 47)	36(77%)	9(19%)	2(4%)		
Social class V					
≤1750g					
Boys (N = 27)	7(26%)	9(33%)	11(41%)	0.72	NS
Girls (N = 31)	11(36%)	8(26%)	12(39%)		
1751-2041g					
Boys (N = 29)	11(38%)	8(28%)	10(34%)	3.85	NS
Girls (N = 25)	14(56%)	8(32%)	3(12%)		

*1 = at grade level, 2 = below grade level, 3 = special class, school, institution.

TABLE 11-XIII

Placement of SGA and preterm AGA children in year 3 in school within social-class categories

		*School placement**				
		1	*2*	*3*	χ^2	*p*
Social class I-IV (N = 164)	SGA	36(55%)	18(28%)	11(17%)	8.41	<0.02
	AGA preterm	69(70%)	26(26%)	4(4%)		
Social class V (N = 89)	SGA	16(39%)	10(24%)	15(37%)	1.78	NS
	AGA preterm	16(33%)	18(38%)	14(29%)		

*1 = at grade level, 2 = below grade level, 3 = special class, school, institution.

However, far fewer (12 per cent) girls in the heavier LBW group were in special settings.

SGA vs. preterm AGA within social class

The school placement of SGA *vs.* preterm AGA caucasian LBW children in year 3 was compared with social-classes I to IV combined and social-class V (Table 11-XIII). There was a statistical significant difference between the SGA and preterm AGA children within classes I to IV combined, 70 per cent of the AGA preterm being at or above grade level compared to 55 per cent of SGA children. Only 4 per cent of the AGA preterm group were in a special class, school or institution. Within social-class V there was no statistically significant difference between SGA and preterm AGA children: 29 per cent of the AGA preterm and 37 per cent of the SGA children were in special settings. This suggests that in social-class groups I to IV the AGA preterm have a considerable advantage over the SGA children. In social-class V both groups were doing poorly, with only approximately one-third of the children in either group performing at or above grade level. Any advantage the AGA preterm group may have had over the SGA children appears to be outweighed by the drawbacks of being in the lowest social-class.

Neurological status

It was of interest to compare the school performance of neurologically normal FBW and CC children. The teacher ratings for reading, arithmetic, spelling and writing levels in years 2 to 5 in school were re-analyzed, excluding LBW and FBW children with neurological abnormality (including minimal brain dysfunctions) and children with a WISC Full-scale IQ <80 at 6½ years of age. Comparisons of neurologically normal LBW and FBW children, and of total CC group*, following analysis of variance, are shown in Table 11-XIV. Scores for the LBW group were statistically significantly lower than for the CC group for reading in years 3 and 4. There were no statistically significant differences between the LBW and FBW children.

Comparisons were also made of the neurologically normal LBW children by birthweight and sex. There was no longer any statistically significant difference between birthweight groups, nor between sexes (Table 11-XV).

Reading disability

The frequency of reading disability in school year 5 was estimated for the LBW and FBW children, using an index designed to identify children who were reading below the level expected for their IQ score (Bond and Tinker 1967):

$$\text{Reading expectancy} = \text{years in school} \times \frac{\text{IQ score}}{100} + 1$$

Reading level = grade level at which child is actually reading

Reading expectancy minus reading level = reading discrepancy

Teacher ratings in school year 5 were used as the measure of reading level, and again, children with a Full-scale IQ <80 at 6½ years were excluded. The child was considered to have a reading disability when the discrepancy between reading expectancy and reading level was two years or more.

As can be seen from Table 11-XVI, 44 (22 per cent) of 197 LBW children and 27 (29 per cent) of the 93 FBW children with a Full-scale WISC IQ ≥80 were rated as reading-disabled by this method. 26 (59 per cent) of these 44 LBW children with a reading disability were boys, as were 18 (67 per cent) of the FBW children. The frequency of reading disability was not significantly different for the LBW and FBW groups; however, there were differences in the distributions of social class (Table 11-XVII), neurological status (Table 11-XVIII) and WISC Full-scale IQ (Table 11-XIX), which suggest that quite different problems underlie the IQ-reading level discrepancies in the two groups. The difference in social-class ranges did not reach statistical significance, but with 25 per cent of the LBW reading-disabled in the highest social-classes (I to III), compared to only 7 per cent of the FBW group, there

*Neurological status not available for CC children.

TABLE 11-XIV

Comparisons of teacher's check-list for reading, arithmetic, spelling and writing levels of neurologically normal LBW and FBW children and total classroom control (CC) group in school years 2 to 5

	(a) LBW			(b) FBW			(c) CC					
Teacher's check-list	*N*	*Mean*	*SD*	*N*	*Mean*	*SD*	*N*	*Mean*	*SD*	*F*	*p*	*Newman-Keuls Test Homogeneous subsets*
Year 2												
Reading	62	8.1	1.4	113	8.3	1.9	107	8.4	1.4	<1	NS	
Arithmetic	62	8.2	1.1	113	8.2	1.4	107	8.3	1.4	<1	NS	
Spelling	62	8.1	1.4	111	8.1	1.6	107	8.2	1.5	<1	NS	
Writing	62	8.0	1.3	113	8.2	1.6	107	8.2	1.3	<1	NS	
Year 3												
Reading	94	11.0	1.8	102	11.4	2.5	138	11.8	1.9	4.25	<0.02	(a)<(c)
Arithmetic	95	11.0	1.6	102	11.3	1.7	138	11.4	1.2	<1	NS	
Spelling	92	11.0	1.8	101	11.0	2.5	136	11.3	2.1	<1	NS	
Writing	94	11.0	1.7	101	11.0	2.0	137	11.3	1.9	<1	NS	
Year 4												
Reading	111	14.1	2.5	98	13.9	2.9	155	14.8	2.2	4.25	<0.008	(a)<(c) (b)<(c)
Arithmetic	111	14.0	1.8	95	13.8	2.0	155	14.5	1.7	4.64	<0.01	(b)<(c)
Spelling	111	14.0	2.2	97	13.8	2.9	154	14.5	2.0	<1	NS	
Writing	111	14.0	1.9	97	14.1	2.5	155	14.4	2.6	<1	NS	
Year 5												
Reading	145	17.0	2.6	87	16.8	3.2	165	17.5	2.3	2.90	NS	
Arithmetic	146	16.8	1.9	87	17.0	2.4	165	17.3	2.0	2.17	NS	
Spelling	145	16.9	2.5	89	16.7	3.2	167	17.3	2.5	1.04	NS	
Writing	143	17.0	2.4	87	16.8	2.7	165	17.3	2.7	<1	NS	

TABLE 11-XV

Comparisons of teacher's check-list for reading, arithmetic, spelling and writing levels of neurologically normal LBW children with birthweight ≤1750g *vs.* 1751-2041g in school years 2 to 5

	≤1750g			1751 to 2041g				
Teacher's check-list	*N*	*Mean*	*SD*	*N*	*Mean*	*SD*	*F*	*p*
Year 2								
Reading	19	8.1	2.0	43	8.2	1.1	<1	NS
Arithmetic	19	7.9	1.3	43	8.3	0.9	<1.44	NS
Spelling	19	8.1	2.0	43	8.1	1.2	<1	NS
Writing	19	7.6	1.7	43	8.1	1.2	<1	NS
Year 3								
Reading	36	11.1	2.0	58	10.9	1.7	<1	NS
Arithmetic	36	11.0	1.8	59	11.0	1.5	<1	NS
Spelling	35	11.1	2.0	57	10.9	1.6	<1	NS
Writing	36	11.2	1.8	58	10.9	1.6	<1	NS
Year 4								
Reading	41	14.0	2.5	70	14.2	2.5	<1	NS
Arithmetic	41	13.9	1.7	70	14.1	1.9	<1	NS
Spelling	41	13.9	2.2	70	14.1	2.3	<1	NS
Writing	41	14.0	1.5	70	14.0	2.1	<1	NS
Year 5								
Reading	57	17.0	2.6	88	17.0	2.6	<1	NS
Arithmetic	57	16.8	2.1	89	16.8	1.8	<1	NS
Spelling	56	16.9	2.6	89	16.8	2.4	<1	NS
Writing	55	17.4	2.8	88	16.7	2.1	<1	NS

TABLE 11-XVI

Reading discrepancy for LBW and FBW children based on WISC Full-scale IQ at 6½ years and reading level in school year 5

	<2 years	*≥2 years*	χ^2	*p*
LBW (N = 197)	153(78%)	44(22%)	1.53	NS
FBW (N = 93)	66(71%)	27(29%)		

TABLE 11-XVII

Social-class distribution of LBW and FBW children with reading discrepancy ≥2 years

	Social class				
	I-III	*IV*	*V*	χ^2	*p*
LBW (N = 44)	11(25%)	18(41%)	15(34%)	3.72	NS
FBW (N = 27)	2(7%)	12(45%)	13(48%)		

was a clear trend towards lower social-class placement of the FBW reading-disabled children. The difference in WISC Full-scale IQ bordered on significance ($p<0.06$), with a trend for higher IQs among the FBW reading-disabled children.

There was a significant difference in the neurological status of the LBW and FBW groups, with more than half (24 of 44, or 54 per cent) of the LBW group showing signs of neurological abnormality at 6½ years of age, compared to only five of 27 (19 per cent) of the FBW group. Among these 24 neurologically abnormal reading-disabled LBW children, by far the most common problem was MBD (21 of the 24): of the other three, one had cerebral palsy, one more than minimal MBD and one MBD and cerebral palsy. Four of the five FBW children had MBD and one had more than minimal MBD.

Classroom behaviour

The Haggerty-Olson-Wickman Behaviour Rating Scale was completed by teachers in school year 3. This scale consists of Schedule A, which rates behaviour problems, and Schedule B, which includes a combination of ratings on over-all social maladjustment*.

For some analyses, scores on Schedule A were grouped to form three categories (low, moderate and high) of degree of behaviour problems. This was derived from examination of the score distribution: low (0 to 8), moderate (9 to 27) and high (28 and above).

LBW VS.FBW

When scores for the LBW (48 boys, 62 girls) and FBW (35 boys, 48 girls) groups were compared for Schedule A, there were significantly higher misbehaviour ratings for the LBW group, and significant sex differences favouring girls. On Schedule B, the LBW *vs.* FBW group difference, but not sex, also was significant. To examine these findings, controlling for the effects of social class, mother's education and the child's IQ at six years of age, analysis of covariance was performed. There were no longer any significant differences between the LBW and FBW children when these factors were controlled, but highly significant sex differences remained on ratings of behaviour problems ($p<0.001$). Analysis of the significance of the three covariates showed that the difference in misbehaviour ratings between the LBW and FBW groups was accounted for by a highly significant difference in IQ scores at age six (Schedule A $p<0.005$, Schedule B $p<0.001$), rather than by birthweight. The effects of social class and mother's education were not significant, but presumably were at least partially reflected in the large differences in IQ scores between the groups. This indicates that the higher frequency of misbehaviour observed among the LBW children as a group could be accounted for by IQ differences.

COMPARISONS WITHIN THE LBW COHORT

School placement. For boys, this was found to be significantly related to ratings of behaviour problems derived from Schedule A (Table 11-XX). In school year 3, 26

*A log. transformation was performed on scores used in analysis of variance and analysis of covariance for statistical reasons.

TABLE 11-XVIII

Neurological status at 6½ years of LBW and FBW children with a reading discrepancy ≥2 years

	Normal	*Abnormal*	χ^2	*p*
LBW (N = 44)	20(46%)	24(54%)	8.99	<0.003
FBW (N = 27)	22(81%)	5(19%)		

TABLE 11-XIX

Ranges of WISC Full-scale IQ at 6½ years of LBW and FBW children with a reading discrepancy ≥2 years

	80-89	*90-109*	*≥110*	χ^2	*p*
LBW (N = 44)	8(18%)	20(46%)	16(36%)	5.62	NS
FBW (N = 27)	—	16(59%)	11(41%)		(<0.06)

TABLE 11-XX

School placement of LBW boys with low, moderate or high degrees of behaviour problems

	Behaviour-problem ratings		
School placement	*Low*	*Moderate*	*High*
At grade level	10(37%)	10(37%)	7(26%)
Below grade level	2(18%)	4(36%)	5(46%)
Special class, school or institution	—	—	10(100%)

$\chi^2 = 16.69$; $p<0.002$.

TABLE 11-XXI

Comparisons of neurologically normal *vs.* abnormal SGA and preterm AGA LBW children with low, moderate and high degrees of behaviour problems in school year 3

	SGA			*Preterm AGA*				
Neurological status at 6½ years	*Low*	*Moderate*	*High*	*Low*	*Moderate*	*High*	χ^2	*p*
Normal (N = 58)	10(40%)	9(36%)	6(24%)	13(39%)	14(42%)	6(19%)	0.38	NS
Abnormal (N = 40)	3(20%)	—	12(80%)	9(36%)	6(24%)	10(40%)	7.13	<0.03

TABLE 11-XXII

Social maladjustment scores for neurologically normal and abnormal LBW children following analysis of covariance

	Neurological status at age 6½ years					
	Normal			*Abnormal*		
	N	*Mean*	*SD*	*N*	*Mean*	*SD*
Boys	23	64.3	18.4	23	83.3	16.9
Girls	33	69.7	16.1	16	77.1	18.9
SGA	25	63.6	18.5	15	89.9	17.8
Preterm AGA	31	70.6	15.6	24	75.1	15.5
Over-all	56	67.5	17.1	39	80.8	17.8

per cent of boys who were at grade level were rated high in misdemeanours, compared to 46 per cent of those below grade-level and 100 per cent of those in special placements. Only four girls were in special placement in school year 3, too few for analysis, but two were rated low in misbehaviour and two were rated high.

SGA vs. preterm AGA LBW children in two birthweight categories. Analysis of covariance compared the misbehaviour scores (Schedule A) of 40 SGA *vs.* 55 preterm AGA LBW* boys and girls in two birthweight categories (≤1750g and 1751 to 2041g). After controlling for the factors of social class, mother's education and IQ scores at 6½ years, SGA children had higher misbehaviour scores than preterm AGA children ($p<0.03$) and boys had higher scores than girls ($p<0.001$). There was no difference between the two birthweight categories and no statistically significant interaction between the main factors.

Neurological status. The behaviour ratings derived from Schedule A (low, medium, high) for neurologically normal and abnormal (at 6½ years) SGA and preterm AGA LBW children were compared (Table 11-XXI). There was no difference in the degree of misbehaviour between the two groups who were neurologically normal, but misbehaviour ratings were significantly higher among the neurologically abnormal SGA group compared to the corresponding preterm AGA group.

Analysis of covariance was used to examine the effect of neurological status (normal *vs.* abnormal) in relation to social-adjustment scores (Schedule B) for the SGS *vs.* preterm AGA boys and girls controlling for social class, mother's education and IQ scores at age 6½ years (Table 11-XXII) Neurologically abnormal children over-all had significantly higher ratings of poor social development compared to the neurologically normal children ($F = 16.08$, $p<0.001$). There were no over-all differences in social adjustment between boys and girls, SGA and preterm AGA children, or the two birthweight categories ≤1750g *vs.* 1751 to 2041g. However, there were significant interactions between neurological status and sex ($F = 4.71$, $p<0.03$), and neurological status and SGA *vs.* preterm AGA grouping ($F = 12.58$, $p<0.001$). Whether they were neurologically normal or abnormal made less difference to social adjustment for girls than for boys; in other words, neurologically abnormal boys had

*15 LBW children of unknown gestation were excluded.

significantly more social-adjustment problems than the other children. Neurologically abnormal SGA children had higher ratings of behaviour maladjustment than neurologically abnormal preterm AGA children. Neurological status was less related to behaviour for preterm AGA children than for SGA children.

Discussion

Reading disabilities have been estimated as affecting between 5 and 20 per cent of the school-age population (Erickson 1977). A survey of reading achievement of all grade 5 students was carried out by the Vancouver School Board (Ellis 1975), which found that 14 per cent of the children were more than two years below grade-level in reading comprehension and 9 per cent in vocabulary, as measured by Gates-MacGinitie Reading Test. Our estimates of 22 per cent of LBW and 29 per cent of FBW children reading two or more years below the level expected for their IQ are high in comparison with the Vancouver School Board figures, and with other samples. However, the FBW reading-disabled children in the present study show a trend towards being of even lower social-class than the LBW children. Perhaps the very high proportion of apparently reading-disabled FBW children merely reflects a large number who are reading below capacity because of poor motivation from low SES environments. Rutter and Yule (1975) have pointed out that discrepancy methods of determining reading disability, based on discrepancy between ability (IQ) and grade level of reading achievement, tend to over-estimate the frequency of reading problems among children with above-average IQs. This is because such children are expected to read above their grade level. If the environment does not encourage reading above grade level, such a child would be considered to have a reading problem when a discrepancy method is used. Of the apparently reading-disabled children in our sample, 35 per cent of the LBW and 41 per cent of the FBW groups had a WISC Full-scale IQ of 110 or above at 6½ years. The use of a discrepancy method may lead to suspicion of reading problems in a relatively high proportion of these children. Although poor motivation and other factors associated with low social-class may partially account for the low reading level of these FBW children, they are unlikely to account for the reading level of the LBW group, in which 25 per cent of the children are in the highest social-class group (I to III).

There was one highly significant difference between the two groups, namely frequency of neurological problems at 6½ years. Qualitatively different underlying factors may be operating for the LBW and FBW children, but it appears that reading below the level expected for IQ is related to neurological problems, especially MBD, for the LBW children, and significantly less so for the FBW children.

Although many FBW children (22 per cent) were below grade level in school-work, very few (1 to 3 per cent) were in special educational settings. In contrast, among the LBW group, 15 per cent in year 1 and 17 per cent in year 3 were in a special class or school. It is interesting that the proportions of LBW and FBW children who were performing below grade level, but in the regular stream, were almost the same. The significant difference between the two groups is the proportion in special educational settings: *i.e.* very few of the FBW children were in a special class, school or institution, compared to the relatively high proportion of special placements among the LBW group.

It should be recalled that in analyses of the Stanford Achievement Test Battery, children with a WISC Full-scale IQ <80 were excluded. Therefore these comparisons are of particular interest in considering how LBW children who have escaped major intellectual impairment perform academically in comparison with the full-birthweight (FBW and CC) children. The classroom control group had significantly better scores than the LBW children on every subtest of the Stanford Battery. In addition to children of low IQ, when neurologically abnormal children were excluded from re-analysis of teacher ratings of key subjects, there were still some significant differences in mean scores between the LBW and CC groups. Therefore it appears that for this LBW sample, even when only the children who had no observable neurological or intellectual problems were compared, there were still some differences favouring the classroom control children. This supports the view of Pasamanick and Knobloch (1960) of 'a continuum of reproductive casualty', extending from death *in utero* to minimal cerebral damage.

In general, throughout the analyses, where both FBW and CC children were available for comparison with LBW children the CC group performed best, the LBW group were lowest and the FBW group fell in between. The FBW control children were selected so that their mean social-class would be similarly low to that of the LBW group. The social class of the CC children was unknown; however, it was assumed that selecting a child from the same classroom would control not only for teacher curriculum differences, but also for social-class differences.

The findings with respect to sex differences in this study are largely as one would expect. In analysis of school placement in school year 3, significantly more boys were in special classes, schools and institutions, reflecting their greater vulnerability. Teacher ratings of key subjects showed some significant differences in reading, spelling and writing, but not arithmetic. These findings are consistent with previous studies which have found that girls performed better than boys on verbal tests (Davie *et al.* 1972, Maccoby and Jacklin 1974). In arithmetic performance, the majority of American studies on representative samples show no sex differences up to adolescence, but when differences are found in the age-range of nine to 13 years they tend to favour boys (Maccoby and Jacklin 1974). Davic and colleagues (1972) analyzed a large British sample at elementary-school age and found boys superior to girls in arithmetic problem-solving, but those authors suspected that this might be influenced by cultural factors. Our finding of no statistically significant differences between the sexes in arithmetic achievement is consistent with the American studies.

Neligan *et al.* (1976) carried out a longitudinal study in Newcastle, aimed at comparing outcomes for SGA and preterm AGA children. The follow-up results to seven years of age found no differences in reading between the two groups. Davie *et al.* (1972) also reported on a British sample at a similar age and found differences in the proportion of educationally backward children among these two groups of children, with a smaller proportion among the preterm AGA than the SGA children. In the present study, significantly more SGA than preterm AGA children were placed in special classes, schools or institutions in school year 3. On the Stanford Achievement Test Battery there was a consistent trend toward better performance by the preterm AGA children, though the differences were not statistically significant. It is possible that if SGA infants escape serious damage there may be no residual differences between SGA and preterm AGA children. However, the number of children available for the Stanford analyses was small (33 SGA, 52 preterm AGA): if the sample had been larger there might have been significant differences. Unfortunately the Stanford test was only introduced to the study in 1970, at which time many of the LBW children had already passed beyond year 3. Our results are consistent with those of Davie and colleagues, rather than Neligan and co-workers. This difference in findings may be due to the birthweights of the sample in the Newcastle study: the mean birthweight for the lightest group, *i.e.* the 'very light-for-dates', was 2397g, whereas the LBW children in our sample were all at or below 2041g at birth. Therefore our comparisons of SGA *vs.* preterm AGA children were carried out on samples of children with lower birthweights than in the Newcastle Study.

It is interesting that for reading and arithmetic, differences between birthweight categories within the LBW sample appeared to assume increasing rather than decreasing importance over the school years. Perhaps teacher expectations of achievement differ in the primary grades (kindergarten to grade 3) compared to later elementary school, when a certain standard would be expected. Moreover, the tasks themselves change; by year 5 the concepts required of the child are more complex, and may be more sensitive indicators of cognitive peformance. When social class and mother's education were controlled, many differences between birthweight categories remained. However, when children with an IQ <80 or with neurological problems were excluded, differences between children born weighing $\leq$1750g *vs.* 1751 to 2041g disappeared. These findings support the suggestion that the effect of very low birthweight may be to increase the proportion with neurological damage, which results in poorer school performance.

Many studies over the years have found LBW children to be educationally disadvantaged to varying degrees compared to FBW children (Drillien 1961, Robinson and Robinson 1965, Wiener 1968). However, there have been differences in the implications of concomitant variables, and thus in interpretation of the nature and degree of such educational impairments. Robinson and Robinson (1965) concluded that poorer reading in their LBW than their FBW samples probably was due to social class rather than birthweight. Wiener (1968), on the other hand, found as we did that birthweight contributed to reading and arithmetic scores independently of social class. However, concluding that the effect of birthweight is still present after allowing for social-class differences is not to minimize the importance of social class in relation to the educational outcomes of LBW children. Davie and colleagues (1972), among others, found social class to be an important factor among educationally backward children. Detailed studies on the Hawaiian island of Kauai also demonstrated the enormous effect of ethnic-social factors on school performance (Werner *et al.* 1971). Concern has been expressed as to whether LBW children of lower SES may be disproportionately impaired compared to LBW children of higher SES (Robinson and Robinson 1965, Caputo and Mandell 1970). Douglas (1956) and Drillien (1964) found that LBW children of higher social-class were relatively less impaired than those of lower social-class. Only the Baltimore study of Wiener *et al.* (1965) did not find a significant interaction between birthweight and social class.

In the present study it is interesting to note how few children in either birthweight category in the upper social-classes were in special educational settings in year 3, in contrast to the relatively large proportion of social-class V children. A large proportion (36 per cent) of the lighter LBW children (≤1750g) in social-classes I to IV were below grade level but were in regular classes. Of the equivalent children in social-class V, 29 per cent were below grade level in regular classes and 40 per cent were in special classes, schools or institutions. In contrast, only 9 per cent of children in this category in social-class I to IV were in special placements. Among the children weighing 1751 to 2041g at birth, almost one-quarter (24 per cent) of the social-class V group were in special classes, schools or institutions, whereas only 8 per cent of the higher social-class categories were. It appears that children with birthweights 1751 to 2041g in social classes I to IV have a relatively good chance of performing close to grade level. It may be that more serious medical problems interact with poor environmental conditions, with the result that a child cannot be placed in the regular stream. Whether poor environmental conditions depress potential, or better conditions facilitate reaching potential, cannot be determined from these data. However, the greatly increased chance of performing at or near grade level for the LBW group of higher social-class, and the similarly increased chance of special class placement of LBW children of low social-class, certainly warrant further investigation. The results, although not statistically significant, also suggest that boys and girls may be differentially affected by social-class variables. There was a larger proportion of boys among the social class V 1751 to 2041g birthweight children in special placements than girls. This suggests a complex interplay between birthweight, sex and social class.

The findings on school placement reported here clearly indicate a disproportionate effect of low birthweight in children of low social-class, as was noted by Douglas (1956) and Drillien (1964), but not by Wiener (1968). Kruuse (1976), in Denmark, similarly found low social-class and LBW to be a most unfortunate combination, as reflected in frequency of special class placement and reading clinics. They concluded that there was a need for social-educational efforts, rather than special education, to change such tendencies.

Summary

The main findings on the educational outcome of LBW children in this sample may be summarized as follows:

(1) Significantly more LBW than FBW children have been placed in special classes, special schools or institutions. LBW children scored lower than CC children on standardized achievement tests and teacher rating scales.

(2) Significantly more SGA than preterm AGA children have been placed in special classes, special schools or institutions. When children with a Full-scale WISC

IQ ≥80 (at 6½ years) were given standardized achievement tests at year 3 in school, there was a consistent trend in favour of the preterm AGA children.

(3) When LBW children who weighed ≤1750g at birth were compared with those who weighed 1751 to 2041g, the lighter children had significantly poorer school performance, and more frequent placement in special classes.

(4) When analyses were conducted adjusting the two birthweight groups to equate them for any differences in social class and mother's education, the results for the lighter LBW group were still significantly poorer for teacher ratings of reading, arithmetic, spelling and writing. This indicates an effect of birthweight, independent of social class and mother's education.

(5) Low social-class was of considerable importance in adversely affecting the educational outcome of LBW children to a significant extent, in addition to the birthweight effect.

(6) When children diagnosed at 6½ years of age as neurologically abnormal (including MBD) or with a Full-scale WISC IQ <80 were excluded from analysis, teacher ratings of reading, arithmetic, spelling and writing no longer showed significant differences between LBW and FBW children. However, a statistically significant difference remained between the LBW and CC groups in reading at school years 3 and 4. The differences between the lighter and heavier LBW children disappeared when these exclusions were made.

(7) Higher misbehaviour ratings among the LBW than the FBW children appeared to be related to IQ scores rather than birthweight. Neurological status was less related to behaviour for preterm AGA children than for SGA children.

12
Environmental Factors and Neurological and Intellectual Functioning in Relation to Social Growth

Annetta K. McBurney and Ruth V. E. Grunau

In this prospective study of LBW infants the Vineland Social Maturity Scale was included in the psychometric test battery at 2½ years and four years to evaluate the children's developing adequacy in meeting social tasks. This scale represents an attempt to provide 'a broad detailed inventory of performances which seemed distinctive for successive age-periods and a generalized categorical evaluation of behavior throughout the life-span' (Doll 1953, p. 55). The underlying assumption is that children's individual social responsibility develops progressively from dependency to acceptance of responsibility for others, and that this matures as one facet of individual growth and adjustment. The child's mastery of representative aspects of social competence in the areas of self-help, locomotion, occupation, self-direction and socialization is noted. The information may be obtained by self-report, or from someone familiar with the subject's habitual behaviour. In the case of children it is customary for the mother or care-giver to provide the required simple, concrete information. A Social Age (SA) and a Social Quotient (SQ) can be derived from the total score.

In early studies the Vineland test most often was used diagnostically and prognostically with the mentally handicapped (*e.g.* Morales 1942) and with 'problem' children—the deprived, maladjusted or delinquent (Lurie *et al.* 1941, Dunsdon 1947). It is still used most frequently in investigations of deviant children, *e.g.* those with mental retardation (Heber 1961, McIntosh and Warren 1969), infantile autism (DeMyer *et al.* 1971) or other handicapping disorders (McFie and Robertson 1973, Fishman and Palkes 1974). In clinical practice it is widely used as an easily administered developmental estimate for younger children whose physical disabilities or deviant behaviour may preclude other testing techniques. Doll (1953, p. 420) claimed significant social-age/mental-age correlations between birth and 14 years. Support for this association appeared in a number of studies in which positive and usually significant relationships were shown (Hurst 1962, Werner and Simonian 1966). Clinicians are also interested in the meaning of psychometric scores which place a child in one category on intellectual grounds (IQ) and in another relating to social behaviour (SQ). However, this interest is reflected only minimally in published findings. Clinical psychologists feel that items used in the very early years of childhood offer a more reliable indication of social competence than can be obtained at later stages, since the abilities tapped seem much less subject to specific training and somewhat less dependent on social-class mores. This issue has still to be clarified.

Gambaro (1944) and Pringle (1966) appear to concur that selection of subjects and procedures of item validation have ensured a scale which is independent of sex and social-class grouping, although Werner (1957) found evidence of some rural-urban differences in SQ. At five years city children obtained higher scores, while at the age of 10 years the position was reversed, rural children having achieved independence in more areas.

A distinct tendency for SQ-IQ discrepancies to be negatively correlated with IQ has been suggested (Doll 1953, Hurst 1962). Substantial differences between IQS and SQS usually are 'explained' as indicating that children with low IQS tend to compensate by accelerated social maturity in relation to their intellectual maturity, whereas the social development of those with higher IQS tends to be more consistent with their intelligence. In some instances the social competence of retarded children also may be viewed optimistically by their parents.

One of the major concerns in this study was the identification of predictive factors for the children's later neurological and intellectual functioning. The Vineland Social Quotient was used in conjunction with other diagnostic techniques to identify defects, and as one of the measures which might reveal developmental differences between birthweight/gestation groups. At the same time, however, it was of interest to note some of the characteristics of SQ and of SQ-IQ discrepancies which might be applicable to other populations.

Excluded from this part of the study were children who failed to return for examination after the neonatal one, blind children, and children with major congenital anomalies. The numbers vary slightly from test to test, since not all children were available for every examination. A Vineland SQ was obtained at 2½ years for 145 preterm AGA and 103 SGA children, and for 81 FBW controls. The numbers for the four-year Vineland test were 154 preterm AGA, 112 SGA and 74 FBW controls.

One purpose of this part of the study was to find out whether Vineland SQS at 2½ and four years (1) discriminated between AGA preterm, SGA and FBW children, between boys and girls and between socio-economic groups; and (2) were associated with IQ at 2½ and four years (Stanford-Binet) and at 6½ years (WISC) and with Haggerty-Olson-Wickman behaviour ratings in Grade 1. Other purposes were to see whether score differences at 2½ and four years (1) discriminated between AGA preterm, SGA and FBW control groups, and between boys and girls; and (2) were associated with antecendant factors to do with the family and maternal history, nursery history and the children's physical and intellectual characteristics. The family factors were ethnic background, socio-economic status, plurality, serial position in the family (first child/other), relationship of child to parents (natural/foster/adopted) and proportion of time spent with the mother. The maternal factors were mother's age, education and emotional status, past history of neuromuscular and psychiatric disorders, neuropsychiatric disorders during the pregnancy, her response to the child's physical needs, her attitude to the child's performance, her care of the child, her focus of attention while the child was being examined, and the method of feeding at three, six, 12 and 18 months. The nursery history included series of three Apgar scores, the number of days incubated, the number of days in hospital and the method of oral feeding.

The physical and intellectual characteristics, clinical abnormalities and affective responses assessed were body length/height (neonatal, three months, six months, 18 months, 2½ years, four years); unusual activity and unusual cry in the nursery; and at 2½ years and four years: response to comforting, affective response to mother, to other familiar persons and strangers, to cuddling, to bathing, feeding, dressing and rough play; convulsions (six, 12, 18 months and 2½ and four years); clinical impression (neonatal); EEG abnormalities at one and about 6¾ years; neurological abnormalities at 1½, 2½ and four years; neurological status at 2½ and four years; 'organic behaviour syndrome' (attention deficit disorder) at four years; IQ range; performance of a task involving spatial abilities at four years; and body image at four years.

We also wanted to ascertain whether Vineland SQs were associated with later psychomotor and other scores, including IQ, perceptual-motor tasks, repetition of an observed motor task, vocal encoding and sentence repetition, 'organic behaviour disorder' (attention deficit disorder), EEG abnormalities, response to parental directions, focus of mother's attention while the child was being examined, and Haggerty-Olson-Wickman behaviour ratings in Grade 1.

The tests used were the Vineland Social Maturity Scale at 2½ and four years, Stanford-Binet (Form L-M) at 2½ and four years, Goodenough-Harris Draw-a-Person at four and 6½ years, Porteus Maze at four years, Haggerty-Olson-Wickman Behavioural Guide, Wechsler Intelligence Scale for Children (WISC)*, Bender Gestalt, Knox Cubes, Benton Sentence Repetition and Vocal Encoding (Illinois Test of Psycholinguistic Ability).

We also used the records for prenatal history, labour and delivery, socioeconomic family history and neurological/developmental examinations (neonatal, three and six months, one, 1½, 2½, four and 6½ years).

Results

Vineland SQs at 2½ and four years

The groups (AGA preterm, SGA and FBW) were examined for homogeneity. While the two LBW groups obtained a similar spread in their SQ scores, the FBW group differed significantly at both 2½ and four years in showing less spread in their scores ($F = 20.47$, $p<0.001$; $F = 14.35$, $p<0.001$). With IQ partialled out, significantly higher mean SQs were still found among FBW controls than the LBW group (*i.e.* AGA preterm and SGA group) at 2½ years: $r = 0.130$, $p<0.025$. At four years, however, these differences were non-significant. Tests of SQ differences between AGA preterm SGA and FBW controls, using IQ as a covariate, also showed non-significant differences.

Significant sex differences in SQ were found in the total sample at both 2½ and four years, in favour of the girls ($t = -4.31$, $p<0.001$; $t = -2.77$, $p<0.005$) (Table 12-I). Further analysis revealed no significant difference between the AGA preterm, SGA and FBW control groups in this respect.

Social-class differences were non-significant at 2½ and at four years.

*Verbal (VIQ), Performance (PIQ) and Full-scale (FSIQ) scores.

TABLE 12-I

Sex differences in Vineland Social Quotient (SQ)

SQ	*N*	*Mean*	*SD*	*t*	*p (one tailed)*
At 2½ yrs					
Boys	162	108.77	18.16	−4.31	<0.001
Girls	167	117.59	18.95		
At 4 yrs					
Boys	167	115.21	17.99	−2.77	<0.005
Girls	173	120.54	17.43		

SQ at 2½ and four years in relation to IQ at 2½, four and 6½ years

In the total population, SQs at both the 2½-year and the four-year examinations were positively and significantly correlated with IQ at 2½, four and 6½ years, and with WISC Verbal IQ and Performance IQ at 6½ years (Tables 12-II and III).

Broken down according to sex and birthweight/gestation categories, these findings hold up for the LBW groups in 36 of 40 subgroupings, the exceptions being in tests of association between: *(a)* SQ at 2½ years and Verbal IQ at 6½ years for SGA boys; and *(b)* SQ at four years of preterm AGA girls and their IQ at 2½ years and Verbal and Performance IQs at 6½ years (Tables 12-II and III).

The FBW controls, however, present less consistent results. The boys' SQ at 2½ years is not significantly related to global IQ at 2½, four and 6½ years, nor to Verbal or Performance IQ, although the association is a positive one. For the control girls, on the other hand, the 2½-year Vineland score is significantly correlated to each of the measures, while the four-year Vineland score is not significantly related to any of them. For the boys, the 2½-year Vineland score is significantly correlated only with the two early IQ scores. It is among these FBW control boys that the only negative association appears in their SQ at four years and Verbal IQ at 6½ years, but this is not significant. It appeared, therefore, with certain reservations, that the clinical use of the Vineland test would be justified as an indicator and predictor of IQ. It was highly efficient in this respect for the total cohort, and for the great majority of the sex/birthweight subgroups of LBW children. It was similarly effective at 2½ years for FBW girls. As an IQ approximation measure, the 2½-year SQ was slightly more efficient than that at four years.

Haggerty-Olson-Wickman behaviour ratings

For the total population and for each of the sex/birthweight subgroupings, negative correlation coefficients were found in 60 of 84 comparisons between both the 2½- and four-year SQs and each Haggerty-Olson-Wickman (HOW) subscale and total score. This indicated an over-all tendency for immaturity of social competence, as measured by the Vineland Social Maturity Scale at these ages, to be associated with misbehaviour scores during the first year at school. The negative associations between SQ at 2½ years and all six of the HOW categories were significant for the total group and for preterm boys. Fewer areas of significant association, however, were found between the 4½-year SQ and HOW scores.

TABLE 12-II

Correlations between SQ at 2½ years and IQ scores

	IQ									
	Stanford-Binet (2½ yrs)		*Stanford-Binet (4 yrs)*		*WISC FSIQ (6½ yrs)*		*WISC PIQ (6½ yrs)*		*WISC VIQ (6½ yrs)*	
Group	*r*	*p*	*r*	*p*	*r*	*p*	*r*	*p*	*r*	*p*
Total sample (N = 316-325)	0.539	<0.001	0.524	<0.001	0.513	<0.001	0.424	<0.001	0.330	<0.001
Preterm AGA boys (N = 77-79)	0.497	<0.001	0.557	<0.001	0.462	<0.001	0.494	<0.001	0.348	<0.001
Preterm AGA girls (N = 63-66)	0.481	<0.001	0.375	<0.001	0.339	<0.005	0.274	<0.025	0.529	<0.001
SGA boys (N = 48-50)	0.607	<0.001	0.60	<0.001	0.594	<0.001	0.392	<0.005	0.086	NS
SGA girls (N = 50-54)	0.544	<0.001	0.418	<0.001	0.402	<0.001	0.470	<0.001	0.346	<0.005
FBW boys (N = 40-42)	0.206	NS	0.163	NS	0.225	NS	0.148	NS	0.188	NS
FBW girls (N = 34-37)	0.639	<0.001	0.427	<0.025	0.503	<0.001	0.510	<0.001	0.418	<0.005

TABLE 12-III

Correlations between SQ at four years and IQ scores

	IQ									
	Stanford-Binet (2½ yrs)		*Stanford-Binet (4 yrs)*		*WISC FSIQ (6½ yrs)*		*WISC PIQ (6½ yrs)*		*WISC VIQ (6½ yrs)*	
Group	*r*	*p*	*r*	*p*	*r*	*p*	*r*	*p*	*r*	*p*
Total sample (N = 297-335)	0.374	<0.001	0.415	<0.001	0.435	<0.001	0.372	<0.001	0.30	<0.001
Preterm AGA boys (N = 78-88)	0.288	<0.005	0.324	<0.001	0.362	<0.001	0.346	<0.001	0.295	<0.005
Preterm AGA girls (N = 59-67)	0.145	NS	0.347	<0.025	0.435	<0.001	0.151	NS	0.195	NS (p = 0.058)
SGA boys (N = 47-52)	0.510	<0.001	0.403	<0.025	0.50	<0.001	0.407	<0.025	0.234	<0.05
SGA girls (N = 51-61)	0.277	<0.025	0.505	<0.001	0.551	<0.001	0.540	<0.001	0.499	<0.001
FBW boys (N = 39-44)	0.514	<0.001	0.430	<0.025	−0.028	NS	0.161	NS	−0.204	NS
FBW girls (N = 30-32)	0.287	NS	0.135	NS	0.092	NS	0.142	NS	0.011	NS

TABLE 12-IV
SQ-IQ difference scores: preterm AGA, SGA and FBW control groups

	SQ-IQ difference scores at 2½ yrs			*SQ-IQ difference scores at 4 yrs*		
Group	*N*	*Mean*	*SD*	*N*	*Mean*	*SD*
Preterm AGA	138	19.667	16.920	151	23.675	18.964
SGA	99	21.303	17.640	110	23.018	19.105
FBW controls	73	20.973	16.725	72	15.764	17.298

Analysis of variance: preterm AGA + SGA *vs.* controls at four years $F = 9.15$, $p<0.005$.

TABLE 12-V
SQ-IQ differences *vs.* sex

SQ-IQ		*N*	*Mean*	*SD*	*t*	*p (one-tailed)*
Total group						
At 2½ yrs	Boys	153	18.08	16.18	−2.48	<0.005
	Girls	157	22.85	17.63		
At 4 yrs	Boys	165	21.01	19.49	−0.70	NS
	Girls	168	22.47	18.28		
Preterm AGA						
At 2½ yrs	Boys	73	16.88	16.12	−2.07	<0.025
	Girls	65	22.80	17.37		
At 4 yrs	Boys	84	22.62	18.50	−0.76	NS
	Girls	67	25.00	19.58		
SGA						
At 2½ yrs	Boys	47	18.89	16.65	−1.30	NS
	Girls	52	23.48	18.38		
At 4 yrs	Boys	51	21.65	19.89	−0.69	NS
	Girls	59	24.20	18.49		
FBW controls						
At 2½ yrs	Boys	33	19.61	15.94	−0.64	NS
	Girls	40	22.10	17.46		
At 4 yrs	Boys	30	15.43	21.13	−0.13	NS
	Girls	42	16.00	14.22		

In subsequent correlation coefficients in which IQ was controlled, associations between HOW scores and SQ at 2½ and four years were also mainly found to be negative, but non-significant. For example, the partial correlation coefficient between SQ at 2½ years and HOW B score was −0.091, and at four years it was −0.066. In other words, while a low SQ seems to be associated with later misdemeanour scores, once the effect of IQ has been removed such correlations tend to be of a very low order.

SQ-IQ scores at 2½ and four years

Scattergram analyses of differences in SQ-IQ scores at both ages indicated an underlying continuum, *i.e.* there was no qualitative difference between positive and negative scores (intercept = 99.276, slope = −0.286, $p<0.001$; intercept = 105.898, slope = −0.445, $p<0.001$).

SQ-IQ difference scores were most often positive ones, *i.e.* SQ exceeded IQ. At 2½ years only 22 of the total 310 children (7.1 per cent) obtained negative scores ranging from −1 to −14. At the four-year examination the proportion, although somewhat greater, was still a small one: 42 of 333 (12.6 per cent) of the scores were negative, ranging from −1 to −25. In addition to the significant negative relationships between IQ and SQ-IQ difference scores, the scattergrams also clearly showed that no child at 2½ years and only one child at four years (whose IQ exceeded 105) obtained a difference score in the scattergram sextant referring to the greatest SQ-IQ differences, *i.e.* children in the average and lower IQ ranges are likely to show the largest differences between SQ and IQ.

Difference scores at 2½ years did not discriminate between the birthweight/gestation groups. At the four-year examination they were not significantly different in the two LBW groups but were highly so ($F = 9.15$, $p<0.005$) when the combined LBW groups were compared to the FBW controls, larger difference scores appearing in the LBW children (Table 12-IV).

Because of the finding in a later part of this study that there appears to be a dependent relationship between SQ-IQ difference scores and the IQ measure itself, the analysis of several variables was extended. As appropriate to the data, partial correlations, analyses of covariance and multiple regression analyses were run, controlling for IQ at each age-level. With IQ partialled out, significant differences no longer appeared in birthweight/gestation comparisons at four years, and non-significant differences were found when the separate categories of preterm AGA, SGA and FBW were considered. At the 2½-year level, however, significant differences were found between the three groups ($r = 0.132$, $p<0.025$). It appeared, therefore, that the difference score at 2½ years discriminates between preterm AGA, SGA and FBW control children, while the four-year one does not.

In the analysis of sex differences, although the mean difference score at 2½ and four years was found to be greater for girls in each birthweight category, statistical significance was reached only in the case of preterm AGA children ($t = -2.07$, $p<0.025$) and for the total cohort at the time of the 2½-year examination ($t = -2.48$, $p<0.005$) (Table 12-V). Analysis of variance showed no birthweight-sex interaction on difference scores at 2½ or four years. An inspection of mean difference scores, however, does indicate that while LBW boys and girls obtain a larger SQ-IQ difference score at four years than at 2½ years, the reverse is true for both boys and girls in the FBW control group.

Family group factors

A significant association was found between SES and difference scores at 2½ years ($F = 4.419$, $p<0.01$) and at four years ($F = 2.779$, $p<0.05$), with an increasing positive SQ-IQ difference appearing at the lower end of the socio-economic index. A test of linearity showed only non-significant deviations from linearity in this relationship. With IQ controlled, however, no such association appears. At 2½ years the results do not support the findings of a negative linear relationship between social status and difference score. At four years the correlation, while negative, is very low and highly non-significant. It appeared, therefore, that in the

TABLE 12-VI
SQ-IQ difference scores: singletons and twins

	SQ-IQ difference scores					
		At 2½ yrs			*At 4 yrs*	
Group	*N*	*Mean*	*SD*	*N*	*Mean*	*SD*
Singletons	251	20.016	17.183	269	19.784	18.545
Twins	58	22.542	16.566	64	30.000	18.136
Analysis of variance		F = 1.047, NS			F = 15.819, $p<0.001$	

case of social class also the residual was non-significant once the effect of IQ had been removed.

Twins obtained larger positive difference scores than did singletons, and this was highly significant at four years (F = 15.819, $p<0.001$) (Table 12-VI). With IQ controlled, this trend remained non-significant at 2½ years, but at four years twins were significantly more likely than singletons to have greater difference scores ($r = 0.136$, $p<0.01$), independently of IQ scores.

The child's legal status within the family was also significantly associated with positive difference scores at 2½ years (F = 5.651, $p<0.01$), the difference scores of natural and adopted children being similar to each other but greater than those of the foster children. This finding was further examined in view of the observed relationship between difference scores and IQ range. It appeared that while the four-year difference scores of foster children were only slightly lower than those of the other two groups, their mean IQ, significantly lower at 2½ years (F = 7.90, $p<0.001$), maintained its relatively lower standing at the age of four years (F = 6.88, $p<0.01$). In other words, the SQs of foster children, but not their IQs, were markedly higher at four years than at 2½ years, while no corresponding SQ increment occurred for natural and adopted children.

The ethnic background of the parents, the child's serial position in the family, and the amount of time spent with the mother were not found to be associated with differences in 2½- or four-year SQ scores.

Maternal factors

There appeared to be no relationship between SQ-IQ differences and the mother's age, marital status, her feeding methods at three, six, 12 and 18 months, assessment of her care of the child at six months and 2½ years, neuropsychiatric disorders during pregnancy, or her past history of neuromuscular and psychiatric disorders. However, significant associations were seen in the other areas. There was a negative association between the four-year difference score and the physician's estimate of the mother's responsiveness to the child's physical needs at the four-year examination (F = 2.803, $p<0.025$). Assessment of her care of the child at four years also was negatively associated with the four-year difference score (F = 2.750, $p<0.05$). The mother's level of education and the difference score at 2½ and four years were found to be negatively associated (F = 3.67, $p<0.01$; F = 3.546, $p<0.01$).

In a further examination of the various educational levels of the mothers *vs.* SQ-IQ difference scores, an analysis of variance using the child's IQ as a covariate did not reveal a significant association. Scanning the adjusted means, however, suggested a possible difference between mothers who had received university education and those who had not. This difference was indeed found at both 2½ and four years, although significance was reached only at the 2½-year examination ($F = 7.58$, $p<0.01$). A similar trend appeared between the focus of the mother's attention during the four-year examination and the four-year difference score ($F = 3.297$, $p<0.05$), and the association was significant when the focus of the mother's attention during the 6½-year examination was studied in relation to the four-year difference score ($F = 3.297$, $p<0.05$). In other words, lower difference scores were obtained by the children of mothers whose attention was appropriately directed to the over-all situation rather than exclusively to either herself or her child. A positive association was seen between neuropsychiatric disorders in pregnancy and the four-year difference score ($\chi^2 = 28.641$, $p<0.05$).

Nursery history

No association was found between the 2½- or four-year difference scores and the number of days spent in an incubator, the number of days in hospital or the oral feeding method in the nursery. The third of the series of Apgar scores, however, was associated with difference scores at 2½ years ($\chi^2 = 28.223$, $p<0.05$). This association no longer appeared in subsequent analyses taking account of IQ, although a significant association was found between the first Apgar score and SQ-IQ difference score at 2½ years ($r = 0.191$, $p<0.005$).

Physical and intellectual characteristics, clinical abnormalities and affective responses

Body-length measurements at six months were negatively correlated with 2½-year difference scores ($r = -0.116$, $p<0.05$), while a highly significant negative relationship appeared between four-year difference scores and body-length/height at each age level: neonatal ($r = -0.211$, $p = 0.001$); three months ($r = -0.190$, $p = 0.002$); six months ($r = -0.158$, $p = 0.007$); 18 months ($r = -0.196$, $p = 0.001$); 2½ years ($r = -0.243$, $p = 0.001$); and four years ($r = -0.185$, $p = 0.001$).

Controlled for IQ, however, these results no longer held. Of all body-length/height comparisons with difference scores, significant negative correlations appeared only in the case of neonatal body-length *vs.* four-year difference scores ($r = 0.111$, $p<0.05$).

Abnormal EEG patterns at one year were not clearly related to difference scores, but abnormal patterns at 6¾ years were significantly associated with difference scores at 2½ years ($F = 5.566$, $p<0.025$).

Neurological abnormalities at 2½ years were significantly associated with difference scores at 2½ years ($F = 4.015$, $p<0.01$) and at four years ($F = 3.451$, $p<0.025$). Neurological status at 2½ years was similarly associated with difference at both ages ($F = 6.486$, $p<0.01$; $F = 5.002$, $p<0.01$). Significant association was

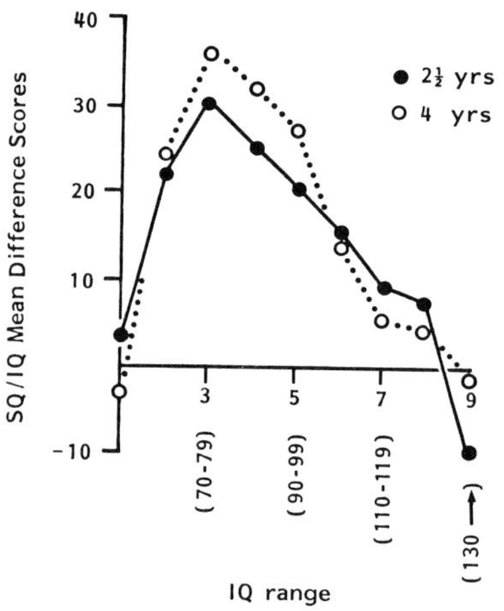

Figure 12-1. SQ-IQ mean difference scores at 2½ years and four years.

shown between specific deficits at four years and difference scores at four years (F = 5.778, $p<0.01$). 'Organic behaviour syndrome' (attention deficit disorder) at four years and difference scores at four years were also significantly related (F = 7.450, $p<0.001$).

A statistically significant negative association was found between 2½-year difference scores and the 2½-year IQ (F = 7.89, $p<0.001$), and between four-year difference scores and the 2½-year IQ ($p<0.05$) and four-year IQ (F = 22.41, $p<0.001$). When this association was studied further, however, it appeared that the relationship tended to be non-linear at both age-levels, but reached significance only at the time of the four-year examination (F = 22.41, $p<0.001$) (Fig. 12-1).

Analysis of variance revealed significant differences at both 2½ years and four years between the nine IQ ranges and SQ/OQ discrepancies (F = 7.89, $p<0.001$; F = 22.41, $p<0.001$). The IQ ranges were collapsed to form two categories, and significant differences were shown between the categories in each case at the 0.001 level (Table 12-VII).

With IQ controlled, no association was found between SQ-IQ difference scores and the performance at four years of a task involving spatial abilities (Porteus Maze test), or body image as measured by Goodenough-Harris scores.

SQ-IQ difference scores as predictors of responses at 6½ years

Controlling for IQ, the Goodenough-Harris, Bender Gestalt, Knox Cube, Sentence Repetition and Vocal Encoding tests were examined for association with SQ-IQ difference scores. WISC subtests were also studied. This did not prove to be a fruitful area of study. No consistent pattern emerged, nearly all correlations being of a low order.

No association was found between difference scores and unusual amounts of activity, unusual cry noted in the nursery and at 2½ and four years, convulsions recorded at six, 12, 18 months and 2½ and four years, or the physician's clinical

TABLE 12-VII

SQ-IQ difference scores *vs.* IQ range

	IQ Range	*N*	*Mean SQ-IQ*	*SD*	*IQ Range*	*N*	*Mean SQ-IQ*	*SD*
	1-50	2	2.00	5.66				
	51-69	14	22.50	20.25				
	70-79	32	30.84	17.40				
	80-89	83	25.59	15.86	Lowest-99	208	24.58	16.83
2½ yrs (N = 312)	90-99	77	21.86	16.33				
	100-109	58	15.38	13.88	100-highest	104	12.20	14.28
	110-119	35	9.26	13.41				
	120-129	9	7.89	15.37				
	130-highest	2	−9.00	8.49				
	Analysis of variance F = 7.895, p<0.001				Analysis of variance F = 41.356, p<0.001			
	Test of linearity F = 2.858, NS							
	1-50	2	−3.50	2.12				
	51-69	13	24.08	20.69				
	70-79	32	36.56	19.00				
	80-89	65	32.37	14.65	Lowest-99	198	30.17	17.04
4 yrs (N = 335)	90-99	86	27.84	16.20				
	100-109	66	14.24	15.20	100-highest	137	9.66	14.12
	110-119	43	6.88	11.07				
	120-129	20	4.70	11.37				
	130-highest	8	−0.88	14.16				
	Analysis of variance F = 22.409, p<0.001				Analysis of variance F = 134.55, p<0.001			
	Test of linearity F = 7.827, p<0.05							

impression at the time of the neonatal examination. The child's affective responses to the mother, to other familiar persons, to a stranger, to cuddling, bathing, feeding, dressing or rough play (variables which had been examined in the attempt to understand large differences between the mother's estimate of her child's social competence and his intelligence-test scores) did not appear to be associated with difference scores.

Despite the several indications noted above that the difference between SQ and IQ is functionally associated with the IQ, informant bias might be one possible explanation for the finding that girls obtained higher SQs relative to their IQs than did boys. Because such 'overestimation' could not be directly examined in the present study, the problem was approached in terms of the 'self-fulfulling prophecy' model. An examination was made of the later achievement of 'highly overestimated', 'neutral' and 'highly underestimated' groups. Since SQ-IQ difference scores had been clearly shown in negative relationships with the IQ itself, a not unexpected finding emerged. Non-significant correlations appeared in each case, suggesting that for the children in this study, at least, one of the possible effects of maternal 'overestimation', *i.e.* higher than expected later achievement, was not observed.

Discussion

Vineland Social Quotient

While SQs did not discriminate between SGA and preterm AGA children, the LBW children, as a group, obtained lower SQs than their FBW controls at both 2½ and four years. These differing developmental patterns were still apparent when statistical tests taking account of IQ were applied, although the trend was less marked and non-significant at the four-year examination.

Sex differences in SQ were observed in favour of the girls at both 2½ and four years, a finding in oppostion to the results of previous investigators (*e.g.* Pringle 1966). This may reflect sex-differentiated patterns of social behaviour or the greater proportion of boys (82/163) than girls (56/172) reported to be 'abnormal' in the course of their follow-up examination because of mental retardation, minimal brain dysfunctions, cerebral palsy, epilepsy, blindness or deafness.

Social-class differences in SQ, on the other hand, were non-significant in this study, as in previously reported ones. This may lend some support to the general impression among clinicians that the items included in the Vineland Social Maturity Scale are more reliable for young children because they are less dependent on teaching than are the items used for later ages.

SQ certainly appears to be associated with global IQ at four years and 6½ years, and with WISC Verbal and Performance IQ at 6½ years in this group of LBW children. The 2½-year SQ of FBW boys, but not girls, was a good predictor of subsequent IQ measures. It would seem, then, that for many children (particularly boys) to whom an intelligence test cannot be administered, a Vineland SQ may be a useful predictive or diagnostic alternative. SQ may also have some worth as an early indication of later behaviour problems in school. This predictive tendency was maintained even after IQ had been accounted for.

SQ-IQ difference scores

For most of the areas examined in the course of this study the findings tend to support the belief that this scale is relatively free of informant bias (Doll 1953, p. 470). The extent of the discrepancy between a child's SQ and IQ appears to be functionally associated with the IQ range. Statistical tests which took account of IQ revealed non-significant relationships between the degree of the SQ-IQ difference and the variables of social class, ethnic background, serial position in the family, proportion of time spent with the mother, feeding methods, the mother's age, her psychiatric disorders preceding and during the pregnancy, and the number of days the infant spent in an incubator or in hospital. Similarly no association was found with body length at any period between three months and four years, with neonatal clinical impression, unusual amounts of activity or of crying, or the four-year Porteus Maze and Goodenough-Harris scores.

Significant association between SQ-IQ difference scores did appear in other comparisons. Large differences were positively associated with plurality, fostering, abnormal EEG at 6¾ years, abnormal neurological signs at 2½ years, abnormal neurological status at 2½ years, and 'organic behaviour syndrome' (attention deficit disorder) at four years. Large SQ-IQ differences were *negatively* associated with the mother's responsiveness to her child's physical needs, with her care of the child at four years, her university education, and her appropriate focus of attention at the time of the four-year examination; and also with the child's IQ at 2½, four and 6½ years. On the whole, therefore, it appears that the frequently noted discrepancies between a child's SQ and IQ may be more a function of factors inherent in the child's own developmental pattern than the outcome of some presumed 'halo' or other maternal effect. Nonetheless, the intelligent mother (*e.g.* with university education) may be more accurate and realistic in assessing her child's ability.

General comments

There is concern about the long-term effects of parental response to the infant in intensive care and of extended early hospitalization. Ross (1980), in a comprehensive review of the literature on maternal-infant bonding and parental response to infants in intensive care, concluded that claims for a critical period for bonding and a biological basis of attachment have not been borne out by empirical evidence, and that the emphasis should be on the importance of facilitating positive maternal responses to the high-risk infant. She delineated some factors, other than separation, which may be important in parental response to the high-risk infant, including emotional reaction to the birth of an unwell baby, the behavioural competence of the infant, the intensive care milieu, and the availability of family support. Maternal behaviour continuously accommodates the changing characteristics of the child in a reciprocal process. There is evidence that the attitudes and behaviour of mothers of LBW infants become indistinguishable from those of mothers of fullterm normal babies as the LBW children 'catch up' developmentally (Leiderman and Seashore 1975).

From 1935 until the late 1960s the Vineland scale was the undisputed tool for assessing social competence. Since then a number of new scales have been developed, most of them specifically for evaluation of disabled children and adults (usually the mentally retarded). Examples are the Cain-Levine Social Competency Scale (Cain *et al.* 1963), Balthazar Scales of Adaptive Behavior (Balthazar 1971), and the AAMD Adaptive Behavior Scale (Nihira *et al.* 1974). In these newer scales competence is assessed in specific sub-areas, such as self-help, communication, social and occupational skills, giving more detailed information for implementing training programmes than the single Vineland scores.

Alpern and Boll (1972) published a test for developmental evaluation of specific skills—physical, self-help, social, academic and communication—which give age equivalents for each area separately, based on report by an adult who knows the child well. An IQ equivalence score can also be derived. In a review of the Alpern and Boll scale, Hunt (1978) concluded that this test was best used as an aid for teachers who needed some estimate of a retarded child's level of functioning in practical skills. She pointed out that the test was not designed to be an instrument for professionals assessing suspected developmental delays, and implied caution in using it for this purpose. Although the Alpern and Boll scale was designed specifically to replace the Vineland, the latter test has continued to be widely used (Buros 1978, Achenbach 1980).

Rosen (1978), in a review of five competence scales (not including Alpern and Boll), concluded that the newer scales are the preferred tools for planning specific behavioural objectives, but that for purposes of diagnosis and classification according to developmental level the Vineland seems the most useful measure. It also has the general advantage of ranging from infancy to adulthood.

It had been noted that the norms for children aged two weeks to 36 months needed adjustment, since the social ages in the original norm tables tended to be consistently higher than the chronological ages of normal controls (Werner and Simonian 1966, Song and Jones 1982). A revision of the Vineland Scale, with updated norms and separate assessment of communication, daily living, socialization and motor skill areas, is now available.

Summary

In a prospective study of 267 preterm AGA, 190 SGA and 203 FBW control children, the Vineland Social Maturity Scale was administered at 2½ and four years, in conjunction with other diagnostic techniques, to investigate developmental patterns within each birthweight/gestation category. It was also hoped that neurological and intellectual functioning might be identified.

Mean social quotients (SQ), with IQ partialled out, were higher in the FBW group than in the combined preterm AGA and SGA group at four years. This tendency was significant at 2½ years. Sex differences in favour of girls were significant at both ages, but no social-class SQ differences were found. For AGA preterm and SGA children and for FBW boys, the SQ appeared to be predictive of IQ at 6½ years, and for the total cohort it appeared to be predictive of behaviour problems at school.

SQ-IQ difference scores were positively associated with plurality, fostering, neurological and EEG abnormalities, attention deficit disorder and Bender Gestalt error score. They were associated negatively with intelligence, the mother's educational status and her care of the child. It is concluded that the Vineland test, at least up to the age of four years, has some value as a supporting or alternative technique of assessment.

13
Electroencephalograms

Henry G. Dunn, Norman L. Auckland and Morton D. Low

Electroencephalographic (EEG) patterns of newborn infants have been studied extensively in recent years. Dreyfus-Brisac and her associates first demonstrated that the features of the normal EEG are related to the gestational age of the neonate (Dreyfus-Brisac *et al.* 1962; Dreyfus-Brisac 1962, 1966). Like the clinical neurological findings, therefore, they may serve as an index of the maturity of the nervous system, and this is known to be more closely related to the length of gestation than to birthweight.

The maturational changes of neonatal EEG activity before and after term are now fairly well documented (Kellaway and Crawley 1964, Dreyfus-Brisac 1966, Satran and Rosen 1967, Parmelee *et al.* 1968, Dreyfus-Brisac and Minkowski 1969, Nolte *et al.* 1969, Monod *et al.* 1972, Werner *et al.* 1977, Ellingson and Peters 1980, Lombroso 1982). However, more work is required to elucidate the long-term evolution of the EEG patterns of LBW children and the prognostic significance of neonatal EEG abnormalities.

Lubchenco and colleagues (1963*b*) recorded EEGs for 55 children at approximately 10 years, who had had birthweights of ≤1500g. 33 (60 per cent) were considered to have abnormal records, in contrast to only 6 per cent of fullterm infants studied longitudinally by one of the co-authors. Of these 33 with abnormal EEGs, six had no abnormality other than 6- and 14-per-second spikes during sleep, and nowadays these might be passed as normal. Nonetheless, the residual proportion of abnormal records in this weight-group was strikingly high. Fráter and Wohlmuth (1965) examined the EEGs of 140 children at six to seven years who had been 'prematurely born': 62 per cent were considered to show abnormal features. These included occipital slow-waves, occasionally only after hyperventilation, and again the criteria of abnormality were somewhat arguable, but the high proportion of abnormal records was noteworthy.

With regard to neonatal EEG patterns in general, some authors have noted the prognostic significance of distinctly abnormal features in infants with prenatal illness or perinatal brain-insults (Schulte and Herrmann 1965, Karch *et al.* 1977, Watanabe *et al.* 1980), or with neonatal convulsions (Tibbles and Prichard 1965, Rose and Lombroso 1970, Ellison *et al.* 1981, Holmes *et al.* 1982). On the other hand, Ellingson *et al.* (1964), Torres and Blaw (1968) and Bergman *et al.* (1983) found that *routine* neonatal EEGs had no significant prognostic value for subsequent clinical development. In a 'premature' group, Ellingson *et al.* (1964) noted that so-called suspicious features in the neonatal EEG appeared to be as common among normally as among abnormally developing children. The authors concluded that such features might better be considered signs of immaturity than of pathology.

These conflicting findings have been clarified to some extent by more detailed analysis. Monod and associates had noted in 1962 that many abnormalities of the neonatal EEG resolved by the second trimester of life, but that severe abnormalities, like irregular suppression-burst patterns ('tracé paroxystique') were liable to lead on to continuing abnormal patterns (Monod and Dreyfus-Brisac 1962, Monod *et al.* 1962). All the markedly abnormal records at three to six months belonged to infants who also had had grossly abnormal EEGs at birth. Similarly, Schulte and Herrmann (1965) concluded that inactive EEGs, repeated paroxysms, and continuous theta or delta sharp-wave activity were severe neonatal abnormalities with mostly poor outcome, and that unilateral or localized depression of voltage persisting over several days also had an adverse prognosis. However, low-voltage records, transient sharp and slow waves, and abnormal rhythmicity had little prognostic significance. Subsequently, Monod *et al.* (1972) analyzed 691 neonatal EEGs of 270 children whose course was followed for from three to 14 years. They concluded that the following features in the neonatal EEG were related to subsequent abnormal development:

(1) inactive EEGs (voltage continuously below 5μv);

(2) irregular suppression bursts ('tracé paroxystique');

(3) continuous and diffuse delta-waves at 0.5 to 1Hz;

(4) low-voltage EEGs (maximal 25μv during quiet sleep) if persisting after the second week in fullterm babies or if combined with abnormal patterns;

(5) monorhythmic records without change in amplitude or shape of pattern;

(6) absence of spatial organization or occipital activity if persisting after the second week;

(7) gross asymmetry and asynchrony between the two hemispheres during the first two weeks in fullterm babies;

(8) abnormal superimposed patterns, *e.g.* bursts of monomorphic sharp frontal transients after the first week in fullterm babies, and non-Rolandic alpha-like rhythms during the first month;

(9) focal spikes, especially if persisting for at least two weeks;

(10) clinical seizures without paroxysmal electrical discharges.

On the other hand, diffuse synchronous bursts of sharp waves and abundant non-Rolandic theta were not considered significant, and non-focal spikes were even assessed as prognostically favourable. Like Harris and Tizard (1960), Monod and co-workers thought that inter-ictal discharges had more prognostic significance than the record during seizures. They concluded that neonatal EEGs could give useful information for fullterm or preterm babies but primarily for predicting a severely unfavourable outcome: 'Very few EEG patterns raise the probability of minor sequelae, and only in fullterm babies'.

In 1981 Tharp and co-workers revised these statements slightly with respect to preterm infants. From a retrospective analysis of 184 neonatal EEGs of 81 infants born at or before 36 weeks gestation, and subsequent clinical examinations of 64 survivors, they concluded that 'a single recording was of prognostic value only if it was markedly abnormal'. EEGs were classified as markedly abnormal if they contained at least one of the following patterns: isoelectric or paroxysmal background; positive Rolandic sharp-waves; electrographic seizures; marked interhemispheric voltage asymmetry (>50 per cent) or asynchrony; excessively slow background with reduction or absence of patterns expected at the particular conceptional age. Moderately abnormal features like low voltage with normal background, with asymmetry of less than 50 per cent or with asynchrony, and low voltage posteriorly with poorly developed occipital activity, were not thought to be of significant prognostic value.

The value of the serial study of maturation from the neonatal EEG has already been noted. Several authors found that persistent severe dysmaturity in relation to conceptional age during the first few months was liable to be associated with subsequent mental retardation or motor dysfunction (Lombroso 1975, Tharp *et al.* 1981, Ellison *et al.* 1982). Such serial investigations may include observation of the spindle-like fast rhythms in LBW infants (Watanabe and Iwase 1972), which Lombroso (1975) calls 'brushes'. He warned that disruption or dysmaturity in such bioelectric patterns may be temporary and may be seen not only in newborns with diseases of the central nervous system, but also in those with systemic disease.

Methods of EEG polygraphy have also been refined. For example, the behavioural 'state' of the infant at the time of the recording has to be noted (Anders *et al.* 1971, Michaelis *et al.* 1972, Prechtl *et al.* 1973, Prechtl 1974). The mechanism maintaining quiet (non-REM) sleep appears to be particularly vulnerable in the immature brain (Schulte *et al.* 1971), and ideally the EEG should include periods of both quiet and active sleep. Lombroso (1981) finds that lability or absence of recognizable states in the neonatal period, as well as persistence of early neonatal states during the first year, are likely to be associated with abnormal neurological outcome.

Further, evoked potentials may be helpful in demonstrating brain injury. For instance, absence of waves IV and V from the brainstem auditory evoked responses may indicate involvement of auditory pathways in asphyxia (Lütschg *et al.* 1980), although such absence may be reversible (Perlman *et al.* 1983). Mapping of brain electrical activity (BEAM), including a topographic display of evoked potentials in sequences of time, frequency and space, has come into use as a promising technique (Duffy *et al.* 1979). Neonatal EEG abnormalities also can be weighted according to their severity and combined with other variables in a scoring system. Multiple regression analyses can then be used to predict neurological abnormality (Ellison *et al.* 1981).

Material and method

As previously described, 501 children with birthweights ≤2041g were admitted to the study as newborns between 1959 and 1965, and 203 control infants with a similar social-class distribution who weighed >2500g at birth in the same hospital were also followed (see Chapter 2). All surviving children had reached school-age by 1972.

The protocol called for all the LBW infants to have 'late neonatal' EEGS recorded after completion of incubator treatment and before discharge from the nursery, but for various reasons this was not always accomplished. It was also planned that both LBW and FBW control children would have further EEGS at about

TABLE 13-I

Results of EEGs

	Total	*Normal*	*Borderline*	*Abnormal*	*Borderline plus abnormal*
LBW children					
Nursery records	276	202	44	30 (10.9%)	26.8%
6 mths to 2 yrs	222	181	23	18 (8.1%)	18.5%
5½ to 8 yrs	251	138	17	96 (38.2%)	45.0%
FBW control children					
6 mths to 2 yrs	99	97	2	—	2.0%
5½ to 8 yrs	117	88	7	22 (18.8%)	24.8%

LBW vs. *FBW*
6 mths-2 yrs: normal *vs.* borderline *vs.* abnormal—$\chi^2 = 16.28$, $p<0.001$; normal *vs.* borderline + abnormal—$\chi^2 = 13.06$, $p<0.001$.
5½-8 yrs: normal *vs.* borderline *vs.* abnormal—$\chi^2 = 14.8$, $p<0.001$; normal *vs.* borderline + abnormal —$\chi^2 = 8.11$, $p<0.01$.

TABLE 13-II

Abnormal EEG features in 'late neonatal' records of LBW children

Low amplitude (less than 25μV, even during quiet sleep)	12
Abnormal rhythm:	
Runs of bisynchronous slow waves, often of high voltage (>200μV)	15
'Alphoid' spindles	1
Excessive fast activity	1
Persistent excessive 'tracé alternant' at conceptional age of 40 and 41 wks	2
Little difference between waking and sleeping patterns at 36 and 38 wks conceptional age	2
Marked asymmetry	15
Focal abnormalities:	
Intermittent sharp waves	32
Intermittent spikes	12
Intermittent slow waves	5
Suppression bursts ('tracé paroxystique')	1

TABLE 13-III

'Late neonatal' EEGs of 276 LBW infants

	N	*Normal*	*Borderline*	*Abnormal*	χ^2	*p*
Preterm AGA	159	119 (74.8%)	26 (16.4%)	14 (8.8%)	1.84	NS
SGA	100	69 (69.0%)	17 (17.0%)	14 (14.0%)		
LGA	3	3	—	—		
Uncertain gestational age	14	11	1	2		
Total	276	202	44	30		

one and 6½ years, but many parents were reluctant to permit this, others had moved away, and about 15 per cent of the LBW infants had died during the first year. Of the LBW children, 276 had a total of 283 EEGS recorded in the nursery at a mean chronological age of 38.5 days (SD 21.4 days) and at a mean conceptional age of 39 weeks (SD 3.7 weeks); 222 had a total of 235 EEGS at a mean chronological age of 12.75 months (SD 3.2 months; range six months to two years); and 251 had a total of 260 EEGS at about 6¾ years (mean 81.4 months, SD 5.1 months; range 5½ to eight years). Another 73 EEGS were recorded at other age-levels, *e.g.* because of seizures, or when a child returned to our area after moving away. A full set of three records was available for analysis for 153 children, and at least two traces at the designated times were available for another 92.

Among the FBW controls, 99 children provided 103 EEGS at about one year (mean 14.8 months, SD 2.3 months), and 117 children had 118 EEGS recorded at about 6¾ years (mean 80 months, SD 4.2 months). Only another two records were obtained at other ages, since they were rarely indicated. A pair of EEGS at the intended time-periods (about one and 6¾ years) was available for 76 control children.

In all cases eight-channel EEGS were recorded with 19 electrodes in the standard international 10-20 system positions. In the newborn period and at one year needle electrodes were used; at 6¾ years cup electrodes usually were attached with Bentonite paste or Grass electrode paste. Photic stimulation was routine, and hyperventilation was used at 6¾ years. Sleep records were obtained for approximately 80 per cent of the neonates, 90 per cent of infants at one year and 73 per cent of children at 6¾ years. Nearly all EEGS were interpreted by one of two readers (N.L.A. or M.D.L.).

For purposes of analysis the LBW children were grouped according to their weight and gestational age at birth. The first category were preterm AGA and the second were preterm or term SGA. The third and fourth categories contained quite small numbers; they comprised those who were large for gestational age (LGA) and those whose gestational age could not be stated with certainty. About three-quarters of the FBW control children had a normal birthweight at term, but as one would expect about 10 per cent were SGA and LGA, respectively, though they all had birthweights exceeding 2500g.

Other groupings also were considered, *e.g.* according to social class, IQ and ultimate neurological status. Social class was defined by the Hollingshead Two-factor Index (1957), and IQ at 6¾ years by the Full-scale score of the Wechsler Intelligence Scale for Children (WISC).

Results

Neonatal records

Of the 276 LBW children who had 'late neonatal' EEGS close to term after incubator treatment, 202 were considered to have normal traces, 44 had borderline and 30 had abnormal records (Table 13-I). Thus about 27 per cent were borderline or abnormal. The abnormal features are listed in Table 13-II. Random non-focal sharp waves were not considered abnormal. Several records contained more than one type of abnormality, so the number of abnormal features in Table 13-II is greater than the combined number of abnormal and borderline records. It should be noted, also, that the EEGS were obtained at a mean chronological age of 5½ weeks and after cessation of incubator care; by that time many of the sick LBW infants had died. This may explain why the more severe and ominous abnormalities like inactive traces or *continuous* theta or delta sharp-wave activity (Schulte and Herrmann 1965) were not seen in our series, and 'tracé paroxystique' was observed only once.

Comparing the frequency of abnormal records of 'AGA preterm', SGA and LGA LBW neonates, we obtained the analysis shown in Table 13-III. It can be seen that the SGA infants had a slightly higher frequency of abnormal records than preterm AGA infants, but the difference is not significant.

EEGs at about one year

At about one year (six months to two years) chronological age, 222 LBW children had EEGS recorded. Of these, 181 were considered normal, 23 borderline and only 18 (8.1 per cent) distinctly abnormal (see Table 13-I). The total frequency of borderline plus abnormal records was 18.5 per cent. The abnormal features are listed in Table 13-IV. Again, several records contained more than one type of abnormality, so the total number of abnormal features is greater than the combined number of abnormal and borderline records.

In comparison, none of the 99 FBW control children who had EEGS recorded at about one year had distinctly abnormal traces, and only two had borderline records (see Table 13-I). One of these appeared to be diffusely somewhat slow for the age of 13 months, with background activity mostly at 4HZ in what appeared to be an alert state. The other had possible spike and wave discharges from the right central region and bursts of somewhat sharp slow-waves of high voltage during drowsiness.

When the frequency of abnormal records for AGA preterm, SGA and LGA LBW infants at about one year was analyzed, again there was no significant difference between the first two categories.

EEGs at about 6¾ years

Between 5½ and eight years, 251 LBW children had EEGS recorded. Of these, 138 were considered normal, 17 borderline and 96 (38.2 per cent) distinctly abnormal (see Table 13-I). The total frequency of borderline plus abnormal records was no less than 45 per cent.

In comparison, among the records of 117 FBW control children, 88 were considered normal, seven borderline and 22 (18.8 per cent) distinctly abnormal. The total frequency of borderline plus abnormal records was 24.8 per cent, *i.e.* significantly lower than for the LBW children ($p<0.01$). Further, the proportion of paroxysmal discharges (focal or generalized spikes or spike and wave) among the *abnormal* records was significantly lower for the controls than for the LBW children ($p<0.02$) (Table 13-V).

Among the 96 LBW children with distinctly abnormal EEGS, 40 (41.7 per cent) had definite spike and/or spike and wave discharges, compared with only six

TABLE 13-IV

Abnormal features in EEGs of LBW infants at about 1 year

Low amplitude	1
Abnormal rhythmicity:	
Excessive diffuse slow activity	5
Bursts of slow waves at ⩾4Hz	3
Bursts of slow waves at <4Hz	1
Abnormal sigma activity	6
Consistent asymmetry:	
Mild (25-50%)	11
Moderate (55-75%)	4
Scattered non-persistent sharp waves	2
Spike and/or spike and wave discharges:	
Bisynchronous 0.5-4Hz spike and wave complexes	
abortive or only on photic stimulation	3
during sleep only	1
multiple, spontaneous, without sleep	1
Focal spike or spike and wave discharges	3
Multifocal (⩾3) spike and wave discharges	1

TABLE 13-V

EEG abnormalities at about 6¾ years

	LBW children (N = 251)		*FBW controls (N = 117)*		χ^2	*p*
Low amplitude		1		—		
Abnormal rhythmicity:						
Excessive diffuse slow activity	31		7			
Excessive bi-occipital slow activity	6		3			
Excessive persistence of slowing after hyperventilation	3		1			
Paroxysmal or sharp response to hyperventilation	7		—			
Bisynchronous bursts of slow waves at ⩾4Hz	14		2			
Bisynchronous bursts of slow waves at <4Hz	9		2			
Fast activity with amplitude >50μV	5		3			
Abnormal sigma activity	3		—			
Mild dysrhythmia or monorhythmic record	16	94	4	22	7.7	<0.01
Consistent mild asymmetry (25-50%)		8		2		
Sharp waves:						
Scattered, non-persistent	5		—			
Focal	9	14	4	4	0.05	NS
Slow waves, focal at ⩽4Hz		—		1		
Spike and/or spike and wave discharges:						
Bisynchronous <4Hz spike and wave complexes						
abortive or only on photic stimulation	13		—			
during sleep and/or drowsiness only	9		1			
spontaneous, without sleep	3		—			
nearly continuous	1		—			
Scattered non-persistent spikes	1		—			
Focal spike or spike and wave discharges	15		5			
Multifocal (>3) spike and wave discharges	—	42*	—	6**		

*_i.e._ in 37.2% of 113 abnormal and borderline records of LBW children
**_i.e._ in 20.7% of 29 abnormal and borderline records of FBW controls
} $\chi^2 = 5.84$, $p<0.02$

TABLE 13-VI

EEGs of 117 FBW control children at about 6¾ years

	N	*Normal*	*Borderline*	*Abnormal*
AGA	89	71	5	13
SGA	11	6	—	5
LGA	9	5	2	2
Uncertain gestational age	8	6	—	2
Total	117	88 (75.2%)	7 (6%)	22 (18.8%)

TABLE 13-VII

Neonatal EEGs *vs.* neurological status and IQ at 6¾ years

		Neurological status			*IQ*			
	N	*Normal*	*Abnormal*	*Unknown*	*≥90*	*<90*	*Unknown*	*Mean IQ (when known)*
Neonatal EEG								
Normal	202	94	73	35	103	60	39	93.7
Borderline	44	18	24	2	30	11	3	93.5
Abnormal	30	16	7	7	11	10	9	88.4

(27.3 per cent) of the 22 FBW control children with abnormal records. It may be noted in passing that only seven of these 46 children with paroxysmal discharges had had clinical seizures.

When the frequency of abnormal records for AGA preterm, SGA and LGA LBW infants at about 6¾ years was compared, again there was no significant difference between the first two categories.

With regard to the FBW control children, the most common unusual EEG features were mild abnormalities of background rhythm, such as excessive diffuse slow-activity for the child's age, mild fast dysrhythmia and excessively mono-rhythmic records. In this respect the control children resembled the LBW group. It is also notable that about 5 per cent (six of 117) of the controls had spike or spike and wave discharges at 6¾ years. Further, when the FBW children were divided into percentile groups for birthweight related to gestational age, the results were as shown in Table 13-VI. Nine of the 20 children whose birthweights were known to be above 2500g but at and above the 90th or at and below the 10th percentiles for gestational age had abnormal or borderline records. This proportion of 45 per cent contrasts with only 20.2 per cent (18 of 89) when birthweights corresponded to gestational age ($p<0.05$).

Correlation of neonatal and subsequent EEGs

When the results of the EEGs in the nursery were compared with those at about one year of age for the same infants, the following correlations emerged: (1) of 147 normal 'late neonatal' EEGs, 126 remained normal, 13 became borderline and eight became abnormal; (2) of 33 borderline 'late neonatal' records, 24 became normal, five remained borderline and four became abnormal; (3) of 21 abnormal 'late neonatal' records, 16 became normal, three became borderline and two remained abnormal.

It is evident that most of the suspicious and abnormal features in the EEGs of newborns tended to subside. Individual analysis of the exceptions usually showed no consistent features. However, one boy's very late record (at 59 weeks conceptional age and five months chronological age) was grossly abnormal. There was spontaneous paroxysmal activity from all head regions, consisting of slow waves of high amplitude in varying frequencies, often associated with both single and multiple spikes, both synchronous and asynchronous. Similar activity during sleep assumed a suppression-burst pattern. This abnormal pattern persisted at six months and at 1½ years, and the boy proved to have an organic convulsive disorder, with profound mental retardation. Another boy's recording showed an amplitude asymmetry (higher on the right) at a chronological age of 6½ weeks (conceptional age 44 weeks). This was confirmed at the age of eight months, when the sleep spindles also were of higher voltage on the right side. Later this child developed epilepsy and had focal sharp and slow waves, chiefly in the left parieto-occipital region. One other boy was noted to have a borderline normal record of somewhat low amplitude at six weeks (conceptional age 40 weeks) and again at 14 months. Later he proved to have minimal brain dysfunction and he had an abnormal EEG with semi-rhythmic runs of theta frequency in both temporal leads at 6 years 5 months.

We also checked whether any abnormalities in the nursery record could be correlated with abnormalities in the trace at 6¾ years, even when the intervening record at about one year was normal. In seven cases an abnormality in the nursery record could have re-emerged at 6¾ years, but there was no consistent pattern.

Correlation of neonatal EEG with neurological status and IQ at 6¾ years

The results of the analysis of 'late neonatal' EEGs in relation to subsequent neurological defects and IQ level are shown in Table 13-VII. About 44 per cent of LBW children with normal neonatal EEGs and known outcome were neurologically abnormal at 6¾ years, compared to 48 per cent of LBW children with borderline or abnormal neonatal EEGs. It is evident that the neonatal EEG has little prognostic significance, though grossly abnormal records may be an exception to this rule. If the individual abnormal features of the EEG are analyzed separately, their prognostic value also appears to be very doubtful. Figure 13-1 might suggest that neonatal records of low amplitude are liable to indicate later abnormal neurological status, while the other abnormal features are just as consistent with subsequent normal neurological function as are normal EEGs. Figure 13-2 seems to indicate that even neonatal records of low amplitude are not likely to be associated with any marked subsequent lowering of intelligence, and that intermittent focal sharp or slow waves or spikes might even be favourable features (as suggested for some forms by Monod *et al.* 1972). However, the numbers clearly are too small to draw any definite conclusions.

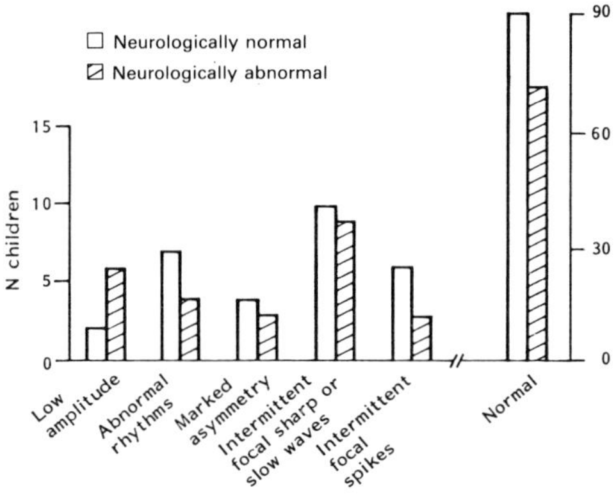

Fig. 13-1. Neonatal EEGs of LBW children and neurological follow-up at 5½ to 8 years.

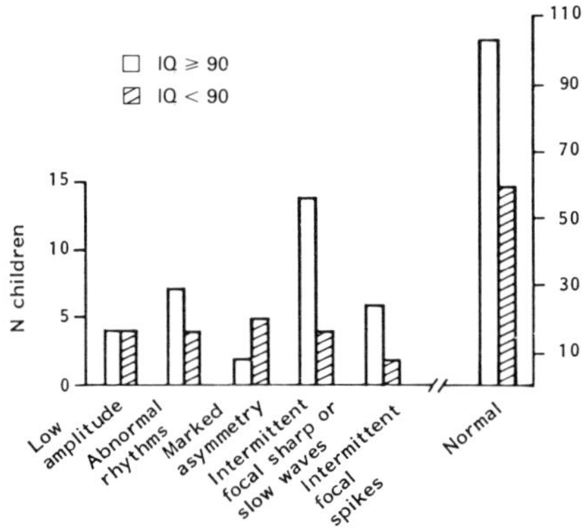

Fig. 13-2. Neonatal EEGs of LBW children and WISC Full-scale IQ at 5½ to 8 years.

Correlation of EEG at about one and 6¾ years

When the EEGS of individual LBW children at about one and 6¾ years were compared, the following correlations emerged: (1) of 137 normal EEGS at about one year, 85 remained normal, four changed to borderline and 48 became abnormal; (2) of 18 borderline EEGS at about one year, five became normal, one remained borderline and 12 became abnormal; (3) of 10 abnormal EEGS at about one year, two became normal, one became borderline and seven remained abnormal.

Thus more than 60 per cent of normal EEGS at one year remained normal, whereas seven of 10 abnormal records remained abnormal. Therefore abnormal records at one year have a much more serious significance than abnormal 'late neonatal' EEGS. The records of children who had had spike or spike and wave discharges at about one year never became normal when repeated at about 6¾ years.

Among the control children, one of the two who had a borderline record at about one year unfortunately moved away and was lost to follow-up. The other had a record which was diffusely somewhat slow, with a dominant rhythm around 4HZ

TABLE 13-VIII

EEGs at about 1 year *vs.* neurological status and IQ at 6¾ years

		Neurological status			*IQ*			
	N	*Normal*	*Abnormal*	*Unknown*	*≥90*	*<90*	*Unknown*	*Mean IQ (when known)*
LBW children:								
EEG normal	181	97 (57.4%)	72	12	109	55	17	94.3
EEG borderline	23	9	12	2	14	7	2	93.4
EEG abnormal	18	2	12	4*	5	8	5	71.3
FBW controls:								
EEG normal	97	77 (90.6%)	8	12	82	—	15	109.7

*One of these died of obstructive hydrocephalus, with delayed behavioural development, at 11 months.

and only small amounts of 5 to 6Hz activity. This infant proved to be mentally retarded, and the later record at 6 years 7 months again was diffusely somewhat slow for the child's age.

Correlation of EEG at about one year with neurological status and IQ at 6¾ years
The results of analysis of EEGS at about one year in relation to subsequent neurological status and IQ level are shown in Table 13-VIII. The normality of the EEG at about one year correlated well with neurological status of LBW children at 6¾ years, and later mean IQ was significantly higher for children with a normal EEG than for those with an abnormal EEG at one year ($t = 4.25$, $p<0.0005$). However, it is also clear that the proportion of children with later normal neurological status among those with a normal EEG at one year was significantly greater among the FBW controls than the LBW children ($p<0.001$), and that later mean IQ also was significantly higher among the FBW controls than the LBW children with normal EEGS at about one year ($t = 7.41$, $p<0.0005$). If a child with a birthweight <2041g had a normal EEG at about one year, there was a nearly 60 per cent chance (97 of 169, *i.e.* 57 per cent) of being neurologically intact at 6¾ years. A child of normal birthweight (>2500g) with a normal EEG at one year in our control series had a chance of about 90 per cent (77 of 85, *i.e.* 90.6 per cent) of being neurologically intact later. Similarly, LBW children with a normal or borderline EEG at one year were likely to have a Full-scale WISC IQ score of about 94 at 6¾ years, compared to a mean score of 110 for controls with normal EEGS.

It will also be noted that an LBW child with an abnormal EEG at one year was likely to be a 'slow learner' later, if not actually retarded. When all the cases of moderate to profound mental retardation (IQ <50) among the LBW children were excluded from the analysis, there was still a notable difference between the subsequent mean Full-scale WISC IQ scores, *i.e.* 95.5 for those with a normal EEG at one year and 81 for those with an abnormal EEG.

Three of the 18 children with an abnormal EEG at about one year were lost to follow-up. 13 of the remaining 15 proved to be neurologically abnormal: one died of obstructive hydrocephalus and had delayed behavioural development; two had an organic convulsive disorder with mental retardation; three had non-specific

TABLE 13-IX

EEGs at about 6¾ years *vs.* neurological status and IQ level

	Neurological status at 6¾ yrs			*IQ at 6¾ yrs*			
	N	*Normal*	*Abnormal*	*≥90*	*<90*	*Unknown*	*Mean IQ (when known)*
LBW children:							
EEG normal	138	93 (67.4%)	45	106	31	1	99.7
EEG borderline	17	10	7	14	3	—	100.9
EEG abnormal	96	40	56 (58.3%)	45	50	1	86.9
FBW controls:							
EEG normal	88	83 (94.3%)	5	87	1		108.6
EEG borderline	7	5	2	7	—		102.9
EEG abnormal	22	15	7 (31.8%)	19	3		105.5

mental retardation; one was autistic, probably due to an organic encephalopathy; three had mild brain dysfunction (following idiopathic hypoglycaemia in one case); two had cerebral palsy (asymmetrical spastic diplegia, left spastic hemiparesis); and one had nerve-deafness. Only two developed normally.

Correlation of EEG at about 6¾ years with neurological status and IQ

Results of the analysis of EEGs at about 6¾ years in relation to neurological status and IQ at the same age are shown in Table 13-IX. Here again, there was close correlation between normality of the EEG and neurological status and IQ. As would be expected, the correlation is even closer ($p<0.001$) than that between EEG at about one year and the later neurological status and IQ ($p<0.01$).

Interestingly, an abnormal EEG appears to be more significantly associated with abnormal neurological status and lowered IQ among the LBW children than the FBW controls. If a child with a birthweight <2041g had a normal EEG at 6¾ years, the chance of neurological normality was about 67 per cent, whereas a control child of normal birthweight and with a normal EEG had a 94 per cent chance of neurological integrity. If the EEG was distinctly abnormal, the LBW child had a 58 per cent chance of neurological abnormality; for FBW controls the chance was less than 32 per cent. Also, for the LBW children an abnormal EEG at 6¾ years was liable to be associated with a significant lowering of IQ (from a mean of about 100 to about 87; $t = 5.57$, $p<0.0005$), while no such significant reduction occurred among FBW controls with an abnormal EEG.

Minimal brain dysfunctions (MBD)

Since minimal brain dysfunctions are the most common neurological abnormality in our follow-up study of LBW children, we analyzed the EEGs of children with this syndrome at 6¾ years. Among the LBW children with MBD, 55 had EEGs recorded at that age, and the FBW controls with MBD supplied another eight.

Table 13-X shows the results of this analysis. The findings are consistent with the view that about half the children with MBD have an abnormal EEG (Capute *et al.* 1968). The frequency of abnormal EEGs is also significantly higher for each

TABLE 13-X

EEGs at about 6¾ years *vs.* minimal brain dysfunctions

	N	*Normal*	*Borderline*	*Abnormal*	*% Borderline plus abnormal with MBD*		*% Borderline plus abnormal in neurologically normal children (Table 13-IX)*	χ^2	*p*
LBW children	55	25	8	22	54.5	$\chi^2 = 1.33$, NS	35.0	6.88	0.05
FBW controls	8	2	2	4	75.0		19.4	13.21	<0.005
Total	63	27	10	26	57.1		28.5	19.05	<0.005

TABLE 13-XI

EEGs at about 6¾ years *vs.* sensorineural hearing-loss

	N	*Normal*	*Borderline*	*Abnormal*	*% Borderline plus abnormal with hearing-loss*	*% Borderline plus abnormal in neurologically normal children (Table 13-IX)*	χ^2	*p*
LBW children:								
Sensorineural hearing-loss	7	3	1	3	57.1	35.0	8.96	<0.01
Min. high-frequency loss	16	10	1	5	37.5			
Total	23	13	2	8	43.5	35.0	0.05	NS
FBW controls:								
Min. high-frequency loss	9	5	—	4	44.4	19.4	13.26	<0.001
Total	32	18	2	12	43.75	28.5	4.40	<0.05

birthweight category than for children who are neurologically normal. However, it must be admitted that this is a somewhat circular argument, since an abnormal EEG contributes to the diagnosis of MBD. The matter is discussed further in Chapter 15.

Sensorineural hearing-defect

Since sensorineural hearing-loss frequently is due to 'brain damage', as from cerebral anoxia or mild kernicterus (see Chapter 9), we analyzed the frequency of associated EEG abnormalities. The group with hearing defects included those with significant sensorineural hearing-loss and those with minimal high-frequency loss. 23 LBW children and nine FBW controls with such hearing losses had EEGs recorded at about 6¾ years (Table 13-XI). Compared to neurologically normal LBW children, the frequency of borderline and abnormal EEGs is significantly higher among children with sensorineural hearing-defects, but not in LBW children with only minimal high-frequency loss.

Strabismus

Since strabismus may be 'neurogenic' and is liable to be associated with clumsiness (Alberman *et al.* 1971) and abnormal EEG (Levinson *et al.* 1951, Stillerman *et al.* 1952), we analyzed the frequency of EEG abnormalities in children with strabismus. 39 LBW and six FBW control children with strabismus had EEGs recorded at about 6¾ years. These could be compared with the results for 229 LBW and 110 FBW control children without strabismus (Table 13-XII). The greater frequency of abnormal and borderline EEGs of the children with strabismus is statistically significant in the LBW group, and even more so in the total series.

EEG abnormalities and social class

EEG abnormalities were examined to see whether their frequency varied with social class (Table 13-XIII). The differences in the frequency of normal records between social classes were not significant, except between classes I to IV (inclusive) and class V among the FBW controls ($p<0.05$). The frequency of normal EEGs is significantly higher in the FBW controls than in LBW children in the total of all social classes ($p<0.001$), and in social-class IV alone ($p<0.01$).

Discussion

As we reported earlier (Dunn *et al.* 1973), one of the main findings of this study is that minor abnormalities in the routine neonatal EEGs of LBW children have very little prognostic significance. This agrees with the conclusion of Monod and colleagues (Monod *et al.* 1972, Tharp *et al.* 1981). It is possible, however, that serial records and more refined techniques of EEG polygraphy may yield more predictive information. As discussed earlier, the infants in our study had EEGs recorded only after completion of incubator treatment (at a mean chronological age of 5½ weeks, and thus near term), so their EEGs are described as 'late neonatal'. The frequency of grossly abnormal EEGs is highest in the first week and becomes progressively less during the first month after birth (Schulte 1966, Monod and Ducas 1968), and many LBW infants with such records die during that time. This may explain why so few

TABLE 13-XII

EEGs at about 6¾ years of children with and without strabismus

	N	*Normal*	*Borderline*	*Abnormal*	*% Borderline plus abnormal*	χ^2	*p*
LBW children:							
with strabismus	39	17	6	16	56.4	6.995	<0.05
without strabismus	229	130	11	88	43.2		
FBW controls:							
with strabismus	6	3	1	2			
without strabismus	110	84	6	20			
Total series:							
with strabismus	45	20	7	18	55.6	10.14	<0.01
without strabismus	339	214	17	108	36.9		

TABLE 13-XIII

EEG *vs.* social class at about 6¾ years

Social class	*LBW children* *N*	*EEG Normal* *N*	*%*	*Borderline + abnormal* *N*	*%*	*FBW controls* *N*	*EEG Normal* *N*	*%*	*Borderline + abnormal* *N*	*%*
I, II and III	61	36	59.0	25	41.0	22	18	81.8	4	18.2
IV	101	61	60.4	40	39.6	53	44	83.0	9	17.0
V	109	52	47.7	57	52.3	42	27	64.3	15	35.7
Total	271	149	55.0	122	45.0	117	89	76.1	28	23.9

babies in our series had any severe abnormalities in their neonatal EEGs. The main groups of abnormalities were intermittent unusual focal-wave forms (sharp waves, spikes or slow waves) in 49 cases, abnormal rhythms in 21, marked asymmetry in 15, and low amplitude in 12 (see Table 13-II). Nearly all these abnormalities had resolved by the age of one year, and the individual abnormal features did not correlate with subsequent abnormal neurological status, with the possible exception of low amplitude (see Fig. 13-1). Ellingson *et al.* (1964) also found that 'suspicious' features in the neonatal EEGs of 'premature' infants were of no consequence. However, depressed background activity in fullterm newborns with perinatal hypoxia was emphasized by Watanabe *et al.* (1980), who found it to have greater adverse prognostic significance than paroxysmal EEG abnormalities. Lombroso (1981) also reported that focal discharges were not significantly ominous unless background activity was depressed or otherwise abnormal.

Monod and colleagues (1972) reported that moderate or even gross asymmetry in neonatal EEGs of preterm infants, and low-voltage records in themselves, had no unfavourable prognostic significance, and that some forms of spikes even appeared to be associated with a favourable outcome. Those authors also noted that diffuse synchronous or localized high-voltage or sharp bursts with normal or subnormal background activity were not prognostically unfavourable. On the other hand, they emphasized the more ominous features listed earlier, which they and others had encountered, particularly in sick babies (Harris and Tizard 1960, Schulte and

Herrmann 1965, Janzen *et al.* 1968, Monod and Ducas 1968). These more severe abnormalities were not seen in our 'late neonatal' records, except for 'tracé paroxystique' in one infant who first had an EEG five months after birth.

We appreciated the importance of obtaining sleep records to detect abnormal electrical phenomena in the newborn (Anderson and Gibbs 1970). However, our EEG recordings mostly were completed by the end of 1972, so the advances in technique since then were only rarely used. Differences between active and quiet sleep in infancy were not analyzed in detail, and serial neonatal records were rarely obtained. Neither were evoked potentials studied. It is probable that persistent focal (and particularly multifocal) discharges on serial tracings for LBW infants are more significant than isolated discharges (Lombroso 1981, Holmes *et al.* 1982, Scher *et al.* 1982).

Monod and associates (1962) investigated the EEG during the second trimester after birth. They found that anomalies are rare during this period, that children who developed normally very rarely showed any significant abnormality at that age, and that major abnormalities in a neonatal record usually persisted and carried a very severe prognosis. We did not obtain EEGs routinely at three to six months, but the one infant who had a grossly abnormal paroxysmal record at five months did very poorly: he had an organic convulsive disorder and profound mental retardation. However, for two other infants in that age-range with abnormal EEGs, the neonatal abnormalities resolved and they did quite well.

Laubichler (1970) analyzed clinical and EEG findings for 104 infants who were at risk for brain damage (*e.g.* after birth asphyxia or encephalitis). They found that whereas the EEG was abnormal in about 60 per cent during the first six months and showed a correlation between hemisyndromes and one-sided or focal EEG changes, it was abnormal in 85 per cent of the infants in the second half of the first year (*i.e.* significantly more often) and showed even better correlation with the clinical findings in distinguishing between unilateral and bilateral anomalies. Hypsarhythmia also was seen only in the second half of the first year. Therefore the second half of the first year may be a more useful period than the second trimester for the prognostic evaluation of EEGs.

Our own experience relates to the prognostic value of EEGs recorded at about 13 months (SD 3.2 months), and there is no doubt of their usefulness at that age. Of 222 LBW children, only 18 (8.1 per cent) had abnormal records and 23 (10.4 per cent) had borderline records. Of the 18 with abnormal records, three were lost to follow-up, one died soon afterwards of obstructive hydrocephalus (with delayed behavioural development) and 12 of the remaining 14 had neurological defects at their final evaluation at 6¾ years. The mean Full-scale WISC IQ score was also significantly depressed in the 13 survivors tested. With regard to the abnormal features of the EEG at about 13 months, it is evident that abnormal spindle (sigma) activity was of little consequence, whereas, for the records available, spike or spike and wave discharges were always followed by abnormal neurological status and EEG at 6¾ years. Dreyfus-Brisac and colleagues (Dreyfus-Brisac *et al.* 1962, Dreyfus-Brisac and Monod 1966) have emphasized the gravity of the clinical significance of focal spikes appearing between one month and two years, and particularly before one year. An exception is frontal spikes: sometimes these are seen in normal children (Monod and Ducas 1968), and Petersen *et al.* (1968) noted a relatively high frequency of focal spikes or sharp waves occurring only during sleep in normal infants of less than six months.

At about 6¾ years, the frequency of abnormal EEGs among 251 LBW children in our study was 38 per cent, which was twice as high as the frequency (18 per cent) for 117 FBW control children. The total proportion of abnormal plus borderline records in the LBW children was 45 per cent; *i.e.* nearly one-half of school entrants with birthweights <2041g had an EEG which was not quite normal. Most of the abnormal features were disturbances of rhythm, including paroxysmal patterns, as has been found in children with behaviour disorders and without epilepsy (Kennard and Willner 1947, Stevens *et al.* 1968, Stevens and Milstein 1970). However, the frequency of focal or generalized spike or spike and wave discharges among the abnormal records was also significantly higher than for the FBW control children. Dreyfus-Brisac and Monod (1966) also found spike foci commonly in the EEGs of the older ex-premature children, and noted that nearly one-quarter of the children with such foci appeared to be clinically normal. The foci had arisen at the age of three years or later and were liable to disappear spontaneously; epilepsy rarely developed. Those investigators found it hard to say whether the spikes were of an organic ('lésionnel') or functional nature. Petersen *et al.* (1968) found focal spikes or sharp waves in the resting EEGs of 15 normal children, but the maximum frequency was less than 5 per cent at six to seven years, whereas in our material focal sharp-waves, spikes and spike and wave complexes occurred in 24 out of 251 children (9.6 per cent). Bisynchronous spike and wave discharges with a frequency of less than 4Hz also occurred spontaneously in many of our cases. The prevalence during sleep was less than the 12 per cent found in normal children of four to seven years by Petersen *et al.* (1968), and might be considered a physiological phenomenon (Monod and Ducas 1968). However, three of our patients had multiple spontaneous discharges of this type even when not sleeping, and in one other case they were almost continuous, so that they could hardly be considered 'normal' in these four children. The total frequency of paroxysmal features in the EEGs of our children can be calculated as 67 out of 251, *i.e.* more than one-quarter and thus significantly higher than the 15 per cent calculated by Eeg-Olofsson (1970) for normal children ($p<0.05$). (14- and 6-per-second positive spikes were excluded from the calculation in both series.)

Only seven of the 46 children with spike or spike and wave discharges in our series had had any clinical seizures. Lairy and Harrison (1968) studied 102 school-age children with EEG foci of spikes or sharp waves, but without epilepsy, and noted no difference in IQ from control patients, but significant inferiority in motor skills and in spatial organization. Zivin and Marsan (1968) found 'epileptiform' discharges in 142 (*i.e.* 2.2 per cent) of 6497 unselected non-epileptic patients of all ages receiving EEG examinations: 14.1 per cent developed seizures during follow-up, *i.e.* a similar proportion to ours. Accordingly, we prefer to think of spike and spike and slow wave discharges as indicative of cerebral dysfunction, whatever the exact pathogenesis may be.

The slightly increased prevalence of EEG abnormalities in children with 'minimal brain dysfunctions' has been documented by Capute *et al.* (1968) and Wikler *et al.* (1970), and again in the present series. Abnormal EEGS have also been encountered in a significant proportion of children with strabismus (Levinson *et al.* 1951, Stillerman *et al.* 1952), and strabismus appears to be unduly common in epilepsy associated with 'brain damage' (Millar 1965). Therefore it is not surprising that children with strabismus in the present series had a significantly higher frequency of abnormal EEGS than those without strabismus. EEG abnormalities were also markedly more common among children with sensorineural hearing-defects. Finally, although it has been suggested that there is an increased frequency of EEG abnormalities among children in the lower social-classes, there was no clear evidence for this in our cases, apart from a significant deficiency of normal EEGS in the FBW controls in social-class V.

Summary

In a prospective study of 501 children with birthweights ≤2041g and of 203 control children with similar social-class distribution and birthweights >2500g born in the same hospital, routine EEGS were analyzed serially. 276 LBW infants had EEGS recorded in the nursery after incubator treatment at a mean conceptional age of 39 weeks; 222 LBW children had EEGS at a mean chronological age of about one year, and 251 had EEGS at about 6¾ years. 99 FBW control children had EEGS recorded at about one year and 117 FBW children had EEGS at about 6¾ years.

Among the 'late neonatal' records of the LBW children near term, about 27 per cent were considered borderline or abnormal. The greater majority of these suspected or definite abnormalities had resolved by the age of about one year; of 54 borderline or abnormal 'late neonatal' records with follow-up, 40 had become normal, only six had become or remained abnormal and eight had remained or become borderline. Also, the correlation between 'late neonatal' EEG abnormalities, neurological status and WISC Full-scale IQ scores at 6¾ years was not significant. However, only one infant had 'tracé paroxystique' (in a first record taken at a chronological age of five months), and there were few grossly abnormal neonatal EEGS in our series which might be considered to have grave prognostic significance.

At about one year, 18.5 per cent of the records of LBW children were considered borderline or abnormal; only two of the 99 FBW control children were thought to have borderline records, while none had definitely abnormal EEGS. The abnormal records of the LBW children appeared to have distinct prognostic significance. Of 28 borderline or abnormal EEGS at about one year, 19 became or remained abnormal at about 6¾ years, and two remained or became borderline. Of 10 distinctly abnormal records at about one year, only two became normal at about 6¾ years, and no EEGS with spike or spike-wave discharges at about one year were found to become normal at about 6¾ years. Also, the correlation between EEG abnormality at about one year and abnormality of neurological status and lowering of mean WISC Full-scale IQ score at about 6¾ years is statistically significant.

At about 6¾ years, 45 per cent of the records of LBW children were considered borderline or abnormal, compared to 24.8 per cent of EEGs of FBW control children. The frequency of definitely abnormal records in LBW children (38.2 per cent) was twice as high as in FBW controls (18.8 per cent). Moreover, the proportion of records with spike or spike and wave discharges among the abnormal EEGs of the LBW children (37.2 per cent) was significantly greater than among the abnormal traces of the FBW controls (20.7 per cent). Only seven of the combined number of 46 children with such discharges had had seizures. There was again a significant relationship between EEG abnormalities and neurological disorders and lowering of mean WISC Full-scale IQ score at this age.

At 6¾ years the preterm AGA among the LBW children had a slightly higher frequency of normal records than the SGA children (59.2 per cent *vs.* 52.3 per cent), but the difference was not significant at this or earlier ages. In general, there was also no significant relationship between EEG abnormality and social class, though the lowest class (V) for both LBW and FBW children had the lowest proportion of normal records and this difference just reached significance ($p<0.05$) in the control children when social-classes I to IV were collectively compared to class V.

Children diagnosed as having MBD and those who were found to have sensorineural hearing-loss had a higher frequency of borderline plus abnormal EEGs at about 6¾ years than those who were considered to be neurologically normal. About half the children with MBD had borderline or abnormal records. Children with strabismus had a higher prevalence of borderline or abnormal EEGs than non-squinting children.

The main conclusion is that a routine EEG at about one year is useful prognostically with regard to future neurological status and intelligence of LBW children, whereas minor abnormalities of the EEG in the 'late neonatal' period after incubator treatment usually tend to resolve. The frequency of EEG abnormality among LBW children is also significantly greater than for FBW controls at about one and 6¾ years, and at the latter age these abnormalities include a greater proportion of spike and spike and wave discharges, usually in the absence of frank seizures.

Acknowledgements: The authors thank Dr. Sherrill T. Purves for her review of the manuscript of this chapter and her helpful comments.

14
Neurological Correlations and Predictions

Henry G. Dunn, Ann-Marie Robertson and Michael Schulzer

In the introductory chapter we reviewed the literature concerning the prognostic value of abnormal neurological signs in LBW newborns and noted that many investigators have found correlations with subsequent abnormalities, but that a high proportion of babies initially considered abnormal seemed to improve spontaneously. It has also become clear that (1) the sequelae may be mild and show themselves in subtle psychological defects, clumsiness, behaviour disturbances and poor school-performance (Graham *et al.* 1962, Drillien 1964, Davies and Stewart 1975, Black *et al.* 1977); and (2) the outcome is influenced by a host of interdependent factors which have to be taken into consideration.

Paine and Donovan (1962) studied the prognostic value of neurological signs in the newborn and found that the most important were the Moro response, the blink response to light, the sucking reflex, and plantar and palmar grasp. Donovan *et al.* (1962) reported that conventional neurological and postural signs were of limited predictive value, but the most ominous combination was depression of automatisms, especially traction and Moro response, with exaggerated tremulousness. Saint-Anne Dargassies (1962) used qualitatively abnormal signs like absence of sucking or Moro response and persistent deviation of the eyes. In the US National Collaborative Perinatal Project, it was found that in prediction the Apgar score could be combined with other perinatal factors like abruptio placentae (Niswander *et al.* 1966) or low birthweight (Drage and Berendes 1966). Prechtl (1967, 1968) went beyond this and established a standardized quantitative neurological examination for fullterm infants; he then analyzed 42 variables in the prenatal and perinatal history and obtained an obstetric risk-score for each baby. Other investigators have used behavioural assessment of newborn infants for prognosis, relating it to either neurological abnormalities or behavioural development later (Graham *et al.* 1962; Rosenblith 1964, 1966; Scarr and Williams 1971, Kurtzberg *et al.* 1979). Neurophysiological findings have also been used, such as neonatal photic response latencies (Butler and Engel 1969) and polygraphic recordings of sleep states (Karch *et al.* 1982). Our experience with neonatal EEGs is summarized in Chapter 13.

For LBW infants, various investigators have emphasized the serious prognostic significance of prolonged initial and/or recurrent apnoea (Fitzhardinge and Ramsay 1973, Stewart and Reynolds 1974, Roberton and Tizard 1975, Ziegler *et al.* 1976, Sheehan *et al.* 1977). Fitzhardinge and colleagues (1976) also showed that major neurological sequelae were closely associated with a neonatal history of seizures and intracranial haemorrhage. Conversely, Nelson and Broman (1977) found that

50 children with moderate or severe cerebral palsy and with more than mild mental retardation (IQ <50) at seven years differed from a large control population with respect to their prospectively ascertained perinatal characteristics; multivariate analysis indicated that intracranial haemorrhage and neonatal seizures were the strongest independent discriminators between the neurologically impaired children and the controls. These dramatic events are more liable to occur among VLBW infants than those with a birthweight between 1501 and 2500g and were rare among survivors in our study. Fitzhardinge and Pape (1981) stated that the infants at highest risk for neurological sequelae are those with (1) birthweight under 1501g or gestational age less than 33 weeks; (2) gestation less than 37 weeks and birthweight more than 2SD below the mean for gestational age; (3) meningitis; (4) seizures or persistent abnormal neurological behaviour; (5) CT or ultrasound evidence of haemorrhage into the ventricles, cerebrum or cerebellum; and (6) bronchopulmonary dysplasia.

In view of these multiple and often interdependent factors, attempts have been made recently to select batteries of significant predictive variables in relation to neurological outcome. Smith *et al.* (1972) arbitrarily defined 'normal' and 'abnormal' criterion groups of children at seven years by use of principal component analysis (rather than clinically) and showed that 83 per cent were already classifiable correctly on the basis of 11 prenatal and perinatal variables. However, this statistical technique may be regarded as dubious from a clinical viewpoint. DeSouza and Milner (1974) observed that apnoeic attacks, absent Moro response, and absent sucking and swallowing one minute after birth were remarkable adverse prognostic indicators. Brown and colleagues (1974) selected 94 asphyxiated newborn infants on the basis of seven criteria—feeding difficulties, apnoeic and cyanotic attacks, apathy, convulsions, hypothermia, persistent vomiting and high-pitched cry. These criteria proved prognostic for subsequent handicaps at a mean age of 21 months. Drorbaugh *et al.* (1975) isolated a high-risk group of LBW newborns by combining four factors, namely gestational age of 33 weeks or less, premature rupture of membranes, low Apgar score at five minutes, and respiratory distress. Pape *et al.* (1978) found a significant association with subsequent neurological impairment only for the neonatal variables of very low birthweight (≤1500g), intracranial haemorrhage, seizures, and severe acidaemia.

It is generally agreed that the predictive value of perinatal data can be improved by adding paediatric neurological and developmental-psychological findings during infancy (Werner *et al.* 1971, Smith *et al.* 1972, Parmelee and Haber 1973, Balow *et al.* 1975-76).

Material and method

The predictive values of different variables for neurological outcome were calculated for 335 LBW children and 139 FBW controls in the present study who were available for neurological examination at 6½ years. In the present chapter we deal with the prediction of neurological status at 6½ years from data in infancy.

We began by determining the degree of association of each single perinatal variable with neurological outcome. A separate analysis of the examination data at birth, 12 months and 18 months was first performed. Initially 127 prenatal and perinatal variables were available, but 27 were eliminated in view of excessively incomplete data. High correlations among some of the remaining variables reduced the total number to 59 at the chronological age of 12 months and to 60 at 18 months (the latter were identical to those at 12 months, with the addition of age at free walking).

For prediction, a stepwise discriminant analysis was then applied to the data at birth, first to reduce the 100 prenatal and perinatal variables for LBW infants to 43 which were marginally significant at $p<0.1$, and then to 11 which jointly were most significant at $p<0.05$. It was then found that the first five gave nearly as good a prediction as the 11 together. Next, a similar discriminant analysis technique was applied to data available at 12 and separately at 18 months chronological age. Variables which had no marginal predictive significance were eliminated. This left about 40 variables each at 12 and 18 months. The discriminant analysis was then repeated separately for the total Griffiths General Quotient (GQ) and for the five subscores, and also separately for abnormal neurological signs and total neurological status at 12 and 18 months, respectively. After this step all the variables with $p>0.05$ were eliminated and the 11 best neonatal predictors were combined in the least correlated way with the best at 12 and 18 months. This gave a total of 35 variables (see Table 14-IV). Then six different discriminant runs were performed at the 5 per cent and another six runs at the 10 per cent levels. Finally, since sex was found to be significant in all runs, different discriminant functions were analyzed for males and females in order to improve prediction for each.

Results

After the univariate step of the discriminant analysis of data available in the newborn period, the 17 most significant variables emerged as shown in Table 14-I. It should be noted that there is a very highly significant correlation between absence or abnormality of the Moro response in the nursery and neurological outcome, as was suspected by Paine and Donovan (1962) and discussed previously in Chapter 5. There are also very important correlations between neurological outcome and birthweight, social class and sex: abnormal outcome tends to be associated with low birthweight, low social-class and male sex (see Table 5-II).

Stepwise discriminant analysis then further reduced the most predictive variables available in the neonatal period to 11, and the five best of these gave nearly as good prediction as the 11. They are shown in Table 14-II. The next best variables were the late Moro response on repeat examination in the nursery, abnormal neurological signs towards the end of the stay in the nursery, persistent hypothermia after admission to the nursery, and abnormalities of truncal tone.

Using only the five best criteria, we were able to show that of 131 LBW children who were neurologically abnormal at 6½ years the abnormality was predictable for 63 per cent, and of 189 LBW normal children the normality was predictable for 76 per cent. Over-all, 70.6 per cent of the children at 6½ years could have been classified correctly (Table 14-III).

When predictor variables at the chronological ages of 12 and 18 months had

TABLE 14-I

Significant antenatal and perinatal variables in relation to neurological status at 6½ years

	p*
Social class	0.002
Maternal education	0.034
Maternal neurological or psychiatric disorder during pregnancy	0.018
Maternal parity (worst outcome in grav. 5+)	0.010
Sex	0.001
Birthweight range (250g categories)	0.000
Cyanosis (general>peripheral>none)	0.006
Concentration of added oxygen	0.009
Oxygen therapy >48 hours	0.003
Intravenous therapy	0.002
Moro response absent in nursery	0.000
Moro response abnormal or suspicious	0.000
Abnormal neurological status on discharge	0.004
Non-neurological abnormality	0.009
Involuntary movements	0.002
Twitching	0.010
Absent or weak sucking	0.002

*Based on univariate step of discriminant analysis.

TABLE 14-II

Five best variables in newborn for prediction of neurological status at 6½ years

	F*
Moro response on initial examination in nursery	0.000
Over-all neurological status on discharge from nursery	0.000
Birthweight	0.002
Sex	0.004
Socio-economic status	0.003

*Based on final step of discriminant analysis.

TABLE 14-III

Number of LBW cases classified by neurological status at 6½ years

Observed		*Predicted from newborn data*			
	N	*Normal*		*Abnormal*	
		N	%	*N*	%
Normal	189	143	76	46	24
Abnormal	131	48	37	83	63

Over-all, 70.6 per cent were classified correctly by the five most discerning variables available in the neonatal period.

been reduced in number by discriminant analyses and were added to the 11 best variables available in the newborn period, the 35 variables in Table 14-IV emerged as most promising.

With further discriminant analyses on uncorrelated sets of the above variables the best predictive batteries were then obtained. These differed for the two sexes. For LBW *girls*, an over-all correct prediction of neurological outcome at 6½ years could be obtained in more than 80 per cent by using five variables: neurological status at 12 months, birthweight range, Moro response on initial examination in nursery, Moro response at one year, and involuntary movements at one year. For LBW *boys*, neurological prediction was not quite so successful but was correct at 6½ years for more than 73 per cent. The best set of variables was neurological status at 18 months, truncal tone in nursery, social class, weight percentile at 12 months, and Landau posture at 12 months (Tables 14-V and VI).

Of the girls and boys who were incorrectly predicted as being abnormal, many were borderline and just failed to qualify as having MBD. In a subset of 23 boys and 15 girls who had been wrongly predicted as normal, no fewer than 26 (68 per cent: 15 boys, 11 girls) had MBD. This represents a significantly higher proportion than in the total sample ($z = 8$, $p = 0.000$). Another six (16 per cent) had 'cerebral dysfunction, more than minimal', *i.e.* similar neurological, behavioural and psychological findings and EEGS as those with MBD, but a Full-scale WISC IQ in the range of 70 to 79. Again this was a significantly more frequent relative occurrence than in the total sample ($z = 2.06$, $p = 0.02$). This suggests that mild forms of cerebral dysfunction are hard to predict. Since the total of 61 cases of MBD in our LBW series comprise 41 males and only 20 females (see Chapter 6), this may also help to explain why prediction of neurological outcome is more certain for girls.

Another way of expressing the prediction from Tables 14-V and 14-VI is that if at one year a girl is predicted from these criteria to be neurologically normal, her chance of actually proving to be normal at 6½ years is 104/124, *i.e.* 83.9 per cent; if she is predicted to be neurologically abnormal, this will prove correct in 35/44, *i.e.* 79.5 per cent of cases. For boys, a similar prediction of normality at 1½ years will prove correct for only 65/94 (69.1 per cent), while a prediction of abnormality will be correct for 47/58 (81 per cent). However, one may also say that if the prediction of normality proves incorrect, there is a two in three chance of a child of either sex having only MBD.

We can then calculate a weighted formula (discriminant function) which would allow the physician to forecast neurological normality at school age from the findings in infancy. This formula needs careful assessment of the criteria in each sex.

(A) *Girls' predictive variables:*

Neurological status at 12 months: expressed as 1 for normal, 2 for suspicious, 3 for abnormal

Birthweight: scored as 1 for 1001 to 1250g, 2 for 1251 to 1500g, 3 for 1501 to 1750g, 4 for 1751 to 2000g, 5 for 2001 to 2041g

Moro response on initial examination in nursery: 1 obtained with ease, 2 obtained with difficulty, 3 no constant pattern, 4 no response

TABLE 14-IV

Thirty-five most useful variables in infancy for prediction of neurological status at 6½ years

Newborn variables	*12-months variables*	*18-months variables*
Moro response at initial examination in nursery	Abnormal neurological signs	Neurological status
Neurological status on discharge from nursery	Combined right and left plantar responses	Griffiths GQ
Birthweight	Weight percentile	Combined right and left plantar responses
Sex	Adequacy of maternal care	Level of mother's care
Social class	Landau posture	Abnormal gait or posture
Moro response on discharge from nursery	Normality of EEG	Performance subscale of Griffiths test
Abnormal neurological signs on discharge from nursery	Type of EEG abnormality	Locomotor subscale of Griffiths test
Hypothermia (rectal temp. <96°F) persisting after admission to nursery	Griffiths GQ	Personal-social subscale of Griffiths test
Truncal tone at first neurological examination in nursery	Parachute response	
Bleeding in nursery	Abnormalities of gait or posture	
Morphine (or heroin) intrapartum	Involuntary movements	
	Presence of abdominal skin reflexes	
	Persistence of Moro response	
	Locomotor subscale of Griffiths test	
	Palmar grasp	
	Tone in right and left leg combined	

TABLE 14-V

Number of LBW girls classified by neurological status at 6½ years

Observed		*Predicted from infant data*			
	N	*Normal*		*Abnormal*	
		N	%	*N*	%
Normal	113	104	92.0	9	8.0
Abnormal	55	20	36.4	35	63.6

Over-all, 82.7 per cent were classified correctly by the five most discerning variables available at one year.

TABLE 14-VI

Number of LBW boys classified by neurological status at 6½ years

Observed		*Predicted from infant data*			
	N	*Normal*		*Abnormal*	
		N	%	*N*	%
Normal	76	65	85.5	11	14.5
Abnormal	76	29	38.2	47	61.8

Over-all, 73.7 per cent were classified correctly by the five most discerning variables available at 1½ years.

Moro response at 12 months: 1 no constant pattern, 2 flexor and extensor components present and symmetrical, or other response
Involuntary movements at 12 months: 1 none, 2 present (choreo-athetosis, tremor, *etc.*)

These five measures, scored in the appropriate numerical units, have to be multiplied by coefficients from the final discriminant function (for weighting) and then added as follows:

Coded variable		*Coefficient*
Neurological status score at 12 months	×	−1.7051
+ Birthweight range score	×	0.4704
+ Moro response score at initial examination in nursery	×	−1.786
+ Moro score at 12 months	×	−2.976
+ Involuntary movement score at 12 months	×	−3.247
+ Constant		10.154

A positive sum predicts neurological normality; a negative sum indicates abnormal neurological outcome.

(B) *Boys' predictive variables:*
Neurological status at 18 months, expressed as 1 for normal, 2 for borderline, 3 for abnormal
Truncal tone in nursery: expressed as 1 normal or questionably hypotonic, 2 hypotonic, 3 hypertonic or questionably hypertonic, 4 other (*e.g.* flaccid, asymmetrical)
Social class: numbered 1 to 5 on Hollingshead scale
Weight percentile at 12 months: 1 below 3rd percentile, 2 for 3rd to 9th percentile, 3 for 10th to 24th percentile, 4 for 25th to 49th percentile, 5 for 50th to 74th percentile, 6 for 75th to 89th percentile, 7 for 90th to 96th percentile, 8 for 97th percentile and above
Landau posture at 12 months: scored as 1 present normally, 2 absent or abnormal

These five measures, scored in appropriate numerical units, have to be multiplied by the corresponding coefficients for the final discriminant function (for weighting) and added:

Coded variable		*Coefficient*
Neurological status at 18 months	×	−1.8661
+ Neonatal truncal tone	×	−1.3386
+ Social class (Hollingshead)	×	−0.4288
+ Weight percentile at 12 months	×	0.3782
+ Landau posture at 12 months	×	−1.311
+ Constant		6.923

A positive sum predicts neurological normality; a negative sum indicates abnormal neurological outcome (see Dunn 1984). For instance a boy with a birthweight of 1559g has a normal neurological status at 18 months (score 1) after having had truncal flaccidity in the neonatal nursery (score 4). His social class is V on the Hollingshead scale. At 12 months his weight was between the 50th and 74th percentiles (score 5) and his Landau reflex was normal (score 1). The calculation of the sum would be as follows:

$$\begin{aligned} 1 \times -1.87 &= -1.87 \\ 4 \times -1.34 &= -5.36 \\ 5 \times -0.43 &= -2.15 \\ 5 \times +0.38 &= 1.90 \\ 1 \times -1.31 &= -1.31 \\ \text{Constant} &= 6.92 \\ \hline &= -1.87 \end{aligned}$$

Since the sum is negative, an abnormal neurological outcome would be expected.

Discussion

As indicated in the introductory chapter, serious motor and mental handicaps among LBW children tend to be preceded by fetal distress and difficulties during delivery, and as a group such neonates differ from control infants, particularly in initiating and maintaining respiration, more frequently having Apgar scores of 3 or less at five minutes or later, having intracranial haemorrhage and/or neonatal seizures (particularly in the VLBW range), a lower mean birthweight than the neurologically normal, and abnormal over-all neurological status (Nelson and Broman 1977, Nelson and Ellenberg 1979). Abnormal head circumference, low haemoglobin and low haematocrit (Churchill *et al.* 1974) are also found significantly more often in these neonates. In newborns with birthweights below 1001g, acidaemia (pH<7.20) also has been correlated significantly with an adverse neurological outcome (Pape *et al.* 1978). Nelson and Broman (1977) found no significant difference between such seriously handicapped children and control subjects with respect to 60 prenatal factors. Low birthweight and short gestation have been found to be important risk-factors for cerebral palsy but were uncommon (McDonald 1967, Ellenberg and Nelson 1979). We have also shown in Chapter 5 that the antecedents of cerebral palsy and mental retardation in LBW children differ somewhat. For mental retardation the most highly significant early variables were an abnormal Moro response in the nursery, abnormal neurological examination at 12 and 18 months, low Griffiths GQ score at 12 and 18 months, abnormal posture or delayed walking at 18 months, and low socio-economic status. LBW children with cerebral palsy also tended to have an abnormal Moro response in the nursery and abnormal neurological examinations and low Griffiths scores at 12 and 18 months, and abnormal posture or gait at 18 months, but they differed in that they did not have a significantly low mean social-class and did have a significantly shorter mean length of gestation than other LBW children, more respiratory difficulties and bleeding as neonates, persistence of Moro response and asymmetrical tonic neck response at 12 months and persistence of variable or extensor plantar response at 18 months (Dunn *et al.* 1982*b*).

When one considers neurological sequelae among LBW children generally, and includes milder abnormalities, the perinatal antecedents tend to be less dramatic. The interplay of several variables, such as perinatal anoxia, low socio-economic status, sex and even genetic and antenatal factors needs to be studied. Detailed neurological assessments may reveal subtle abnormalities, both in the newborn period and during later development (Prechtl 1968, Touwen 1979, Njiokiktjien and Kurver 1980). Several authors have noted that abnormalities of muscle tone, asymmetries and involuntary movements may subside during infancy (Drillien 1972, Minkowski *et al.* 1977, Bierman-van Eendenburg *et al.* 1981), and even cerebral palsy may be 'outgrown' (Nelson and Ellenberg 1982). The question whether 'soft signs' and MBD may ensue in such cases is still open and needs further investigation (Drillien *et al.* 1980, Hertzig 1981).

In view of the multiple interacting, and often interdependent, variables responsible for brain dysfunction in LBW children, the use of predictive batteries appears to be essential, and our results show that discriminant analysis proved useful in sorting out which variables may best be combined to obtain maximum information with the smallest number of relatively independent factors. A somewhat similar approach with scoring and weighting of several variables was used by Ellison and co-workers (1981) to predict outcome after neonatal seizures.

It was interesting to note the usefulness of the Moro response in this respect, which had been pointed out previously by Paine and his colleagues in 1962. Clearly the clinical neurological examination also remains a valuable predictor, both in the nursery and at 12 and 18 months. The batteries of five variables for boys and girls which emerged from our studies should be of practical usefulness in predicting future neurological status, particularly for healthy infants and for those who have marked handicaps. They are less able to predict minimal brain dysfunctions, including learning disabilities. In future, predictive formulae inevitably will require revalidation as new techniques of diagnosis and intervention are used, and it may well be found that new measures are more helpful, *e.g.* ultrasonogram of LBW children's heads (Pape *et al.* 1979, Bejar *et al.* 1980, Thorburn *et al.* 1981, Harvey *et al.* 1982). Meanwhile it is encouraging that neurological normality at 6½ years can be predicted with a probability of 83.9 per cent for girls at one year, and 69.1 per cent for boys at 1½ years on the basis of five fairly simple variables, while abnormality (including even MBD) can be predicted with a probability of 79.5 per cent for girls at one year and 81 per cent for boys at 1½ years.

It is of incidental interest that birthweight was one of the five most useful predictors for girls, whereas social class did not reach that final battery. For boys, social class did enter the predictive battery, along with weight percentile at one year, suggesting that both contribute to the prediction. Further, it will be recalled that the FBW control children in the present study were selected from a somewhat low social group in hospital so as to make their mean social class comparable to that of the LBW cohort (see Chapter 2). In comparison to these FBW children, and also to a separate group of classroom controls, the LBW group had a much higher proportion of neurological and intellectual handicaps. Moreover, Pape *et al.* (1978) found that the prognosis for infants with a birthweight below 1001g was not significantly correlated to social class. For all these reasons it seems clear that these handicaps are at least partly associated with the biological risks of low birthweight.

Summary
Among VLBW infants (birthweight ≤1500g), severe motor and mental handicaps frequently are preceded by perinatal cerebral (particularly intraventricular) haemorrhage and/or anoxic-ischaemic encephalopathy, and in such cases the resulting cerebral palsy may be accompanied by mental retardation and seizures. Mental retardation without cerebral palsy in LBW children is correlated more with low social-class and factors operating earlier in gestation, including maternal neurological or psychiatric disease, as shown in Chapter 5. The correlations between neurological findings in infancy, including postural responses, and neurological outcome are also emphasized again. In attempts to predict such outcome, batteries of variables have demonstrated that even in an unselected population it is possible to identify infants at markedly increased risk for cerebral palsy in the newborn period. In the present study stepwise discriminant analysis was used to determine small batteries of variables which were most highly predictive of abnormal neurological status at 6½ years in LBW neonates and infants.

APPENDIX

Two related studies concerning prediction of outcome for LBW children will be published in detail separately, but may be summarized here.

Prediction of IQ at 6½ years

Linda C. Eaves and Annetta K. McBurney

(1) When simple correlations were made between variables from the newborn period to age 6½ years and IQ at the latter age, the cognitive variables, particularly from the age of 2½ years, were most highly correlated with the Full-scale WISC-R IQ at 6½ years, while socio-economic, neurological and other measures were correlated less closely.

(2) Multiple regression analysis from ages 12 months, 18 months, 2½ and four years, predicting IQ score at 6½ years was performed using psychological, neurological and other variables. The results from each level were similar, scores from the Griffiths or Stanford-Binet tests being the chief contributors, while social class, neurological status and being AGA preterm *vs.* SGA were also important.

(3) Prediction was better for LBW than for control FBW children.

(4) When neurological and psychological variables from ages one to four years were combined to predict IQ at 6½ years, the Stanford-Binet IQ at four and neurological status at one year combined to account for over half the variance in the later IQ score.

(5) Discriminant analysis was used to classify children with IQs of 70 and below *vs.* greater than 70. Correct classification was possible for 83 to 90 per cent of cases, with varying subsets of variables being the best predictors at each age.

Prediction of school achievement from measures in infancy and early childhood
Ruth V. E. Grunau

(1) Prediction of placement during school year 3 as 'at grade level', 'below grade level' or 'special placement' resulted in over-all correct identification of only 65 per cent from measures at 12 months of age and 80 per cent from 6½-year data. Prediction was best for identifying children who later required special placement, with correct identification increasing from 71 per cent from 12-month data to 83 per cent from data at 6½ years.

(2) Prediction of outcome for children in the middle group was poor. Including the 'below grade level' children either with those 'at grade level' or in 'special placement' to form two criterion groups instead of three gave a better rate of correct identification.

(3) The best predictor variables at 12 and 18 months were Griffiths GQ, neurological status and sex, plus whether the child was SGA or preterm AGA at birth. The Stanford-Binet IQ score at 2½ and four years, WISC Full-scale IQ at 6½ years, plus neurological status at each age, were the most significant indices of outcome from the set examined.

(4) Identification of children at 6½ years who later in school year 3 would be 'at grade level' compared to 'below grade level' showed that a task of fine-motor dexterity predicted outcome, in addition to neurological status and WISC Full-scale IQ.

(5) From the 6½-year test battery, the variables significantly related to achievement in reading, spelling and arithmetic in school year 5 were WISC Full-scale IQ, neurological status, and the Crawford Dexterity Test for all three subjects. In addition, Draw-a-Person score and social class were related to reading and spelling level, and WISC Block Design subtest to arithmetic. Writing achievement was related to WISC Performance IQ, neurological status, Draw-a-Person score and sex.

15
Evolution of Minimal Brain Dysfunctions to the Age of 12 to 15 Years

Henry G. Dunn, Helena H. Ho, John U. Crichton, Ann-Marie Robertson, Annetta K. McBurney, Ruth V. E. Grunau and P. Susan Penfold

In Chapter 6 we outlined our definitions of minimal brain dysfunctions (MBD) and noted the clinical usefulness of this unitary concept for LBW children, provided the individual features of these dysfunctions are analyzed in each case (and can then be remedied, if possible). MBDs were found to be the most common sequel of LBW, occurring in 61 (18.2 per cent) of 335 children with birthweights ≤2041g followed to the age of 6½ years, in contrast to only 10 (6.5 per cent) of 139 FBW control children. Accordingly, we decided to study the further development of these children by re-assessing as many as possible at the age of 12 to 15 years, *i.e.* after an interval of six to nine years, together with suitable controls.

Previous follow-up studies of children with MBDs have been reviewed by Helper (1980). He found that 33 studies had adequate diagnostic criteria (including hyperactivity and learning disabilities, a follow-up interval of at least two years, and a sample size of at least 10). All the samples were predominantly male. The average age at diagnosis was about eight years and the duration of follow-up ranged up to about 24 years (Menkes *et al.* 1967, Rawson 1968). Many studies lacked adequate control groups. Interestingly, Borland and Heckman (1976) used brothers as controls for 20 men, which had the obvious advantage of ideal matching for intelligence, familial and social factors in childhood, but on average the brothers were two years younger and had not been evaluated systematically at the time of diagnosis of the MBD child. Nonetheless, it emerged that the brothers did significantly better in high-school and that after 20 to 25 years the MBD men had not achieved a socio-economic status equal to that of their fathers and brothers.

All the studies reviewed by Helper (1980) indicated that the school performance of MBD children was poor. About one-half had to repeat one or more grades (Hinton and Knights 1971, Minde *et al.* 1971). Minde and colleagues studied the possibility that lower mean IQ rather than hyperactivity accounted for these children's grade-failure. A subgroup of hyperactive children was matched for IQ with normal classmates and did not exceed the controls in the number of grades repeated, but had significantly lower marks and less favourable behaviour ratings by the teachers. Several studies showed that hyperactivity diminished after the age of eight to 12 years, but social-emotional maladjustment and difficulties in learning continued (Laufer 1962, Minde *et al.* 1971, Mendelson *et al.* 1971, Weiss *et al.* 1971, Riddle and Rapoport 1976).

With respect to educational outcome, Riddle and Rapoport (1976), in a two-year follow-up of 72 hyperactive eight-year-old boys from middle-class families, found that reading and arithmetic remained significantly poorer than in a non-hyperactive control group, but only the mathematics scores for the hyperactive group were below the national average for this test. Those authors also found depressive tendencies in 17 of the 72 boys at 10 years. Rourke and Orr (1977) performed a four-year follow-up of boys who were retarded readers in Grades 1 or 2. The boys tended to show increases ranging from 12 to 14 percentile points on reading tests but remained well below the 50th percentile for the tests and below the level of the control group, though they reached the average range.

In a follow-up study of hyperactive children into adolescence, Weiss and associates (1971) actually found a small but significant increase in Full-scale and Verbal IQ scores, while mean scores on the Lincoln-Oseretsky Motor Development Scale declined very significantly. The over-all rate of EEG abnormalities in a subsample of 30 children remained constant at about 40 per cent. Behaviour ratings showed a substantial reduction in hyperactivity, distractability, aggression and excitability over the five years, but over-all the behaviour remained abnormal, with a shift from gross overactivity to 'fidgeting' and restlessness. The mothers commented on the emotional immaturity of the teenagers and their inability to concentrate or to persist in working towards major goals. In the study by Mendelson *et al.* (1971) the mothers reported a shift to antisocial rather than immature behaviour. 59 per cent had had at least one contact with police. The same group of investigators also found that the teenagers persisted in impulsivity, aggressiveness and failure to complete projects and were frequently depressed (Stewart *et al.* 1973).

In a prospective study of boys aged eight to 11 years with learning disabilities, Ackerman *et al.* (1977) showed that at 14 years academic achievement remained deficient and two-thirds had repeated grades. The boys remained particularly deficient on four WISC subtests, Digit Span, Arithmetic, Coding and Information. Neurological functioning also remained deficient, despite significant improvement. Attention was still impaired on complex tasks. Emotional and behaviour problems were much more frequent than among control children, but problems involving overt conflict with parents and other authorities appeared to be largely confined to the subgroup of the learning-disabled sample who were identified earlier as hyperactive. Gillberg and Gillberg (1983) followed 42 children from the age of seven to 10 years who had been diagnosed as having MBD on the basis of concomitant attention deficit disorder and motor/perceptual dysfunction. According to teachers', parents' and self-rating questionnaires, the majority of the MBD children showed severe behavioural/experiential problems at follow-up.

In this connection, Cantwell (1972) found that the *parents* of 50 hyperactive children had increased rates of alcoholism (predominantly in males), hysteria (in females) and sociopathy, compared to the parents of 50 matched control children. 10 per cent of the parents of the hyperactive children were thought to have been hyperactive themselves in childhood, and *all* these 10 per cent were psychiatrically ill with alcoholism, hysteria or sociopathy. Weiss *et al.* (1971) noted that 25 per cent of hyperactive children had a history of overt antisocial behaviour at five-year follow-up, and having parents with 'poor mental health' was one of three factors which distinguished this ultimately delinquent group from the other hyperactive children at the initial evaluation.

Neuropsychological re-assessments of teenagers have demonstrated significant residual deficits in such functions as figure-ground discrimination, visual-motor skills (Silver and Hagin 1964) and complex reaction time (Dykman *et al.* 1973).

Special remedial education has often been provided for MBD children. Psychotherapy generally was considered valuable but no study with randomized or controlled evaluation of its effect was found by Helper (1980). Stimulant medications were used widely but often for variable periods and in variable dosage. Although they appeared to calm hyperactive children and to make their classroom behaviour more attentive and socially acceptable, the ultimate outcome in terms of academic achievement and emotional adjustment did not appear to be significantly improved (Weiss *et al.* 1975, Riddle and Rapoport 1976).

There is disagreement in the literature about the social and vocational adjustment of adolescents with MBD after the school years. Menkes *et al.* (1967) found that of 14 patients who were hyperactive with short attention-span, neurological abnormalities and an IQ of at least 70 at five to 15½ years, four had been admitted to institutions as psychotic, two others were retarded, and only eight were self-supporting after a mean interval of 24 years. A major prognostic factor was IQ; all but one of the people who were self-supporting had an IQ above 90. On the other hand, Rawson (1968) demonstrated very high levels of achievement among dyslexic patients of high socio-economic status who had been followed for a similar period. Borland and Heckman (1976) found that the large majority of their 20 formerly hyperactive men had completed high-school and more than 20 years later were self-supporting. They had a mean IQ of 102.4, but nearly one-half had psychiatric problems and 20 per cent were sociopathic. It seems to be generally agreed that drug treatment for hyperactivity has little effect on behaviour after medication is stopped.

In general, high IQ, high social status, supportive concerned parents in a profession and intensive systematic educational efforts appear to be favourable prognostic factors for the academic and vocational success of children with MBD. The significance of low birthweight for the long-term prognosis has not yet been assessed in detail, to our knowledge.

Material and method

In order to clarify the course and significance of MBDs in LBW children we re-established contact with 40 of the 61 LBW survivors in our study for whom that diagnosis had been made at 6½ years and re-examined them at a mean age of about 13 years (range 11 years 10 months to 15 years 8 months). Of the remaining 21 children with MBDs, nine were not in the age-range of 12 to 15 years at the time of the study or were unsuitable for other reasons such as drug therapy; eight had moved away; and four refused to be re-examined, mostly because the parents feared that some 'labelling' at this age might be harmful. Many of these 21 children were still having educational problems according to school data and correspondence, but no delinquency was evident so far. We also re-assessed 38 LBW children in our study who had been considered neurologically normal at 6½ years and who were matched with 38 of the LBW children with MBD for birthweight (within 250g), sex and social class. 25 normal FBW control children from the project were also examined in the same manner, and the school progress of the LBW children with and without MBDs was compared to that of classroom control children of the same sex and grade.

The following areas were investigated: (1) physical examination, with emphasis on neurological development; (2) psychological assessment at 12 to 15 years, as compared to earlier findings; (3) social and emotional relationships and behavioural abnormalities; (4) evolution of EEG, now including frequency analysis and evoked responses; and (5) educational achievements.

In the neuropaediatric examination the full-scale clinical assessment was supplemented by the Harris Tests of Lateral Dominance and also by 16 motor tests adapted from the Lincoln-Oseretsky Motor Development Scale (Sloan 1955) by Rutter *et al.* (1970), as well as tests for grip strength, timing of dressing and heel-toe walking, six tests of motor persistence (also adapted from Rutter *et al.* 1970), and the Crawford Small Parts Dexterity Test.

The psychological examination at 6½ years had included the WISC, the Bender Gestalt Test of Visual-Motor Perception and the Goodenough-Harris Draw-a-Person Test. For scoring MBD a half-point was given for a discrepancy of 20 or more between the Verbal and Performance scores of the WISC, a full point for an error score of 2 SD or more, and a half-point for an error score of 1 SD or more in the Bender Gestalt test, and a half-point for a Goodenough-Harris IQ score (man/woman average) 15 or more below the Full-scale IQ score of the WISC.

At 12 to 15 years the WISC was used again. The Bender test was performed with the Background Interference Procedure (Canter 1966, 1973). The first presentation was scored for the number of errors. At the end of the psychometric examination the Bender figures were again copied, but on this occasion the designs were drawn on background interference papers (BIP). Scores were then obtained for the Bender test under normal conditions, as well as the test using BIP paper; the different scores were noted and the Bender class was determined. In addition, the Porteus Maze and the Embedded Figures tests were administered. The WISC was scored for MBD as before. On the Bender Gestalt Test a half-point was given for a B-class (borderline) record or for more than 30 errors, and a full point was allotted for a C-class record ('organic brain disorder'). In the Porteus Maze Test a half-point was allotted for a TQ less than 80, and in the Embedded Figures Test a half-point was given for a score less than 25. In addition, the Fist-Ring Test of Oseretsky and Luria was used in the adaptation described by Crinella (1973), but was not considered in scoring for MBD.

With respect to attention deficit disorder (ADD), a full point towards MBD was given if all or nearly all the features listed were encountered, and a half-point if a significant minority of the features were present, *e.g.* mood swings, perseveration and impulsiveness. A full point was given for an abnormal EEG and a half-point for a borderline record. Moreover, 50 of our alumni aged 12 to 15 years, including 14 with MBD, had special EEG investigations, which included measurement of visual evoked potentials to word and pattern stimuli, study of contingent negative variations in response to speech, and power spectral data during a variety of specially designed tests.

In order to assess their social and emotional relationships, 98 of the 103 teenagers were seen at home by a social worker, and the parents were interviewed separately and asked to complete specially designed questionnaires. The Devereux Adolescent Behaviour Rating Scale was also completed in accordance with answers given by the father and mother; poorly correlated ideas from the father and mother were excluded from the results. On the basis of this information Dr. P. S. Penfold, a child psychiatrist, classified the emotional characteristics of the children according to psychiatric diagnoses.

The following educational data were collected at 12 to 15 years: Stanford Achievement Test, Advanced Partial Battery, Form W; Academic Promise Test, Abstract Reasoning and Verbal Reasoning subtests; High-school Personality Questionnaire, Form A; Semantic Differential School Attitude Scale*; Word Association Test*; and Teacher check-list*, *i.e.* ratings of 16 items of learning and behaviour at school, plus letter grades from the school reports. Results from the Stanford Achievement Test Primary II Battery administered earlier in school year 3 were used for comparison.

Results

The mean age of the 103 children (40 LBW with MBD, 38 LBW considered neurologically normal and 25 FBW controls) at the 6½-year examination had been 78.1 months or 6½ years (SD 0.59) and at the re-examination was 13 years (SD 0.90). All children were re-scored with respect to the presence of MBD. At 12 to 15 years eight of the 40 MBD children were re-categorized as being within normal limits, since they failed to obtain two points on the scoring system (see Chapter 6). The over-all status for six others was unclear or suspicious of MBD, because diagnostic tests had been refused, particularly the EEG, so that the scoring could not be completed. On the other hand, six of the 38 LBW and two of the 25 FBW children considered normal at 6½ years of age had to be re-classified as having MBD at 12 to 15 years, since they now reached two full points on the scoring system.

The evolution of MBD in 40 LBW children diagnosed by the age of 6½ years is shown in Table 15-I: 28 were boys and 12 were girls; 30 were singletons, and the 10 twins included three pairs and four whose co-twin was not in this study. All weighed less than 2200g at birth.

On the basis of the tests used at 12 to 15 years, the psychological abnormalities were even more frequent than earlier. On the other hand, ADD and neurological abnormalities diminished in nearly half the children. There was relatively little change in the frequency of EEG abnormalities.

Neurological abnormalities

The evolution of neurological findings for 40 children with MBD is shown in Table

*Unpublished tests.

TABLE 15-I

Evolution of MBD in 40 children between 6½ and 12 to 15 years

	Diminished	*Unchanged*	*Increased*	*Not re-tested*
Psychological abnormalities	11	12	16	1
Attention deficit disorder	17	14	9	—
Neurological abnormalities	19	19	2	—
EEG abnormalities	7	18	7	8

TABLE 15-II

Evolution of neurological abnormalities in 40 children with MBD between 6½ and 12 to 15 years

	N at 6½ years	*Subsiding*	*Remaining*	*Newly noted*	*N at 12-15 years*
Hypertonus and/or hyperreflexia	15	8	7	7	14
Involuntary movements and/or motor impersistence	11	8	3	4	7
Poor co-ordination of gross movements	15	14	1	1	2
Poor co-ordination of fine movements	25	20	5	6	11
Poor finger localization (more than one error)	27	23	4	2	6
Right-left confusion	25	16	9	2	11
Astereognosis	3	3	—	2	2
Visual and/or auditory perceptual defect	10	8	2	5	7
Dyslalia and mild dysarthria	16	13	3	3	6

15-II. It will be seen that co-ordination of gross movements of clumsy children tends to improve in the great majority, while co-ordination of fine movements is still abnormal in about one-third in their teen years. Right-left confusion and finger localization, which normally are often still imperfect at 6½ years, also have a marked tendency to improve. Similarly, mild speech defects are usually overcome in time. On the other hand, increased muscle tone or tendon reflexes are still about as frequent in the teen years as before, and visual and/or auditory perceptual defects and involuntary movements (*e.g.* synkinesis or tremors) are still present in the teen years in nearly one-half of the children who exhibited such symptoms.

*Motor proficiency testing**

Testing of motor skills was carried out on 38 LBW children who had been diagnosed as having MBD at 6½ years, and on 38 matched LBW and 25 FBW control children who had been considered to be neurologically normal at that age. The ages of the children at the time of the motor testing were: for 76 LBW children, range 12 years to 15 years 8 months (mean 13 years 3 months); for 25 FBW children, range 11 years

*The authors are indebted to Miss Sheila Cox, B.Sc., O.T., for her assistance with the motor proficiency testing.

TABLE 15-III

Balance scores

	N	Mean	SD	F test (p)	Duncan Multiple Range Test
(a) LBW MBD	38	12.9	4.7		
(b) LBW normal	38	15.3	3.6	0.01	a<b = c
(c) FBW normal	25	15.8	3.9		

TABLE 15-IV

Hand-finger co-ordination scores

	N	Mean	SD	F test (p)	Duncan Multiple Range Test
(a) LBW MBD	38	8.5	0.9		
(b) LBW normal	38	8.9	0.4	0.03	a/b
(c) FBW normal	25	8.8	0.6		

TABLE 15-V

Eye-hand co-ordination scores

	N	Mean	SD	F test (p)	Duncan Multiple Range Test
(a) LBW MBD	38	18.0	2.4		
(b) LBW normal	38	19.1	1.5	0.046	a/b
(c) FBW normal	25	19.0	2.3		

10 months to 12 years 6 months (mean 12 years 2 months).

Significant or nearly significant differences between the LBW MBD group and the others were found in five tests:

(1) *Balance:* standing on one foot; standing heel-to-toe; jumping in the air with about-face, landing on tiptoes and holding balance for three seconds; balancing on tiptoe; standing on one foot with eyes closed (Table 15-III). LBW teenagers diagnosed as having MBD at 6½ years had significantly worse mean balancing skills than LBW or FBW teenagers who had been considered neurologically normal at that age.

(2) *Hand-finger co-ordination:* closing and opening hands alternately; touching finger tips (Table 15-IV).

(3) *Eye-hand co-ordination:* hand tapping; placing coins and matchsticks; drawing lines; catching a tennis-ball (Table 15-V).

Thus LBW teenagers diagnosed as having MBD at 6½ years had significantly worse mean scores for hand-finger and eye-hand co-ordination than LBW teenagers who had been considered neurologically normal at that age, but did not differ significantly from FBW controls.

(4) *Foot-hand co-ordination:* jumping and clapping; tapping with feet and fingers (Table 15-VI). LBW teenagers diagnosed as having MBD at 6½ years had

TABLE 15-VI

Foot-hand co-ordination scores

	N	Mean	SD	F test (p)	Duncan Multiple Range Test
(a) LBW MBD	37	4.5	1.6		
(b) LBW normal	37	5.3	1.3	0.03	a = c<b
(c) FBW normal	25	4.5	1.4		

TABLE 15-VII

Comparison of LBW MBD, LBW normal and FBW normal children on various psychological measures

Psychological test	*(a) LBW MBD (N = 38)*		*(b) LBW normal (N = 38)*		*(c) FBW normal (N = 25)*		*Significant findings*	
	Mean	*SD*	*Mean*	*SD*	*Mean*	*SD*		
WISC-R Verbal IQ	96.3	13.0	108.0	11.2	107.5	13.4	a/b; a/c;	p = 0.000
Performance IQ	96.0	13.3	107.0	8.7	109.7	12.2	a/b; a/c;	p = 0.000
Full-scale IQ	95.9	13.0	107.8	9.2	109.4	12.3	a/b; a/c;	p = 0.000
Porteus Maze	116.2	18.7	122.6	15.0	124.7	13.2		
Bender Standard Mode	22.0	14.8	14.9	9.9	18.4	10.4	a,b,c;*	p = 0.002
Bender difference scores	4.8	10.3	3.7	8.3	4.0	5.6		
Bender class	1.9	1.0	1.5	0.9	1.3	0.7	a,b,c;*	p = 0.010
Fist-ring	10.0	2.7	10.0	2.2	10.6	2.1		
Embedded Figures	28.1	2.9	29.4	2.2	30.0	2.1	a/c	p = 0.015

*In analyses of (a) *vs.* (b) *vs.* (c) an over-all significant difference was found.

TABLE 15-VIII

Difference in Block Design scores at about 6½ and 13 years (later *vs.* earlier score)

	N	Mean	SD
LBW MBD	38	−0.97	3.28
LBW normal	38	−0.71	2.22
FBW normal	25	+0.84	3.30

significantly worse foot-hand co-ordination than LBW teenagers who had been diagnosed as neurologically normal at that age, but did not differ significantly from FBW controls (who were on average one year younger).

(5) *Crawford Dexterity Tests.* Pins: tests with pins and collars showed a trend to better skills among the non-MBD children but the difference was not statistically significant. Screws: tests with screws showed differences of borderline significance between the LBW MBD and the LBW normal groups in favour of the latter (p = 0.052).

No significance was found in comparisons of rapid finger-tapping (each hand), strength of hand-grip (each hand), closing and opening hands, touching finger-tips or persistence tests.

Psychological assessment
Thirty-eight matched pairs of LBW children with and without MBD and 25 FBW control children were analyzed on the various psychological measures.

Comparison of LBW MBD (a) vs. *LBW normal* (b) vs. *FBW normal* (c) *groups.* Analysis of variance was used to test for over-all differences, allowance by blocking being made for matching in groups (a) and (b). The Duncan Multiple Range Test was applied to examine the significance of differences between the various pairs of groups. The results are shown in Table 15-VII. It will be noted that the LBW children with MBD have significantly lower mean Verbal, Performance and Full-scale WISC IQ scores than the other two categories. They also tend to have more errors on the Bender Gestalt tests, and they have significantly lower scores than the FBW control teenagers on the Embedded Figures Test.

Sex differences. Analysis of covariance was used to test for differences between various gestation-birthweight categories, MBD and control groups, and sexes. Significant differences at the 0.05 level were found only in the following WISC-R comparisons: *VIQ*—LBW MBD males/LBW normal males*, LBW MBD females/LBW normal females*; LBW MBD females/FBW females*; *PIQ*—LBW MBD males/LBW normal males*; LBW MBD females/LBW normal females*; LBW MBD females/FBW females*; *FS IQ*—LBW MBD males/LBW normal males*; LBW MBD females/LBW normal females*; LBW MBD females/FBW females*.

Analysis of covariance with social class as covariate supported all these findings of differences between the three main groups and between males and females, and also revealed further differences: *Porteus Maze*—LBW MBD/FBW*; LBW MBD males/FBW females*; *Bender Class*—LBW MBD/FBW*; LBW males/FBW males*.

It appears, therefore, that of the psychological tests used, those most sensitive to significant group differences are WISC-R VIQ, PIQ and FS IQ, Bender Standard Mode, Bender Class and Embedded Figures.

All significant differences were in the hypothesized direction.

Differences between the 6½-year and subsequent scores. The scores obtained at 6½ years and at the follow-up at about 13 years were examined for differences in WISC Verbal, Performance and Full-scale IQ, for changes in the Verbal minus Performance discrepancy, and for differences in WISC subtest and Bender Gestalt Test scores. The only instance of significant change in mean score over the time-period was found in the Block Design subtest, in which the LBW MBD and LBW normal children differed from the FBW controls. The mean scores of the LBW groups declined, whereas those of the FBW control children rose (see Table 15-VIII).

The Duncan Multiple Range Test found two homogeneous subsets (LBW MBD children and LBW normal). Analysis of variance indicated that the FBW group was significantly different ($F = 3.17$; $p<0.05$) in degree and direction of score change, *i.e.* in that group an improvement occurred during the years between the tests.

Social and emotional relationships
Ninety-eight of 103 children were interviewed by the social worker, with one or

*Better mean score.

TABLE 15-IX

Social and emotional problem scores at about 13 years

	(a) LBW MBD			(b) LBW normal			(c) FBW normal					Duncan Multiple
	Mean	*SD*	*N*	*Mean*	*SD*	*N*	*Mean*	*SD*	*N*	*F*	*p*	*Range Test*
Mental health	5.33	3.46	39	3.46	2.38	37	2.32	2.29	25	F = 9.44	0.000	b = c<a
Physical health												
Hospitalization (wks) in first 4 yrs	5.50	8.96	37	5.97	14.32	36	2.13	3.19	24	NS		
Hospitalization (wks) after first 4 yrs	0.78	2.29	37	0.17	0.45	36	0.42	1.53	24	NS		
Sleeping problems	0.59	0.91	39	0.59	0.93	37	0.32	1.64	25	NS		
Family stability	4.23	1.60	39	4.19	1.35	37	4.36	1.50	25	NS		
Life problems of child	2.82	2.53	39	1.73	1.79	37	0.84	1.07	25	F = 6.61	0.002	b = c<a
Housing	3.58	1.78	36	3.84	1.84	38	3.83	1.49	24	NS		
Satisfaction of school placement viewed by parents	0.83	1.16	35	0.43	0.99	35	0.27	0.49	24	NS		
Attitude of child to school	3.78	0.58	37	4.17	0.81	36	4.37	0.58	24	F = 5.15	0.008	a<c
Maladaptive behaviour	1.23	3.14	37	−0.39	2.05	36	−1.17	2.26	24	F = 8.31	0.001	b = c<a
Co-operation with interviewer	2.06	1.37	36	1.63	1.48	35	0.92	1.12	24	NS		
Global rating of emotional adjustment of family and child	13.25	2.43	28	13.87	2.98	31	13.86	2.85	21	NS		
Global rating of emotional adjustment of child only	2.76	0.90	37	3.22	0.90	36	3.55	0.72	24	F = 5.26	p = 0.007	b = c>a

TABLE 15-X

Psychiatric diagnoses for various categories of children

Psychiatric diagnosis	*(a)LBW MBD* *N*	*%*	*(b) LBW normal* *N*	*%*	*(c) FBW normal* *N*	*%*	*Duncan Multiple Range Test*
Normal or borderline:							
(1) Normal	17	46.0	23	65.7	21	87.5	
(2) Adjustment reaction	5	13.5	5	14.3	—	—	
Total	22	59.5	28	80.0	21	87.5	a/c
Abnormal:							
(1) Behaviour disorder	6	16.2	3	8.6	1	4.2	
(2) Neurosis	6	16.2	4	11.4	2	8.3	
(3) Organic brain syndrome	3	8.1	—	—	—	—	
Total	15	40.5	7	20.0	3	12.5	

both parents present. On the basis of the reports from the social interview, the father's and mother's questionnaires, and the Devereux Adolescent Behaviour Rating Scale, the aspects shown in Table 15-IX were studied. With the exception of items 7, 10 and 11 (child's attitude, global ratings of emotional adjustment), a negative observation or answer was given one point, so a low score in the other items indicates few problems.

It is evident that the mental and emotional health of MBD children and their families were significantly poorer than the others. The MBD children had more life problems in school or at home and more maladaptive behaviour in general, and were less happy in school. Parental satisfaction of school placement, housing, family stability and certain aspects of physical health (such as length of admission to hospital and sleep problems) did not show significant differences among the three groups. The global ratings of emotional problems in the parents and their marriage in the 12 months prior to assessment were also similar. The global rating of emotional problems in the child was found to be higher in the LBW MBD children than in the others.

Table 15-X shows that over half of the LBW MBD children were considered to be emotionally within normal limits or to have merely an adjustment reaction, whereas 40 per cent were given a diagnosis of abnormality according to the classification of the American Psychiatric Association. There were significantly more abnormal children in the LBW MBD category than in the other two groups ($\chi^2 = 7.327$, $p = 0.026$). The greatest differences were between the LBW MBD and the FBW normal control-group. It may seem surprising that 12.5 per cent of the FBW control children were judged to have a psychiatric disorder, but it must be remembered that most of these children were diagnosed on the basis of interviews and parent questionnaires and had not been brought to medical attention. A similar prevalence was found on the Isle of Wight by Rutter *et al.* (1975).

Twelve of 37 LBW MBD children (32.4 per cent) reported having used medication at some time to calm their nerves. Only two of the 36 neurologically normal LBW (5.6 per cent) and none of the 25 FBW controls had done so ($\chi^2 = 7.194$, $p = 0.066$).

TABLE 15-XI

Evolution of 'organic behaviour syndrome' (attention deficit disorder) in 40 children between the ages of 6½ and about 13 years

	N at 6½ years	*Subsiding*	*Remaining*	*Newly noted*	*N at 12-15 years*
Brief attention-span and/or distractability	34	16	18	2	20
Hyperkinesis	32	23	9	1	10
Irritability and/or low frustration tolerance	24	10	14	4	18
Perseveration	20	16	4	2	6
Unpredictability	15	10	5	5	10
Temper tantrums	18	16	2	2	4
Impulsiveness	12	9	3	6	9
Mood swings	11	7	4	6	10
Destructiveness	4	4	—	2	2

TABLE 15-XII

Evolution of 'organic behaviour syndrome' (attention deficit disorder) between the ages of 6½ and about 13 years, according to IQ

	WISC Full-scale IQ		
	≥100	*<100*	
ADD diminished to half or less features	10/12	11/25	$\chi^2 = 5.111$ $p<0.025$
Hyperkinesis subsided	9/10	13/22	$\chi^2 = 2.60$ NS

Four of 39 MBD children were known to have played truant from school; two of these were also delinquent, requiring residential management, and in both cases the mothers also had emotional problems. However, the true proportions may be higher, since all the information was volunteered by the parents and false negative impressions may mask the true proportion of delinquency.

Attention deficit disorder. This syndrome, usually associated with hyperactivity, to which we refer in Chapter 6, represents the present concept of the hyperkinetic impulse disorder which has long been thought to occur commonly in children with 'brain damage' (Strauss and Werner 1942, Strauss and Lehtinen 1947, Laufer *et al.* 1957) and has been considered a characteristic behavioural aspect of minimal brain dysfunction (Paine 1962, Clements 1966, Clements and Peters 1981, Small 1982, Shaywitz *et al.* 1982). In our study this was originally referred to as the 'organic behaviour syndrome', with the features listed in Table 15-XI.

Among the 40 LBW MBD children who were re-assessed, 37 had at least some features of this syndrome at 6½ years. This is not surprising, since the presence of the syndrome represented one of the criteria for the diagnosis of MBDs. The frequency of the various features in this behaviour syndrome is shown in Table 15-XI, which also demonstrates the evolution of the components. Hyperkinesis had indeed subsided in about two-thirds of cases by the age of about 13 years, and temper tantrums and perseveration were also subsiding markedly, whereas brief attention-span, distractability, irritability and low frustration tolerance, impulsiveness and mood swings still represented major problems.

Further analysis showed that the syndrome as a whole and hyperkinesis by itself had a greater tendency to subside if the WISC Full-scale IQ at about 13 years was 100 or more than if it was below 100 (Table 15-XII). The difference in favour of the more intelligent teenagers was significant when the proportions of children were compared in whom the number of features of the syndrome was reduced to one-half or less, but did not reach significance with respect to the proportion in whom hyperkinesis subsided.

Other emotional abnormalities. 37 of the 40 LBW children with MBDs had abnormal behaviour other than ADD, such as nervousness, fears, disobedience, unhappiness, masturbation, finger-sucking, enuresis, encopresis and sleep disturbances. The nature of the symptoms was liable to change from the age of 6½ to about 13 years, *e.g.* from thumb-sucking to disobedience, and poor motivation for schoolwork frequently supervened, but there was nearly always continuing evidence of emotional disturbance, particularly anxiety. This was reflected in the finding that the LBW children with MBD tended to have poorer mental health and emotional adjustment and more maladaptive behaviour in general than the LBW and FBW control children who were neurologically normal (see Table 15-IX).

Evolution of EEGs

Ninety-five EEGS were obtained for the 103 children at a mean of 6¾ years (range 5½ to eight years), and 88 were repeated at a mean of about 13 years (range 12 to 15 years). The LBW MBD group had a higher number of abnormal or borderline EEGS than the full-birthweight group at both age levels (Table 15-XIIIa,b). At about 6¾ years the LBW children who were neurologically normal also had a significantly larger number of abnormal or borderline EEGS than the FBW control group, but at about 13 years the difference was no longer significant.

Table 15-XIIIc summarizes the changes in the EEGS during the intervening years in the children who had records at both age-levels. Thus the EEG records remained in the same category for 51.6 per cent of the LBW children with MBD, while 22.6 per cent of the records improved and 25.8 per cent worsened. These proportions are not greatly different from those for the LBW children who were neurologically normal. The lower proportion of improved records in the FBW control group may be explained by the fact that 96 per cent of the records in this group were normal at 6¾ years, so there were few that could get better. The proportion of abnormal and borderline EEGS (48.7 per cent) among the 37 LBW children with MBD at 6¾ years is very similar to that in the total group of 55 LBW MBD children (54.5 per cent) in our follow-up study who had the EEG recorded at that age (see Table 13-X). It will be noted that the proportion of borderline and abnormal records rises to 58.1 per cent in the present sample of LBW MBD children at about 13 years.

At about 6¾ years epileptiform discharges were found in two of the 37 records

TABLE 15-XIII(a)

EEG results at age of about 6¾ years

EEG	*(a) LBW MBD*		*(b) LBW normal*		*(c) FBW normal*		*Total*		
	N	*%*	*N*	*%*	*N*	*%*	*N*	*%*	
Normal	19	51.3	20	60.6	24	96.0	63	66.3	$\chi^2 = 14.052$ $p<0.001$
Abnormal and borderline	18	48.7	13	39.4	1	4.0	32	33.6	a = b/c
Total	37		33		25		95		

TABLE 15-XIII(b)

EEG results at age of about 13 years

EEG	*(a) LBW MBD*		*(b) LBW normal*		*(c) FBW normal*		*Total*		
	N	*%*	*N*	*%*	*N*	*%*	*N*	*%*	
Normal	13	41.9	17	53.1	19	76.0	49	55.7	$\chi^2 = 6.6408$ $p<0.05$
Abnormal and borderline	18	58.1	15	46.9	6	24.0	39	44.3	a/c
Total	31		32		25		88		

TABLE 15-XIII(c)

Change of EEG between ages of about 6¾ and 13 years

EEG	*(a) LBW MBD*		*(b) LBW normal*		*(c) FBW normal*		*Total*	
	N	*%*	*N*	*%*	*N*	*%*	*N*	*%*
Improved	7	22.6	6	20.0	1	4.0	14	16.3
Unchanged	16	51.6	18	60.0	18	72.0	52	60.4
Deteriorated	8	25.8	6	20.0	6	24.0	20	23.3
Total	31		30		25		86	

for LBW children with MBD but also in three of the 33 records for LBW children who were neurologically normal, while there were no such discharges in the 25 records of the 25 normal FBW control children at that age. On follow-up at about 13 years epileptiform discharges were noted in three of the 31 records obtained from LBW children with MBD and also in three of the 32 LBW children who had been considered neurologically normal. In addition, one of the FBW control children with previously normal EEG had developed paroxysmal 2½-3HZ slow-wave bursts lasting up to 15 seconds, particularly on hyperventilation, and then exhibited generalized 'absence' (true petit mal) seizures.

Sixteen of the LBW children with MBD (11 boys, five girls), aged 12½ to 15 years, who were all proven dextrals, were studied further by Dr. M. D. Low and his colleagues at the Vancouver General Hospital. They applied a test battery including power spectral analysis, coherence functions in the alpha band and speech-contingent negative variations (CNVs), visual evoked potentials to words and pattern visual evoked potentials. These tests were performed during reading, speech and other tasks presumed to engage primarily the left or right hemisphere and were compared with those for 29 normal control children. Correlations and multivariate analysis of the data showed no consistent intrahemispheric correlations among the different measures, but MBD children showed significantly greater intrahemispheric and interhemispheric ratios than normal children, suggesting reduced cerebral integration in the MBD syndrome (Low *et al.* 1979). For 15 such LBW children aged 11½ to 14 years an attempt was also made to correlate the WISC-R Verbal and Performance IQ figures with the amplitude of visual evoked potentials to word and speech CNVs in the two hemispheres. Canonical correlation analysis indicated that amplitude of the evoked potential at 200 to 300msec in the left hemisphere correlated with Verbal IQ, and amplitude at 100msec in the right hemisphere correlated with a difference between Performance and Verbal IQs, with Performance emphasized. With respect to the diagnosis of MBD, the analysis indicated that CNV variables might be more relevant than WISC Verbal and Performance scores (Rogers *et al.* 1980).

Educational achievements

Performance on the Stanford Achievement Test Advanced Partial Battery Form W, the Academic Promise Test (APT) and a word association test were compared across the following five groups of children:

(1) LBW MBD (N = 35);
(2) LBW normal (N = 38);
(3) FBW normal (N = 25);
(4) classroom controls for LBW MBD (CC for MBD, N = 34);
(5) classroom controls for LBW normal (CC for LBW N, N = 37).

An analysis of covariance was performed on each of the subtests: the independent variables were group 1 to 5 above and sex; the covariate was age of the child at time of testing. The means, standard deviations and results of Duncan Multiple Range Tests for the group variable, following analysis of covariance, are presented in Table 15-XIV. In each of the Stanford Achievement subtests and in the Abstract Reasoning APT subtest, there was a statistically significant difference between the LBW MBD group and the other four groups, the LBW MBD group performing significantly below the level of the others. Moreover, there was a trend in which the means of the LBW N group were consistently lower than the two CC groups, with the FBW group tending to fall in between. In the Verbal Reasoning APT subtest and the word association test there was a statistically significant difference between the LBW MBD group and each CC group, but not between LBW MBD and LBW normal children.

There was only one statistically significant over-all sex difference (the girls

TABLE 15-XIV

Educational achievement and aptitude tests at age 12 to 15 years

		(a) LBW MBD (N = 35)	*(b) LBW normal* (N = 35)	*(c) FBW normal* (N = 25)	*(d) CC* for LBW MBD* (N = 34)	*(e) CC for LBW normal* (N = 37)	*F*	*p*	*Duncan Multiple Range Test*
Stanford Achievement Test									
Paragraph meaning	Mean	23.8	32.7	32.1	33.2	35.5	6.67	<0.0001	a/b, a/c, a/d, a/e
	SD	11.2	10.6	10.8	13.1	9.1			
Spelling	Mean	24.0	31.2	30.2	32.2	34.9	5.08	<0.0008	a/b, a/c, a/d, a/e
	SD	11.4	11.9	11.2	10.5	10.2			
Language	Mean	72.8	90.7	93.4	92.0	94.4	9.87	0.0000	a/b, a/c, a/d, a/e
	SD	19.8	16.0	16.5	18.7	16.2			
Arithmetic computation	Mean	11.6	17.8	19.7	18.2	19.8	6.55	<0.0001	a/b, a/c, a/d, a/e
	SD	6.6	8.2	8.0	9.2	7.5			
Arithmetic concepts	Mean	13.4	18.0	18.6	19.3	22.4	9.20	0.0000	a/b, a/c, a/d, a/e
	SD	6.2	6.7	6.5	7.6	6.2			
Arithmetic applications	Mean	10.9	14.6	14.3	15.8	17.1	8.35	0.0000	a/b, a/c, a/d, a/e
	SD	4.2	4.9	3.9	6.3	4.5			
Academic Promise Test									
Abstract reasoning	Mean	30.5	36.5	41.3	39.3	38.9	4.43	<0.002	a/b, a/c, a/d, a/e
	SD	10.7	11.1	10.8	11.2	12.1			
Verbal reasoning	Mean	25.4	29.6	29.9	31.0	34.1	5.74	<0.0003	a/d, a/e
	SD	9.7	7.8	7.6	10.4	7.7			
Word Association Test	Mean	28.6	32.5	34.1	34.2	35.2	3.13	<0.02	a/c, a/d, a/e
	SD	9.0	8.1	7.2	10.7	8.3			

*CC = classroom control.

TABLE 15-XV

Stanford Achievement Test results in school year 3

Stanford Achievement Test		*(a) LBW MBD (N = 22)*	*(b) LBW normal (N = 23)*	*(c) FBW normal (N = 18)*	*(d) CC* for LBW MBD (N = 14)*	*(e) CC* for LBW normal (N = 12)*	*F*	*p*	*Duncan Multiple Range Test*
Word meaning	Mean	20.4	25.3	25.2	25.8	23.5	2.06	NS	
	SD	7.1	8.0	6.2	4.7	8.1			
Paragraph meaning	Mean	29.5	39.1	40.7	42.2	40.0	3.51	<0.01	a/b, a/c, a/d, a/e
	SD	12.1	12.9	11.9	9.6	13.0			
Spelling	Mean	15.7	21.4	21.3	23.1	22.7	3.17	<0.02	a/b, a/c, a/d, a/e
	SD	7.3	7.8	7.2	7.6	5.7			
Word study skills	Mean	36.0	46.5	45.6	48.5	45.4	3.55	<0.01	a/b, a/c, a/d, a/e
	SD	12.9	10.5	12.8	8.4	12.9			
Arithmetic computation	Mean	21.2	32.0	34.9	33.6	32.8	6.61	<0.0001	a/b, a/c, a/d, a/e
	SD	10.4	9.0	9.2	6.9	11.7			
Arithmetic concepts	Mean	19.6	27.0	26.8	28.6	28.1	2.94	<0.03	a/b, a/c, a/d, a/e
	SD	9.6	8.5	10.1	9.3	9.3			

*CC = classroom control.

were higher in the Stanford Spelling Test) out of the nine analyses. In two other subtests (Stanford Paragraph Meaning and APT Verbal Reasoning) there was a significant group × sex interaction, *i.e.* the pattern of sex differences changed depending on the group.

Test scores at year 3 in school on the Stanford Achievement Primary II Battery Form W were available for some of the children in the follow-up study. Analysis of variance on each subtest of this earlier battery was performed, with group (1 to 5 as above) and sex as independent variables. Means, standard deviations and tests of significance for the group variable are presented in Table 15-XV. There were no statistically significant sex differences or group × sex interactions. In each subtest (except Word Meaning) there were statistically significant differences between the LBW MBD children and each of the other groups. There were no significant differences among the other four groups.

Analysis of the WISC Full-scale IQ scores showed statistically significant differences between the LBW MBD and LBW normal children. Educational test scores were therefore re-analyzed to check whether poorer performance by the LBW MBD compared to LBW normal children might have been due to lower IQ. Results of analysis of covariance indicated that after controlling for IQ, statistically significant differences remained, favouring LBW normal children on every Stanford Achievement subtest except Spelling. There were no residual differences on the Abstract Reasoning subtest of the APT. It was concluded that the poorer educational performance of the LBW MBD childen on the Stanford subtests cannot be attributed solely to lower IQ.

It was of interest to compare changes over time between the five groups of children on the comparable Stanford Achievement subtests from school year 3 to the follow-up study at adolescence. The aim here was to see if the LBW MBD had fallen disproportionately behind the older children, or were perhaps catching up with them. Analysis of variance was performed on the difference scores for each of the following subtests: Paragraph Meaning, Spelling, Arithmetic Computation and Arithmetic Concepts. There were no statistically significant differences for group or sex, or their interaction, for any of the four subtests. These findings suggest that although LBW MBD children performed significantly below the other four groups on school achievement tests at year 3 and were still significantly below them at adolescence, the LBW MBD maintained the same relative position.

Discussion

In Chapters 1 and 6 the concept of MBD has been explained. The arguments levelled against such a wide-ranging syndrome, and particularly against a hyperkinetic impulse disorder as its specific behavioural aspect, have been noted. Nonetheless, children who present with an intricate mixture of learning disabilities, clumsiness, attention deficit and impulsive 'driven' behaviour, and increasing feelings of insecurity at school, are encountered commonly and defy classification into subsyndromes. In our view, the various components of MBD should be analyzed in each case and treated as far as possible. The neurological, psychological, behavioural and electroencephalographic abnormalities all contribute to the diagnosis, and the educational handicaps also have to be assessed. It is agreed that the affected children merge into the normal population, in which it has been conservatively estimated that about 5 to 10 per cent of children, particularly boys, have learning disabilities needing individual attention. This occurrence of MBD in the general population is illustrated by the fact that 6.5 per cent of our FBW control children had MBD by our criteria, and that eight out of 40 LBW children diagnosed as having MBD at 6½ years in our study no longer fulfilled these criteria at 12 to 15 years, whereas six out of 38 LBW children previously considered neurologically normal had amassed a sufficient number of points for the diagnosis of MBD at the re-assessment.

Various authors have pointed out that the clinical features of MBD are liable to change in the school years, partly because of maturation (Laufer 1962, Satz *et al.* 1971), but learning difficulties are likely to persist and the emotional sequelae may become more severe and remain as the main handicap in adolescents and adults (Laufer *et al.* 1957, Wender 1971, Borland and Heckman 1976, Riddle and Rapoport 1976, Milman 1979). This is also illustrated by our findings.

The *neurological* signs in these children are often 'soft', and their diagnostic value has been doubted (Adams *et al.* 1974, Erickson 1977, McMahon and Greenberg 1977). However, although the 'soft signs' are found to a lesser extent in the general population (Kennard 1960, Hertzig *et al.* 1969), a detailed neurological and neuropsychological examination is often revealing and may show abnormalities, *e.g.* in visual perception and visual-motor integration (Cohn 1961, Anderson 1963), which may be amenable to treatment and should be considered in devising suitable teaching techniques. Weiss and colleagues (1971) noted that by the age of 12 years hyperactive children often excelled in activities such as swimming and skiing, yet scored poorly on the Lincoln-Oseretsky Motor Development Scale, which by this age measures primarily fine-motor control. In our study, abnormalities of muscle tone, involuntary movements, poor co-ordination of fine movements, right-left confusion, and auditory or visual perceptual defects, were still encountered commonly at 12 to 15 years in children with MBD. Among many motor-proficiency tests, balance as well as hand-finger, foot-hand and eye-hand co-ordination were still significantly impaired in teenagers with MBD compared to neurologically normal LBW children.

In the *psychological* sphere it was noted in Chapter 6 that children with MBD tend to have significantly lower mean Verbal and Performance scores at 6½ years than LBW and FBW control children who were considered neurologically normal. We also found that the Bender Visual-Motor Gestalt Test yielded higher mean error scores for the MBD group than for the control children. This is confirmed again at 12 to 15 years, and at this age the Embedded Figures Test also yielded a significantly lower mean score for the LBW children with MBD than for FBW controls. The mean Verbal and Performance IQ scores on the WISC were close together for each category of children. There was little evidence that discordance between Verbal and Performance scores on the WISC was greater for LBW children with MBD than for controls. Rutter *et al.* (1970) and Minde *et al.* (1971) were also sceptical about Verbal-Performance discrepancies as indicators of brain dysfunction. On follow-up in our study, the only instance of significant change of mean subtest scores during the intervening seven to eight years was in the Block Design subtest; in this the mean scores of the LBW groups declined, while those of the FBW control children rose and came to differ significantly from those of the LBW teenagers.

With regard to *social and emotional* relationships, it is noteworthy that the LBW MBD children had significantly more mental-health and life problems and more maladaptive behaviour than the other two categories, and that the global rating of the emotional adjustment of LBW teenagers with MBD was significantly lower than that in the other two categories. It is also interesting that the LBW MBD children's attitude to school was less positive than that of FBW control children. On the other hand, physical health of the children, family stability, satisfaction with the school placement as viewed by the parents, and emotional adjustment of the child's family did not differ significantly between the various categories. The global ratings of parents' emotional problems and the state of their marriage in the 12 months prior to the assessment were also similar. One can only speculate whether the parents of LBW MBD children have a lower prevalence of emotional disturbance than parents of hyperactive children in general, as reported by Kenny *et al.* (1971) and Cantwell (1972), perhaps because the LBW children's brain dysfunctions are based more often on perinatal 'brain damage' and less often on genetic factors and abnormal family environment than in other aetiological groups.

The high frequency of psychiatric disorders among the LBW teenagers with MBD corresponds to the findings in follow-up studies of hyperactive and other types of MBD children (Weiss *et al.* 1971, Borland and Heckman 1976, Milman 1979, Gillberg and Gillberg 1983). Of the LBW children with MBD, 40.5 per cent had significant psychiatric disorders, compared to only 20 per cent of the LBW children who had been neurologically normal at 6½ years, and 12.5 per cent of FBW controls. The disorders appear less severe in the LBW group than in the series reported by Menkes *et al.* (1967). In our briefer follow-up of six to nine years none of the 40 children with MBD had yet become psychotic. In our study the rates of children who had required medication to 'calm their nerves', who had played truant from school, or who had been delinquent were also highest in the LBW MBD category.

The presence of a behaviour syndrome including distractability, brief attention-span, emotional lability, low frustration-threshold and either hyper-activity or sluggishness in prematurely-born children, and particularly in boys, was noted by Shirley (1939). These features resemble those subsequently described by Strauss and co-authors (Strauss and Werner 1942, Strauss and Lehtinen 1947) as occurring in children with brain injury. The occurrence of such behaviour in LBW children was noted again by Drillien (1964), Werry (1968) and Neligan *et al.* (1976). In Chapters 1 and 6 we commented that the existence of a specific 'organic behaviour syndrome' or 'hyperkinetic syndrome' is still controversial. Dykman *et al.* (1971) emphasized the attention deficit in learning disabilities, and the American Psychiatric Association (1978) adopted the term 'Attention Deficit Disorder' (with or without hyperkinesis) for a similar constellation of symptoms. It is interesting that of all the features of the 'organic behaviour syndrome' in the 40 LBW children with MBD in our study the most frequent were brief attention-span and/or distractability, which occurred at some time in 36, while hyperactivity (observed by parents and physician) was the second most common, occurring in 33 children. It is notable, too, that hyperkinesis had diminished from affecting 32 children at 6½ to only 10 at 12 to 15 years, whereas brief attention-span and/or distractability persisted (or were newly noted) in 20, or one-half. Irritability and/or low tolerance of frustration were also common and were still present in 18 (45 per cent) of the 40 children at 12 to 15 years; and unpredictability (10), mood swings (10) and impulsiveness (nine) were also still important. This corresponds to previous findings that overactivity tends to diminish in adolescence (Laufer *et al.* 1957, Menkes *et al.* 1967, Weiss *et al.* 1971) but that impulsiveness, learning difficulties and poor social adaptation remain (Minde *et al.* 1971, Cohen *et al.* 1972, Huessy and Cohen 1976). It is also interesting that the proportion of LBW children in our series in whom the number of features indicative of attention deficit disorder diminished to one-half or less by the age of 12 to 15 years was significantly greater for those whose Full-scale WISC IQ was 100 or more than for those with an IQ below 100. One reason for this may be that the more intelligent tend to encounter less emotional stress at school. It may also be recalled that in the long-term follow-up study by Menkes and colleagues (1967), IQ was the only variable from the diagnostic work-up which predicted self-support in adulthood. Milman (1979) observed on follow-up of 73 children with MBD into late adolescence and early adult life that hyperactivity was reduced, but new symptoms of obsessions, depression and tics had appeared. A better outcome was associated with high social-class, good intelligence, male sex and mild symptomatology, *i.e.* qualities that facilitate adaptation and compensation.

With respect to the *EEG*, about one-half (48.7 per cent) of the records for LBW children with MBD at about 6¾ years were abnormal or borderline, and this proportion increased to 58 per cent at about 13 years. At both ages the rate of such abnormal or suspect EEGs was significantly greater than for FBW controls. However, the proportion of abnormal or borderline records for LBW children considered neurologically normal at 6½ years also increased from 39 to 47 per cent during that interval. Capute *et al.* (1968) also found that about one-half of all children with MBD had abnormal EEGs, and Stevens *et al.* (1968) reported abnormal EEGs in 50 to 60 per cent of children with behavioural and learning problems, compared to a 10 to 15 per cent frequency in normal children. EEG abnormalities usually range from mild to moderate, *e.g.* excessive bilateral posterior slow activity, excessive diffuse theta, asymmetries, or paroxysmal responses to intermittent photic stimuli. The last are known to occur in 8.9 per cent of normal children, particularly girls, and to reach their maximum at about 12 to 13 years (Eeg-Olofsson *et al.* 1971). Even central and centro-temporal spike discharges are seen in about 2 per cent of normal children at rest, and more during sleep, and only about half the children with focal spikes have seizures (Graziani *et al.* 1981). Thus, like MBD itself, the EEG abnormalities merge into the findings in the general population.

Abnormalities of sensory evoked potentials in children with learning disabilities and behaviour problems have been described by Satterfield (1973), Preston *et al.* (1974), Njiokiktjien *et al.* (1977) and Symann-Louett *et al.* (1977). Thus, with respect to visual evoked responses, wave-form differences between reading-disabled and normal children have been demonstrated, particularly in the left parietal area (Symann-Louett *et al.* 1977). Topographic mapping has shown more widespread aberrations of electrical brain-activity in children with dyslexia (Duffy *et al.* 1980). Visser *et al.* (1982) suggested that visual evoked potentials are a more sensitive detector of late sequelae of perinatal neurological problems than the EEG itself. It is interesting, therefore, that a sample of the LBW children with MBD in the present study exhibited abnormal responses to speech-contingent negative variation and reversing-pattern visual stimuli, suggesting reduced interaction within and between hemispheres during complex tasks.

As to *educational* achievements, it is evident that learning problems continued for our LBW children with MBD, as they did in studies of hyperactive children (Minde *et al.* 1971, Riddle and Rapoport 1976, Ross and Ross 1982) and those with other manifestations of MBD (Rourke and Orr 1977, Ackerman *et al.* 1977, Helper 1980). As a group, they performed significantly below the level of the LBW children who had been considered neurologically normal at 6¾ years in each of the Stanford Achievement subtests and in the Abstract Reasoning subtest of the APT. The difference from the classroom control groups was even greater. It was also interesting that the statistical difference was most marked ($p = 0.0000$) in the Language, Arithmetic Concepts and Arithmetic Applications subtests of the Stanford Achievement Test. In a recent study of the school performance of 25 children with birthweights $\leqslant$1000g at a mean age of 10.6 years, Nickel *et al.* (1982) found that Arithmetic Reasoning, Mathematics Achievement and Reading Comprehension were specific weaknesses.

Similar differences in educational achievement between the LBW children with MBD and their neurologically normal counterparts were already found in school year 3 in our series, though at that time the most significant deficit appeared to be in arithmetic computation. The relative position of the LBW MBD children in comparison with the other groups had not changed greatly during the intervening years.

We did not find any significant sex differences in school achievement, except for higher mean scores among girls in the Stanford Spelling Test. In this connection Bell *et al.* (1977) claimed that in school populations boys do not have reading problems more often than girls, but their behaviour causes more problems in the classroom and anxiety at home, so that they are referred more speedily for special education. There is also greater concern about boys with learning disabilities becoming delinquent. In our study the greater frequency of behaviour problems among boys was documented with the Haggerty-Olson-Wickman Behaviour Ratings given by teachers (see Chapter 11).

It is important to note that the academic inferiority of the LBW MBD group, compared to the other categories, could not be attributed solely to lower mean IQ, as was also found by Minde *et al.* (1971) with respect to hyperactive children. The inferior learning skills may be attributable partly to behaviour problems and low self-esteem (Weiss *et al.* 1971) and also partly to uneven cognitive patterns.

We agree with Sameroff and Chandler (1975) and with Helper (1980) that the ultimate prognosis for MBD children appears to depend on the interplay of multiple variables, namely the nature and extent of the cognitive and behavioural manifestations of MBD, the child's general intellectual level, the socio-economic status and concern of the parents, and the quality of remedial management. Whether early stimulation and intervention in preschool day-care programmes may forestall MBD, especially in the lower social-classes, remains to be determined (Scarr-Salapatek and Williams 1973, Beckwith *et al.* 1976, Haskins *et al.* 1978).

Finally, the extent of MBD among LBW children should be emphasized. In our study this diagnosis was made for 18 per cent of the children with birthweights mostly below 2041g born between 1959 and 1965. Fitzhardinge and Steven (1972*b*) suspected it in 25 per cent of 96 fullterm SGA children with birthweights below the third percentile who were born between 1960 and 1966 and were followed for a minimum of five years. Francis-Williams and Davies (1974) found learning difficulties at school-age in one-fifth of 120 children with birthweights ≤1500g born between 1961 and 1968. Recently Nickel *et al.* (1982) reported that of 25 children with birthweights ≤1000g, born between 1960 and 1972 and re-assessed at a mean age of 10.6 years, only seven (28 per cent) were achieving at or above grade-level in school. Since another seven (28 per cent) had major neurological or sensory handicaps, this evidently left 11 (44 per cent) with milder handicaps. Our follow-up study shows the legacy of MBD for LBW children. Physicians should take note of this important group of adolescents who have educational and emotional handicaps and are coming into adult life with reduced social competence.

Summary

Among the neurological sequelae of LBW at 6½ years, the most common were minimal brain dysfunctions. As a result of re-examination and re-scoring at about 13 years, eight of 40 LBW children with MBD were found to be within normal limits. However, six LBW and two FBW children considered normal at 6½ years had to be re-classified as having MBD at about 13 years. During the intervening six to seven years psychological abnormalities tended to become more frequent and EEG abnormalities persisted, whereas abnormal neurological findings and the attention deficit disorder diminished in almost half the children.

Co-ordination of gross movements improved more during the intervening years than co-ordination of fine movements. Right-left confusion, finger localization and mild speech defects improved markedly. In contrast, increased muscle tone or tendon reflexes tended to persist, and visual and/or auditory perceptual defects and involuntary movements were noted in the teen years in almost one-half of the children who had exhibited such symptoms at an earlier age. Among 27 tests of motor proficiency, the tests of balance and of hand-finger, eye-hand and foot-hand co-ordination from the Lincoln-Oseretsky battery differentiated most significantly between the LBW MBD children and other categories.

The LBW children diagnosed as having MBD at 6½ years had significantly lower mean Verbal, Performance and Full-scale WISC IQ scores at 12 to 15 years than the other two categories. They also tended to make more errors on the Bender Gestalt Tests and had significantly lower scores than FBW control teenagers on the

Embedded Figures Test. There were no marked sex differences on these tests. There was little change in the differences between the various mean WISC and Bender Gestalt scores of the LBW MBD *vs.* LBW normal and FBW normal children at the earlier and later ages. An exception was that on the WISC Block Design subtest the mean scores of the LBW groups declined, while those of the FBW control children rose.

The mental and emotional health of the MBD children and their families were significantly poorer than for the other categories. In the LBW MBD group, the children's emotional and life problems were significantly greater and maladaptive behaviour was significantly more common. As teenagers, their attitude to school was also more negative. 40 per cent of the LBW MBD children had a behaviour disorder, neurosis or organic brain syndrome. Of the 40 LBW MBD children, 37 had had at least some symptoms of the attention deficit disorder at 6½ years. At about 13 years hyperkinesis, temper tantrums and perseveration had subsided markedly, but brief attention-span, distractability, irritability and/or low thresholds of frustration continued to be major problems. 37 of the 40 LBW MBD children had abnormal behaviour other than attention deficit disorder, such as nervousness, fears, disobedience, unhappiness, enuresis, encopresis and sleep disturbances. These symptoms changed with age and frequently poor motivation for school-work supervened, but almost always there was continuing evidence of emotional disturbance.

The LBW MBD group had a significantly higher number of abnormal or borderline EEGs at both 6½ and 13 years, and the number rose slightly at the later age, as did the proportion in the other groups of children. The EEG findings for the LBW MBD children suggested that there was reduced interaction within and between hemispheres during complex tasks.

In each of the Stanford Achievement subtests and in the Abstract Reasoning subtest of the APT, the LBW MBD groups performed significantly below the level of the other four groups. They also obtained significantly lower scores on the Verbal Reasoning subtest and the Word Association Test than the two classroom control groups. Significant differences remained after controlling for IQ, favouring LBW normal over LBW MBD children, on every Stanford Achievement subtest except Spelling.

The ultimate prognosis for MBD children appears to depend on the interplay of multiple variables, particularly the nature and extent of the cognitive and behavioural manifestations of MBD, the child's general intellectual level, the socio-economic status and concern of the parents, and the quality of remedial management.

REFERENCES

Abramovich, S. J., Gregory, S., Slemick, M., Stewart, A. (1979) 'Hearing loss in very low birthweight infants treated with neonatal intensive care.' *Archives of Disease in Childhood,* **54,** 421-426.

Abramowicz, M., Kass, E. H. (1966) 'Pathogenesis and prognosis of prematurity.' *New England Journal of Medicine,* **275,** 878-885, 938-942, 1001-1006, 1053-1059.

Accardo, P. J. (1980) *A Neurodevelopmental Perspective on Specific Learning Disabilities.* Baltimore: University Park Press. pp. 7-13.

Achenbach, T. M. (1980) 'Behavior disorders of children and adolescents.' *In:* Woody, R. H. (Ed.) *Encyclopedia of Clinical Assessment, Vol. 1.* San Francisco: Jossy-Bass. pp. 113-127.

Ackerman, P. T., Dykman, R. A., Peters, J. E. (1977) 'Learning disabled boys as adolescents.' *Journal of the American Academy of Child Psychiatry,* **16,** 296-313.

Adamkin, D. H., Shott, R. J., Cook, L. N., Andrews, B. F. (1977) 'Nonhyperoxic retrolental fibroplasia.' *Pediatrics,* **60,** 828-830.

Adams, R. M., Kocsis, J. J., Estes, R. E. (1974) 'Soft neurological signs in learning-disabled children and controls.' *American Journal of Diseases of Children,* **128,** 614-618.

Ahmann, P. A., Lazzara, A., Dykes, F. D., Brann, A. W., Schwartz, J. F. (1980) 'Intraventricular hemorrhage in the high-risk preterm infant: incidence and outcome.' *Annals of Neurology,* **7,** 118-124.

Alberman, E. D. (1963) 'Birthweight and length of gestation in cerebral palsy.' *Developmental Medicine and Child Neurology,* **5,** 388-394.

—— Butler, N. R., Gardiner, P. A. (1971) 'Children with squints. A handicapped group?' *Practitioner,* **206,** 501-506.

Albrecht, W. (1930) 'Die geburtstraumatischen Schädigungen des Ohres.' *Zeitschrift für Hals-, Nasen- und Ohrenheilkunde,* **27,** 495-501.

Alden, E. R., Mandelkorn, T., Woodrum, D. E., Wennberg, R. P., Parks, C. R., Hodson, W. A. (1972) 'Morbidity and mortality of infants weighing less than 1000 grams in an intensive care nursery.' *Pediatrics,* **50,** 40-49.

Alm, E. I. (1953) 'The long-term prognosis for prematurely born children. A follow-up study of 999 premature boys born in wedlock and of 1002 controls.' *Acta Paediatrica,* **42,** Suppl. 94.

Alpern, G. D., Boll, T. J. (1972) *Developmental Profile.* Indianapolis: Psychological Development Publications.

Ambrus, C., Weintraub, D., Niswander, K., Fischer, L., Fleishman, J., Bross, I., Ambrus, J. (1970) 'Evaluation of survivors of the respiratory distress syndrome at 4 years of age.' *Journal of Pediatrics,* **120,** 296-302.

American Academy of Ophthalmology and Otolaryngology (1959) 'Guide for the evaluation of hearing impairment.' *Transactions of the American Academy of Ophthalmology and Otolaryngology,* (Mar./Apr.), 234-238.

American Psychiatric Association (1978) 'Attention deficit disorders.' *In: Diagnostic and Statistical Manual of Mental Disorders (3rd edn.).* Washington, D.C.: American Psychiatric Association. pp. 26-33.

Amit, M., Camfield, P. R. (1980) 'Neonatal polycythemia causing multiple cerebral infarcts.' *Archives of Neurology,* **37,** 109-110.

Anderberg, M. R. (1973) *Cluster Analysis for Applications.* New York: Academic Press.

Anders, R., Emde, R., Parmelee, A. (1971) *A Manual of Standardized Terminology, Techniques and Criteria for Scoring States of Sleep and Wakefulness in Newborn Infants.* Los Angeles: UCLA Brain Information Service/BRI Publications Office.

Anderson, E., Gibbs, E. (1970) 'The normal and abnormal electroencephalogram of the neonate.' *Clinical Electroencephalography,* **1,** 30-40.

Anderson, R. P., Halcomb, C. G. (Eds.) (1976) *Learning Disability/Minimal Brain Dysfunction Syndrome.* Springfield, Ill.: C. C. Thomas.

Anderson, U. M. (1967) 'The incidence and significance of high frequency deafness in children.' *American Journal of Diseases of Children,* **113,** 560-565.

Anderson, W. A. D. (1963) 'The hyperkinetic child: a neurological appraisal.' *Neurology,* **13,** 968-973.

Andrews, F. M., Morgan, J. N., Sonquist, J. A. (1967) *Multiple Classification Analysis: a Report on a Computer Program for Multiple Regression Using Categorical Predictors.* Ann Arbor: Survey Research Center, University of Michigan.

Armstrong, D., Norman, M. G. (1974) 'Periventricular leucomalacia in neonates. Complications and sequelae.' *Archives of Disease in Childhood,* **49,** 367-375.

Arnvig, J. (1955) 'Vestibular function in deafness and severe hardness of hearing.' *Acta Oto-*

laryngologica, **45,** 283-288.
Asher, C., Roberts, J. A. F. (1949) 'Study on birth weight and intelligence.' *British Journal of Social Medicine,* **3,** 56-68.
Asher, P., Schonell, F. E. (1950) 'A survey of 400 cases of cerebral palsy in childhood.' *Archives of Disease in Childhood,* **25,** 360-378.
Ashford, J. R., Fryer, J. G., Brimblecombe, F. S. W. (1969) 'Secular trends in late foetal deaths, neonatal mortality and birth weight in England and Wales.' *British Journal of Preventive and Social Medicine,* **23,** 154-162.
Ashton, N., Ward, B., Serpell, G. (1953) 'Role of oxygen in the genesis of retrolental fibroplasia—a preliminary report.' *British Journal of Ophthalmology,* **37,** 513-520.
Avery, G. B., Meneses, L., Lodge, A. (1972) 'The clinical significance of "measurement microcephaly".' *American Journal of Diseases of Children,* **123,** 213-217.
Avery, M. E., Oppenheimer, E. H. (1960) 'Recent increase in mortality from hyaline membrane disease.' *Journal of Pediatrics,* **57,** 553-559.
Babson, S. G. (1970) 'Growth of low-birth-weight infants.' *Journal of Pediatrics,* **77,** 11-18.
—— Henderson, N. B. (1974) 'Fetal undergrowth: relation of head growth to later intellectual performance.' *Pediatrics,* **53,** 890-894.
—— Kangas, J., Young, N., Bramhall, J. L. (1964) 'Growth and development of twins of dissimilar size at birth.' *Pediatrics,* **33,** 327-333.
—— Behrman, R. E., Lessel, R. (1970) 'Fetal growth: liveborn birth weights for gestational age of white middle class infants.' *Pediatrics,* **45,** 937-944.
Bacola, B., Behrle, F. C., Schweinitz, L. de, Miller, H. C., Mira, M. (1966) 'Perinatal and environmental factors in late neurogenic sequelae.' *American Journal of Diseases of Children,* **112,** 359-374.
Baird, D. (1964) 'The epidemiology of prematurity.' *Journal of Pediatrics,* **65,** 909-924.
Balow, B., Rubin, R., Rosen, M. J. (1975/76) 'Perinatal events as precursors of reading disability.' *Reading Research Quarterly,* **1,** 36-71.
Balthazar, E. E. (1971) *Balthazar Scales of Adaptive Behavior for the Profoundly and Severely Mentally Retarded.* Champaign, Ill.: Research Press.
Banker, B. Q. (1967) 'The neuropathological effects of anoxia and hypoglycemia in the newborn.' *Developmental Medicine and Child Neurology,* **9,** 544-550.
—— Larroche, J. C. (1962) 'Periventricular leukomalacia of infancy. A form of neonatal anoxic encephalopathy.' *Archives of Neurology,* **7,** 386-410.
Bard, H. (1978) 'Neonatal problems of infants with intrauterine growth retardation.' *Journal of Reproductive Medicine,* **21,** 359-363.
Barkley, R. A. (1981) 'Specific guidelines for defining hyperactivity in children (attention deficit disorder).' *In:* Lahey, B., Kazdin, A. (Eds.) *Advances in Child Clinical Psychology, Vol. 4.* New York: Plenum Press.
Barnard, D. R, Simmons, M. A., Hathaway, W. E. (1979) 'Coagulation studies in extremely premature infants.' *Pediatric Research,* **13,** 1330-1335.
Barton, M. E. (1964) 'Prematurity and hearing loss.' *In:* Fisch, L. (Ed.) *Research in Deafness in Children.* Oxford: Blackwell Scientific. pp. 32-33.
—— Court, S. D., Walker, W. (1962) 'Causes of severe deafness in school-children in Northumberland and Durham.' *British Medical Journal,* **1,** 351-355.
Baum, J. D. (1971) 'Retinal artery tortuosity in ex-premature infants.' *Archives of Disease in Childhood,* **46,** 247-251.
—— Searls, D. (1971) 'Head shape and size of pre-term low-birthweight infants.' *Developmental Medicine and Child Neurology,* **13,** 576-581.
Bayley, N. (1958) 'Value and limitations of infant testing.' *Children,* **5,** 129-133.
Beargie, R. A., James, V. L., Greene, J. W. (1970) 'Growth and development of small-for-date newborns.' *Pediatric Clinics of North America,* **17,** 159-167.
Beckwith, L., Cohen, S. E., Kopp, C. B., Parmelee, A. H., Marcy, T. G. (1976) 'Caregiver-infant interaction and early cognitive development in preterm infants.' *Child Development,* **47,** 579-587.
Bejar, R., Curbelo, V., Coen, R. W., Leopold, G., James, H., Gluck, L. (1980) 'Diagnosis and follow-up of intraventricular hemorrhages by ultrasound studies of infant's brain through the fontanelles and sutures.' *Pediatrics,* **66,** 661-673.
Bell, A. E., Abrahamson, D. S., McRae, K. N. (1977) 'Reading retardation: a 12-year prospective study.' *Journal of Pediatrics,* **91,** 363-370.
Bender, L. (1956) *Psychopathology of Children with Organic Brain Disorders.* Springfield, Ill.: C. C. Thomas.

Bennett, F. C., Chandler, L. S., Robinson, N. M., Sells, C. J. (1981) 'Spastic diplegia in premature infants.' *American Journal of Diseases of Children,* **135,** 732-736.
Benton, A. L. (1940) 'Mental development of prematurely born children. A critical review of the literature.' *American Journal of Orthopsychiatry,* **10,** 719-746.
Bergman, I., Painter, M. J., Hirsch, R. P., Crumrine, P. K., David, R. (1983) 'Outcome in neonates with convulsions treated in an intensive care unit.' *Annals of Neurology,* **14,** 642-647.
—— Hirsch, R. P., Fria, T. J., Shapiro, S. M., Holzman, I., Painter, M. J. (1985) 'Cause of hearing loss in the high-risk premature infant.' *Journal of Pediatrics,* **106,** 95-101.
Bethenod, M., Bourgeois, J., Sann, L., Cottancin, G., Rigal, D., Fau, M., Vachet, M-F., Saunier, B. (1979) 'Evolution des enfants nés avec un très petit poids de naissance.' *Pédiatrie,* **34,** 573-593.
Bierman-van Eendenburg, M. E. C., Jurgens-van der Zee, A. D., Olinga, A. A., Huisjes, H. H., Touwen, B. C. L. (1981) 'Predictive value of neonatal neurological examination: a follow-up study at 18 months.' *Developmental Medicine and Child Neurology,* **23,** 296-305.
Birch, H. G. (1964) *Brain Damage in Children.* Baltimore: Williams & Wilkins.
—— Gussow, J. D. (1970) *Disadvantaged Children; Health, Nutrition and School Failure.* New York: Grune and Stratton.
Bjerre, I. (1975*a*) 'Physical growth of 5-year-old children with a low birth weight.' *Acta Paediatrica Scandinavica,* **64,** 33-43.
—— (1975*b*) 'Neurological investigation of 5-year-old children with low birthweight.' *Acta Paediatrica Scandinavica,* **64,** 859-864.
—— Hansen, E. (1976) 'Psychomotor development and school-adjustment of 7-year-old children with low birthweight.' *Acta Paediatrica Scandinavica,* **65,** 88-96.
—— Värendh, G. (1975) 'A study of some biological and socio-economic factors in low birth weight.' *Acta Paediatrica Scandinavica,* **64,** 605-612.
Black, B., Brown, C., Thomas, D. (1977) 'A follow-up study of 58 pre-school children less than 1500 grams birthweight.' *Australian Paediatric Journal,* **13,** 265-270.
Black, V. D., Lubchenco, L. O., Luckey, D. W., Koops, B. L., McGuinness, G. A., Howell, D. P., Tomlinson, A. L. (1982) 'Developmental and neurological sequelae of neonatal hyperviscosity syndrome.' *Pediatrics,* **69,** 426-431.
Blakeley, R. W. (1959) 'Erythroblastosis and perceptive hearing loss: responses of athetoids to tests of cochlear function.' *Journal of Speech and Hearing Research,* **2,** 5-15.
Blennow, G., Svenningsen, N. W., Almquist, B. (1974) 'Noise levels in infant incubators (adverse effects?)' *Pediatrics,* **53,** 29-32.
Bloom, L., Hood, L., Lightbown, P. (1974) 'Imitation in language development. If, when and why.' *Cognitive Psychology,* **6,** 380-420.
Bolton, D. P. G., Cross, K. W. (1974) 'Further observations on cost of preventing retrolental fibroplasia.' *Lancet,* **i,** 445-448.
Bond, G. L., Tinker, M. A. (1967) *Reading Difficulties: Their Diagnosis and Correction.* Toronto: Prentice Hall.
Borland, B. L., Heckman, H. K. (1976) 'Hyperactive boys and their brothers.' *Archives of General Psychiatry,* **33,** 669-675.
Bosch, C., Kowalewski, S. (1981) 'Ergebnisse neurologischer Nachuntersuchungen im Alter von 1-7 Jahren bei Frühgeborenen mit Geburtsgewichten unter 1500 Gramm.' *Monatsschrift für Kinderheilkunde,* **129,** 274-278.
Bosher, S. K. (1972) 'Neonatal changes in the endolymph and their possible relationship to peri-natal deafness.' *Acta Oto-laryngologica,* **73,** 203-211.
—— Hallpike, C. S. (1966) 'Observations of the histogenesis of the inner ear degeneration of the deaf white cat and its possible relationship to the aetiology of certain unexplained varieties of human congenital deafness.' *Journal of Laryngology and Otology,* **80,** 222-235.
Bowes, W. A., Halgrimson, M., Simmons, M. A. (1979) 'Results of the intensive perinatal management of very low-birth-weight infants (501 to 1500 grams).' *Journal of Reproductive Medicine,* **23,** 245-250.
Boydstun, J. A., Ackerman, P. T., Stevens, D. A., Clements, S. D., Peter, J. E., Dykman, R. A. (1968) 'Physiologic and motor conditioning and generalization in children with minimal brain dysfunction.' *Conditional Reflex,* **3,** 81-104.
Bradley, C. (1937) 'The behavior of children receiving benzedrine.' *American Journal of Psychiatry,* **94,** 577-585.
—— (1957) 'Characteristics and management of children with behaviour problems associated with organic brain damage.' *Pediatric Clinics of North America,* **4,** 1049-1060.
Brandt, I. (1973) 'Dynamik des postnatalen Schädelwachstums bei Früh und Reif- geborenen bis zum

18. Lebensmonat.' *Monatsschrift für Kinderheilkunde,* **121,** 12-18.
—— (1978) 'Growth dynamics of low-birth-weight infants with emphasis on the perinatal period.' *In:* Falkner, F., Tanner, J. M. (Eds.) *Human Growth, Vol. 2: Postnatal Growth.* New York: Plenum Press. pp. 557-617.
—— Schröder, R. (1971) 'Postnatales Wachstum and Psychische Entwicklung der Frühgeborenen im Vergleich zu den Reifgeborenen.' *Monatsschrift für Kinderheilkunde,* **119,** 275-282.
Bray, P. R., Shields, W. D., Wolcott, G. J., Madsen, J. A. (1969) 'Occipito-frontal head circumference—an accurate measurement of intracranial volume.' *Journal of Pediatrics,* **75,** 303-305.
British Columbia, Ministry of Health Division of Vital Statistics (1972, 1980) *Unpublished statistics from physician's notice of birth and registration of death. (Personal communication.)*
Brown, J. K. (1980) 'Some thoughts on cerebral palsy and perinatal asphyxia.' *In:* Tonkin, R. S. (Ed.) *Child Health Strategies.* Vancouver, B.C.: Alpine Press. pp. 45-55.
—— Purvis, R. J. Forfar, J. O., Cockburn, F. (1974) 'Neurological aspects of perinatal asphyxia.' *Developmental Medicine and Child Neurology,* **16,** 567-580.
Brown, R. (1973) *A First Language.* Cambridge, Mass.: Harvard University Press.
Bruckner, H. L. (1968) 'Retrolental fibroplasia—associated with intrauterine anoxia?' *Archives of Ophthalmology,* **80,** 504-505.
Buch, N. H. (1966) 'The inner ear of newborn infants (a histopathological study).' *Journal of Laryngology and Otology,* **80,** 765-777.
Buros, O. K. (Ed.) (1978) *The Eighth Mental Measurements Yearbook, Vol. 1.* New Jersey: Gryphor Press.
Burstein, J., Papile, L. A., Burstein, R. (1977) 'Subependymal germinal matrix and intraventricular hemorrhage in premature infants: diagnosis by CT.' *American Journal of Roentgenology,* **128,** 971-976.
Butler, B. V., Engel, R. (1969) 'Mental and motor scores at 8 months in relation to neonatal photic respones.' *Developmental Medicine and Child Neurology,* **11,** 77-82.
Butler, N. R., Alberman, E. (1969) *Perinatal Problems.* London: Longman.
Cain, L. F., Levine, S., Elzey, E. F. (1963) *Manual for the Cain-Levine Social Competency Scale.* Palo Alto, Ca.: Consulting Psychologists Press.
Calame, A., Prod'hom, L. S. (1972) 'Pronostic vital et qualité de survie des prématurés pesant 1500 g et moins à la naissance, soignés en 1966-1968.' *Schweizerische Medizinische Wochenschrift,* **102,** 65-70.
—— Reymond-Goni, I., Maherzi, M., Roulet, M., Marchand, C., Prod'hom, L. S. (1976) 'Psychological and neuro developmental outcome of high risk newborn infants.' *Helvetica Paediatrica Acta,* **31,** 287-297.
Camfield, P. R., Camfield, C. S., Allen, A. C., Rees, E. P., Stinson, D. A., Urban, L. E. (1981) 'Progressive hydrocephalus in infants with birth weights less than 1500 g.' *Archives of Neurology,* **38,** 653-655.
Campanelli, P. A., Pollock, F. J., Henner, R. (1958) 'An oto-audiological evaluation of forty-four premature children.' *Archives of Otolaryngology,* **67,** 609-615.
Campbell, S. B., Endman, M. W., Bernfeld, G. (1977) 'A three-year follow-up of hyperactive pre-schoolers into elementary school.' *Journal of Child Psychology and Psychiatry,* **18,** 239-249.
Canter, A. (1966) 'A background interference procedure to increase sensitivity of the Bender-Gestalt test to organic brain disorder.' *Journal of Consulting Psychology,* **30,** 91-97.
—— (1973) Personal communication.
Cantwell, D. P. (1972) 'Psychiatric illness in the families of hyperactive children.' *Archives of General Psychiatry,* **27,** 414-417.
Capper, A. M. (1928) 'Fate and development of immature and premature children: a clinical study and review of the literature, and a study of cerebral hemorrhage in the newborn infant.' *American Journal of Diseases of Children,* **35,** 262-288, 443-491.
Capute, A. J., Niedermeyer, E. F., Richardson, F. (1968) 'The electroencephalogram in children with minimal cerebral dysfunction.' *Pediatrics,* **41,** 1104-1114.
Caputo, D. V., Mandell, W. (1970) 'Consequences of low birth weight.' *Developmental Psychology,* **3,** 363-383.
—— Goldstein, K. M. Taub, H. B. (1979) 'The development of prematurely born children through middle childhood.' *In:* Field, T. M., Sostek, A. M. Goldberger, D., Shuman, H. H. (Eds.) *Infants Born at Risk.* New York: Spectrum.
—— —— —— (1981) 'Neonatal compromise and later psychological development: a 10-year longitudinal study. *In:* Friedman, S. L., Sigman, M. (Eds.) *Preterm Birth and Psychological*

Development. New York: Academic Press. pp. 353-386.
Castrén, J. (1955) 'The significance of prematurity on the eye with reference to retrolental fibroplasia.' *Acta Ophthalmologica Scandinavica,* Suppl. 44.
Centano, P. A., Walter, R., Thelander, H. E. (1956) 'A five-year study of prematurity.' *California Medicine,* **84,** 269-278.
Chadd, M. A., Gray, O. P. (1972) 'Hypothermia and coagulation defects in the newborn.' *Archives of Disease in Childhood,* **47,** 819-821.
Chamberlain, R. N., Simpson, R. N. (1977) 'Cross-sectional studies of physical growth in twins, postmature and small-for-dates children.' *Acta Paediatrica Scandinavica,* **66,** 457-463.
Chaplin, E. R., Goldstein, G. W., Myerberg, D. Z., Hunt, J. V., Tooley, W. H. (1980) 'Posthemorrhagic hydrocephalus in the preterm infant.' *Pediatrics,* **65,** 901-909.
Chase, H. C. (1977) 'Time trends in low birth weight in the United States, 1950-74.' *In:* Reed, D. M., Stanley, F. J. (Eds.) *The Epidemiology of Prematurity.* Baltimore: Urban & Schwarzenberg. pp. 17-37.
Chase, H. P. (1973) 'The effects of intrauterine and postnatal undernutrition on normal brain development.' *Annals of the New York Academy of Sciences,* **205,** 231-244.
Chessells, J. M., Wigglesworth, J. S. (1971) 'Coagulation studies in severe birth asphyxia.' *Archives of Disease in Childhood,* **46,** 253-256.
—— —— (1972) 'Coagulation studies in preterm infants with respiratory distress and intracranial hemorrhage.' *Archives of Disease in Childhood,* **47,** 564-570.
Childs, B., Evans, P. R. (1954) 'Birth weights of children with cerebral palsy.' *Lancet,* **i,** 642-646.
Chiswick, M. L., Johnson, M., Woodhall, C., Gowland, M., Davies, J., Toner, N., Sims, D. G. (1983) 'Protective effect of vitamin E (DL-alpha-tocopherol) against intraventricular hemorrhage in premature babies.' *British Medical Journal,* **2,** 81-84.
Churchill, J. A., Masland, R. L., Naylor, A. A., Ashworth, M. R. (1974) 'The etiology of cerebral palsy in pre-term infants.' *Developmental Medicine and Child Neurology,* **16,** 143-149.
Clark, C., Gibbs, J. A. H., Maniello, R., Outerbridge, E. W., Aranda, J. V. (1981) 'Blood transfusion: a possible risk factor in retrolental fibroplasia.' *Acta Paediatrica Scandinavica,* **70,** 535-539.
Clements, S. D. (1966) *Minimal Brain Dysfunction in Children. NINDB Monograph No. 3.* Washington, D.C.: U.S. Dept. of Health, Education and Welfare.
—— Peters, J. E. (1981) 'Syndromes of minimal brain dysfunction.' *In:* Black, P. (Ed.) *Brain Dysfunctions in Children: Etiology, Diagnosis and Management.* New York: Raven Press. pp. 181-191.
Cohen, N. J., Weiss, G., Minde, K. (1972) 'Cognitive styles in adolescents previously diagnosed as hyperactive.' *Journal of Child Psychology and Psychiatry,* **13,** 203-209.
Cohn, R. (1961) 'Delayed acquisition of reading and writing abilities in children.' *Archives of Neurology,* **4,** 153-164.
Collis, E. (1954) 'Some differential characteristics of cerebral motor defects in infancy.' *Archives of Disease in Childhood,* **29,** 113-122.
Commey, J. O., Fitzhardinge, P. M. (1979) 'Handicap in the preterm small for gestational age infant.' *Journal of Pediatrics,* **94,** 779-786.
Conners, C. K. (1973) 'Psychological assessment of children with minimal brain dysfunction.' *Annals of the New York Academy of Sciences,* **205,** 282-302.
Cooke, R. W. I., Lucas, A., Yudkin, P. L. N., Pryse-Davies, J. (1977) 'Head circumference as an index of brain weight in the fetus and newborn.' *Early Human Development,* **1,** 145-149.
Cooper, J. E. (1965) 'Epilepsy in a longitudinal survey of 5000 children.' *British Medical Journal,* **1,** 1020-1022.
Cornblath, M., Odell, G. B., Levin, E. Y. (1959) 'Symptomatic neonatal hypoglycemia associated with toxemia of pregnancy.' *Journal of Pediatrics,* **55,** 545-562.
Corner, B. (1960) *Prematurity.* London: Cassell.
Cornet, A., Bard, H., Orquin, J., Doray, B. H. (1976) 'Fibroplasie retrolenticulaire et exsanguino-transfusion.' *Union Médicale du Canada,* **105,** 1666-1668.
Corrigan, F. E., Berger, S. I., Dienstbier, R. A., Strok, E. S. (1967) 'Influence of prematurity on school performance.' *American Journal of Mental Deficiency,* **71,** 533-535.
Cox, L. C., Hack, M., Metz, D. A. (1984) 'Auditory brain stem response abnormalities in the very low birthweight infant: incidence and risk factors.' *Ear and Hearing,* **5,** 47-51.
Cox, M., Dunn, H. G. (1967) 'Idiopathic hypoglycaemia and children of low birth-weight.' *Developmental Medicine and Child Neurology,* **9,** 430-447.
Crabtree, N., Gerrard, J. (1950) 'Perceptive deafness associated with severe neonatal jaundice.' *Journal of Laryngology and Otology,* **64,** 482-506.

Crichton, J. U., Mackoff, H. P. (1969) 'A clinical approach to the measurement of cerebral dysfunction.' *Pediatrics,* **44,** 365-374.

—— Robertson, A. M., Tredger, E., Dunn, H. G. (1971) 'The evolution of minimal cerebral dysfunction in children of low birth weight.' *Proceedings of the XIIIth International Congress of Pediatrics, Vienna, Vol. 3.* Vienna: Vienna Academy of Medicine. pp. 135-140.

—— Dunn, H. G., McBurney, A. K., Robertson, A. M., Tredger, E. (1972*a*) 'Long-term effects of neonatal jaundice on brain function in children of low birth weight.' *Pediatrics,* **49,** 656-670.

—— —— —— —— —— (1972*b*) 'Minor congenital defects in children of low birth weight.' *Journal of Pediatrics,* **80,** 830-832.

Crinella, F. (1973) 'Identification of brain dysfunction syndromes in children through profile analysis: patterns associated with so-called "minimal brain dysfunction".' *Journal of Abnormal Psychology,* **82,** 33-45.

Cross, K. W. (1973) 'Cost of preventing retrolental fibroplasia?' *Lancet,* **2,** 954-956.

Crosse, V. M., Hill, E. E. (1975) *The Preterm Baby and Other Babies with Low Birth Weight. 8th edn.* Edinburgh: Churchill Livingstone. pp. 121-245.

Crothers, B., Paine, R. S. (1959) *The Natural History of Cerebral Palsy.* Cambridge, Mass.: Harvard University Press.

Cruise, M. O. (1973) 'A longitudinal study of the growth of low birth weight infants. I: Velocity and distance growth, birth to 3 years.' *Pediatrics,* **51,** 620-628.

Dale, A., Stanley, F. J. (1980) 'An epidemiological study of cerebral palsy in Western Australia, 1956-1975. II: Spastic cerebral palsy and perinatal factors.' *Developmental Medicine and Child Neurology,* **22,** 13-25.

Danish, J. M., Levitan, M. (1967) 'Changing aspects of deafness in school-age children.' *Archives of Otolaryngology,* **86,** 166-171.

Dann, M., Levine, S. Z., New, E. V. (1958) 'The development of prematurely born children with birth weights or minimal postnatal weights of 1000 grams or less.' *Pediatrics,* **22,** 1037-1053.

—— —— —— (1964) 'A long-term follow-up study of small premature infants.' *Pediatrics,* **33,** 945-960.

Daum, C., Danziger, A., Kurtzberg, D., Rugg, H., Vaughan, H. G. Jr. (1981) 'Periventricular low density as a predictor of neurobehavioural outcome in very low birth weight infants.' *Pediatric Research,* **15,** 447. *(Abstract.)*

Davey, P. R. (1962) 'Hearing loss in children of low birth weight.' *Journal of Laryngology and Otology,* **76,** 274-277.

Davie, R., Butler, N., Goldstein, H. (1972) *From Birth to Seven. A Report of the National Child Development Study.* London: Longman.

Davies, D. P. (1980) 'Size at birth and growth in the first year of life of babies who are overweight and underweight at birth.' *Proceedings of the Nutrition Society,* **39,** 25-33.

—— (1981) 'Growth of "small-for-dates" babies.' *Early Human Development,* **5,** 95-105.

—— Beverley, D. (1979) 'Changes in body proportions over the first year of life: comparisons between "light-for-dates" and "appropriate-for-dates" term infants.' *Early Human Development,* **3,** 263-265.

—— Evans, T. J. (1978) 'Nutrition and early growth of preterm infants.' *Early Human Development,* **2,** 383-392.

—— Platts, P., Pritchard, J. M., Wilkinson, P. W. (1979) 'Nutritional status of light-for-date infants at birth and its influence on early postnatal growth.' *Archives of Disease in Childhood,* **54,** 703-706.

Davies, P. A. (1984) 'Follow-up of low birthweight children.' *Archives of Disease in Childhood,* **59,** 794-797.

—— Davis, J. (1970) 'Very low birth-weight and subsequent growth.' *Lancet,* **2,** 1216-1219.

—— Stewart, A. L. (1975) 'Low-birth-weight infants: neurological sequelae and later intelligence.' *British Medical Bulletin,* **31,** 85-91.

—— Tizard, J. P. M. (1975) 'Very low birthweight and subsequent neurological defect (with special reference to spastic diplegia).' *Developmental Medicine and Child Neurology,* **17,** 3-17.

Davis, H., Silverman, S. R. (1970) *Hearing and Deafness (3rd edn.)* New York: Holt, Rinehart & Winston. pp. 255-256.

Dawkins, M. (1965) 'The "small for dates" baby.' *In:* Dawkins, M., MacGregor, B. (Eds.) *Gestational Age, Size and Maturity. Clinics in Developmental Medicine No. 19.* London: Spastics Society with Heinemann.

Dayal, V. S., Kokshanian, A., Mitchell, D. P. (1971) 'Combined effects of noise and kanamycin.' *Annals of Otology, Rhinology and Laryngology,* **80,** 897-902.

de Boer, C., Rice, J. R. (1968*a*) *Least Squares Cubic Spline Approximation I—Fixed Knots. Technical Report CSD TR 20.* Lafayette: Purdue University.

—— —— (1968*b*) *Least Squares Cubic Spline Approximation II—Variable Knots. Technical Report*

CSD TR 21. Lafayette: Purdue University.
de Hirsch, K., Jansky, J. J., Langford, W. S. (1964) 'The oral language performance of premature children and controls.' *Journal of Speech and Hearing Disorders,* **29,** 60-69.
—— —— —— (1966) 'Comparisons between prematurely and maturely born children at three age levels.' *American Journal of Orthopsychiatry,* **36,** 616-628.
de la Cruz, F. F., Fox, B. H., Roberts, R. H. (Eds.) (1973) *Minimal Brain Dysfunction. Annals of the New York Academy of Sciences,* **205.**
de Myer, M. K., Norton, J. A., Borton, S. (1971) 'Social and adaptive behaviours of autistic children as measured in a structured psychiatric interview.' *In:* Churchill, D. W., Alpern, G. D., de Myer, M. K. (Eds.) *Infantile Autism; Proceedings of Colloquium at Indiana University, 1968.* Springfield, Ill.: C. C. Thomas.
Denckla, M. B. (1977) 'Minimal brain dysfunction and dyslexia: beyond diagnosis by exclusion.' *In:* Blaw, M. E., Rapin, I., Kinsbourne, M. (Eds.) *Topics in Child Neurology.* New York: Spectrum Publications. pp. 243-261.
Denhoff, E. (1973) 'The natural life history of children with minimal brain dysfunction.' *Annals of the New York Academy of Sciences,* **205,** 188-205.
—— Hainsworth, P. K., Hainsworth, M. L. (1972) 'The child at risk for learning disorder.' *Clinical Pediatrics,* **11,** 164-170.
—— Stern, L. (1979) *Minimal Brain Dysfunction.* New York: Masson.
de Reuck, J., Chattha, A. S., Richardson, E. P. (1972) 'Pathogenesis and evolution of periventricular leukomalacia in infancy.' *Archives of Neurology,* **27,** 229-236.
DeSouza, S. W., Milner, R. D. G. (1974) 'Clinical and CSF studies in newborn infants with neurological abnormalities.' *Archives of Disease in Childhood,* **49,** 351-358.
Dobbing, J. (1970) 'Undernutrition and the developing brain. The relevance of animal models to the human problem.' *American Journal of Diseases of Children,* **120,** 411-415.
—— (1974) 'The later growth of the brain and its vulnerability.' *Pediatrics,* **53,** 2-6.
Doll, E. A. (1953) *Measurement of Social Competence. Educational Test Bureau.* Minneapolis: Educational Publishers.
Dominion Bureau of Statistics and Department of National Health and Welfare (1960) 'Mortality statistics of childhood.' *In: Canadian Conference on Children.* Ottawa: Queen's Printer.
Donovan, D. E., Coues, P., Paine, R. S. (1962) 'The prognostic implications of neurologic abnormalities in the neonatal period.' *Neurology,* **12,** 910-914.
Douek, E., Bannister, L. H., Dodson, H. C., Ashcroft, P., Humphries, K. N. (1976) 'Effects of incubator noise on the cochlea of the newborn.' *Lancet,* **2,** 1110-1113.
Douglas, A. A. (1961) 'Ophthalmological aspects.' *In:* Henderson, J. L. (Ed.) *Cerebral Palsy in Childhood and Adolescence: a Medical, Psychological and Social Study.* Edinburgh: E. & S. Livingstone.
—— (1963) 'The role of brain damage in the aetiology of squint.' *In:* Smith, V. H. (Ed.) *Visual Disorder and Cerebral Palsy, Little Club Clinics in Developmental Medicine No. 9.* London: National Spastics Society with Heinemann Medical. pp. 9-21.
Douglas, J. W. B. (1956) 'Mental ability and school achievement of premature children at 8 years of age.' *British Medical Journal,* **1,** 1210-1214.
—— (1960) '"Premature" children at primary schools.' *British Medical Journal,* **1,** 1008-1013.
—— Mogford, C. (1953) 'The results of a national enquiry into the growth of premature children from birth to 4 years.' *Archives of Disease in Childhood,* **28,** 436-445.
Dowding, V. M. (1981) 'New assessment of the effects of birth order and socio-economic status on birth weight.' *British Medical Journal,* **1,** 683-686.
Drage, J. S., Berendes, H. (1966) 'Apgar scores and outcome of the newborn.' *Pediatric Clinics of North America,* **13,** 637-643.
Drake, W. E. (1968) 'Clinical and pathological findings in a child with a developmental learning disability.' *Journal of Learning Disabilities,* **1,** 9-25.
Dreyfus-Brisac, C. (1962) 'The electroencephalogram of the premature infant.' *World Neurology,* **3,** 5-12.
—— (1966) 'The bioelectrical development of the central nervous system during early life.' *In:* Falkner, F. (Ed.) *Human Development.* Philadelphia: W. B. Saunders. pp. 286-305.
—— Minkowski, A. (1969) 'Low birth weight and EEG maturation.' *Electroencephalography and Clinical Neurophysiology,* **26,** 638.
—— Monod, N. (1966) 'Les foyers EEG (pointes) détectés par la surveillance systématique prolongée d'enfants nés à terme et prématurés. Etude électro-clinique.' *Revue de Neuropsychiatrie Infantile,* **14,** 899-924.

—— Flescher, J., Plassart, E. (1962) 'L'électroencéphalogramme: critère d'âge conceptionnel du nouveau-né à terme et prématuré.' *Biologia Neonatorum,* **4,** 154-173.
—— Monod, N., Morel-Kahn, F. (1962) 'Pointes focalisées chez l'enfant. Corrélations électrocliniques dans le cadre d'études longitudinales systématiques.' *Revue Neurologique,* **106,** 129.
Drillien, C. M. (1957) 'The social and economic factors affecting the incidence of premature birth. Part 1. Premature births without complications of pregnancy.' *Journal of Obstetrics and Gynaecology of the British Empire,* **64,** 161-184.
—— (1958) 'A longitudinal study of the growth and development of prematurely and maturely born children. I. Introduction.' *Archives of Disease in Childhood,* **33,** 417-431.
—— (1959) 'A longitudinal study of the growth and development of prematurely and maturely born children. Part III: Mental development.' *Archives of Disease in Childhood,* **34,** 37-45.
—— (1961*a*) 'A longitudinal study of the growth and development of prematurely and maturely born children. Part VII: Mental development, 2-5 years.' *Archives of Disease in Childhood,* **36,** 233-240.
—— (1961*b*) 'The incidence of mental and physical handicaps in school-age children of very low birth weight.' *Pediatrics,* **27,** 452-464.
—— (1964) *The Growth and Development of the Prematurely Born Infant.* Edinburgh: Livingstone.
—— (1967) 'The incidence of mental and physical handicaps in school age children of very low birth weight. II.' *Pediatrics,* **39,** 238-247.
—— (1968) 'Causes of handicap in the low weight infant.' *In:* Jonxis, J. H. P., Visser, H. K. A., Troelstra, J. A. (Eds.) *Aspects of Praematurity and Dysmaturity. Nutricia Symposium.* Leiden: H. E. Stenfert Kroese. pp. 287-302.
—— (1969) 'School disposal and performance for children of different birthweight born 1953-1960.' *Archives of Disease in Childhood,* **44,** 562-570.
—— (1970) 'The small-for-date infant: etiology and prognosis.' *Pediatric Clinics of North America,* **17,** 9-24.
—— (1972) 'Aetiology and outcome in low-birthweight infants.' *Developmental Medicine and Child Neurology,* **14,** 563-574.
—— Ingram, T. T. S., Russell, E. M. (1962) 'Comparative aetiological studies of congenital diplegia in Scotland.' *Archives of Disease in Childhood,* **37,** 282-288.
—— Thomson, A. J. M., Burgoyne, K. (1980) 'Low-birthweight children at early school-age: a longitudinal study.' *Developmental Medicine and Child Neurology,* **22,** 26-47.
Drorbaugh, J. E., Moore, D. M., Warram, J. H. (1975) 'Association between gestational and environmental events and central nervous system function in 7-year-old children.' *Pediatrics,* **56,** 529-537.
D'Souza, S. W., Black, P. (1979) 'A study of infant growth in relation to the type of feeding.' *Early Human Development,* **3,** 245-255.
Dubowitz, L. M. S., Dubowitz, V. (1981) *The Neurological Assessment of the Preterm and Fullterm Newborn Infant. Clinics in Developmental Medicine No. 79.* London: S.I.M.P. with Heinemann Medical; Philadelphia: Lippincott.
—— —— Palmer, P., Verghote, M. (1980) 'A new approach to the neurological assessment of the preterm and full-term infant.' *Brain and Development,* **2,** 3-14.
Duffy, F. H., Burchfield, J. L., Lombroso, C. T. (1979) 'Brain Electrical Activity Mapping (BEAM): a new method for extending the clinical utility of EEG and evoked potential data.' *Annals of Neurology,* **5,** 309-321.
—— Denckla, M. B., Bartels, P. H., Sandini, G. (1980) 'Dyslexia: regional differences in brain electrical activity by topographic mapping.' *Annals of Neurology,* **7,** 412-420.
Duke-Elder, S. (1970) *System of Ophthalmology. Vol. 5.* London: Henry Kimpton. p. 227.
Dunham, E. C. (1955) *Premature Infants.* New York: Harper.
Dunn, H. G. (1984) 'Social aspects of low birthweight.' *Canadian Medical Association Journal,* **130,** 1131-1141.
—— Crichton, J. U., Robertson, A. M., Traynor, M. E., Tredger, E. (1971) 'Late prognosis in children of low birthweight.' *In: Proceedings of the XIIIth International Congress of Pediatrics, Vienna.* Vienna: Vienna Academy of Medicine. pp. 33-38.
—— Auckland, N. L., Low, M. D., Crichton, J. U., Robertson, A. M., Tredger, E. M., McBurney A. K. (1973) 'Prospective study of electroencephalograms in children of low birthweight.' *Electro-encephalography and Clinical Neurophysiology,* **34,** 756.
—— Crichton, J. U., Robertson, A. M., McBurney, A. K., Schulzer, M. (1982*a*) 'Antecedents of mental retardation in children of low birthweight.' *Annals of Neurology,* **12,** 218.
—— —— —— —— Grunau, R. V. E., Schulzer, M. (1982*b*) 'Detection and prediction of mental retardation in children of low birthweight.' *In:* Fukuyama, Y., Arima, M., Maekawa, K.,

Yamaguchi, K. (Eds.) *Child Neurology. Excerpta Medica International Congress Series, No. 579.* Amsterdam: Excerpta Medica. pp. 194-201.
—— —— Grunau, R. V. E., McBurney, A. K., McCormick, A. Q., Schulzer, M. (1980) 'Neurological, psychological and educational sequelae of low birthweight.' *Brain and Development,* **2,** 57-67.
Dunsdon, M. I. (1947) 'Notes on the intellectual and social capacities of a group of young delinquents.' *British Journal of Psychology,* **38,** 62-66.
Dykman, R. A., Ackerman, P. T., Clements, S. D., Peters, J. E. (1971) 'Specific learning disabilities: an attentional deficit syndrome.' *In:* Myklebust, H. R. (Ed.) *Progress in Learning Disabilities, Vol. 2.* New York: Grune & Stratton. pp. 56-93.
—— Peters, J. E., Ackerman, P. T. (1973) 'Experimental approaches to the study of minimal brain dysfunction: a follow-up study.' *Annals of the New York Academy of Sciences,* **205,** 93-108.
Eastman, N. J., DeLeon, M. (1955) 'The etiology of cerebral palsy.' *American Journal of Obstetrics and Gynecology,* **69,** 950-961.
Eaves, L. C., Nuttall, J. C., Klonoff, H., Dunn, H. G. (1970) 'Developmental and psychological test scores in children of low birthweight.' *Pediatrics,* **45,** 9-20.
Edwards, W. C., Moran C. T. (1974) 'Esotropia surgery.' *Journal of Pediatric Ophthalmology,* **11,** 177-183.
Eeg-Olofsson, O. (1970) 'The development of the electroencephalogram in normal children and adolescents from the age of one through 21 years.' *Acta Paediatrica Scandinavica,* Suppl. 208, 1-46.
—— Petersén, I., Séllden, U. (1971) 'The development of the electroencephalogram in normal children from the age of one through 15 years. Paroxysmal activity.' *Neuropädiatrie,* **2,** 375-404.
Eichenwald, H. F. (1966) 'Some observations on dosage and toxicity of kanamycin in premature and full-term infants.' *Annals of the New York Academy of Sciences,* **132,** 984-991.
Eisenberg, L. (1957) 'Psychiatric implications of brain damage in children.' *Psychiatric Quarterly,* **31,** 72-92.
Ellenberg, J. H., Nelson, K. B. (1979) 'Birthweight and gestational age in children with cerebral palsy or seizure disorders.' *American Journal of Diseases of Children,* **133,** 1044-1048.
—— —— (1981) 'Early recognition of infants at high risk for cerebal palsy: examination at age four months.' *Developmental Medicine and Child Neurology,* **23,** 705-716.
Ellingson, R. J., Peters, J. F. (1980) 'Development of EEG and daytime sleep patterns in low risk premature infants during the first year of life: longitudinal observations.' *Electroencephalography and Clinical Neurophysiology,* **50,** 165-171.
—— Dutch, S. J., McIntire, M. S. (1964) 'A longitudinal study of EEG development in human prematures.' *Electroencephalography and Clinical Neurophysiology,* **17,** 711.
Ellis, E. N. (1975) *Survey of Achievement in Reading in Grade of Vancouver Schools, February 17-21, 1975. Research Report 75-09.* Vancouver, B.C.: Vancouver School Board, Evaluation and Research Education Services Group.
Ellison, P. H., Largent, J., Bahr, J. (1981) 'A scoring system to predict outcome following neonatal seizures.' *Journal of Pediatrics,* **99,** 455-459.
—— Franklin, S., Jones, M. G. (1982) 'Serial electroencephalography in the preterm infant as a predictor of neurological sequelae.' *Annals of Neurology,* **12,** 213A-214A.
Ennals, D. (1978) *Eleanor Rathbone Memorial Lecture. Health Circular HC (78) 5.* London: H.M.S.O.
Erickson, M. T. (1977) 'Reading disability in relation to performance on neurological tests for minimal brain dysfunction.' *Developmental Medicine and Child Neurology,* **19,** 768-775.
Everitt, B. (1974) *Cluster Analysis.* London: Heinemann Educational.
Falk, S. A. (1974) 'Noise pollution: neonatal aspects.' *Pediatrics,* **54,** 476-479.
—— Farmer, J. C. (1973) 'Incubator noise and possible deafness.' *Archives of Otolaryngology,* **97,** 385-387.
Falkner, F. (1973) 'Velocity growth.' *Pediatrics,* **51,** 746-747.
Fancourt, R., Campbell, S., Harvey, D., Norman, A. P. (1976) 'Follow-up study of small-for-dates babies.' *British Medical Journal,* **1,** 1435-1437.
Fedrick, J. (1969) 'Comparison of birthweight/gestation distribution in cases of stillbirth and neonatal death according to lesions found at necropsy.' *British Medical Journal,* **3,** 745-748.
—— Adelstein, P. (1978) 'Factors associated with low birthweight of infants delivered at term.' *British Journal of Obstetrics and Gynaecology,* **85,** 1-7.
—— Butler, N. R. (1970) 'Certain causes of neonatal death. II: Intraventricular haemorrhage.' *Biology of the Neonate,* **15,** 257-290.
Field, J. G. (1960) 'Two types of tables for use with Wechsler's intelligence scales.' *Journal of Clinical Psychology,* **16,** 3-7.
Field, T. M., Dempsey, J., Shuman, H. H. (1979) 'Bayley behavioral ratings of normal and high risk

infants: their relationship to Bayley mental scores.' *Journal of Pediatric Psychology,* **4,** 277-283.
——— ——— ——— (1981) 'Developmental follow-up of pre- and post-term infants.' *In:* Friedman, S. L., Sigman, M. (Eds.) *Preterm Birth and Psychological Development.* New York: Academic Press. pp. 299-312.
Fisch, L. (1955) 'The aetiology of congenital deafness and audiometric patterns.' *Journal of Laryngology and Otology,* **69,** 479-493.
—— (1964) 'The incidence of known and unknown causes of deafness and the verification of causes.' *In:* Fisch, L. (Ed.) *Research in Deafness in Children.* Oxford: Blackwell. pp. 14-25.
—— Norman, A. P. (1961) 'Hyperbilirubinaemia and perceptive deafness.' *British Medical Journal,* **2,** 142-144.
—— Osborn, D. A. (1954) 'Congenital deafness and haemolytic disease of the newborn.' *Archives of Disease in Childhood,* **29,** 309-316.
Fisch, R., Bilek, M., Miller, L., Engel, R. (1975) 'Physical and mental status at 4 years of age of survivors of the respiratory distress syndrome.' *Journal of Pediatrics,* **86,** 497-503.
—— Gravem, H. J., Engel, R. R. (1968) 'Neurological status of survivors of neonatal respiratory distress syndrome.' *Journal of Pediatrics,* **73,** 395-403.
Fishman, M. A., Palkes, H. S. (1974) 'The validity of psychometric testing in children with congenital malformations of the central nervous system.' *Developmental Medicine and Child Neurology,* **16,** 180-185.
Fitzgerald, G., Hallpike, C. S. (1942) 'Studies on the human vestibular function. I: Observations on the directional preponderance of caloric nystagmus resulting from central lesions.' *Brain,* **65,** 115-137.
Fitzhardinge, P. M., Pape, K. E. (1981) 'Follow-up studies of the high-risk newborn.' *In* Avery, G. B. (Ed.) *Neonatology, 2nd edn.* Philadelphia: Lippincott. pp. 350-367.
—— Ramsay, M. (1973) 'The improving outlook for the small prematurely born infant.' *Developmental Medicine and Child Neurology,* **15,** 447-459.
—— Steven, E. M. (1972*a*) 'The small-for-date infant. I: Later growth patterns.' *Pediatrics,* **49,** 671-681.
—— —— (1972*b*) The small-for-date infant. II: Neurological and intellectual sequelae.' *Pediatrics,* **50,** 50-57.
—— Pape, K., Arstikaitis, M., Boyle, M., Ashby, S., Rowley, A., Netley, C., Swyer, P. R. (1976) 'Mechanical ventilation of infants of less than 1501gm birthweight: health, growth and neurologic sequelae.' *Journal of Pediatrics,* **88,** 531-541.
Fletcher, M. C., Brandon, S. (1955) 'Myopia of prematurity.' *American Journal of Ophthalmology,* **40,** 474-481.
Fledelius, H. C. (1980) 'Ophthalmic changes from age 10 to 18 years. A longitudinal study of sequels of low birthweight. I: Refraction.' *Acta Ophthalmologica,* **58,** 889-898.
Flodmark, O., Becker, L. E., Harwood-Nash, D. C., Fitzhardinge, P. M., Fitz, C. R., Huang, S. H. (1980) 'Correlation between computed tomography and autopsy in premature and full-term neonates that have suffered perinatal asphyxia.' *Radiology,* **137,** 93-103.
—— Scotti, G., Harwood-Nash, D. C. (1981) 'Clinical significance of ventriculomegaly in children who suffered perinatal asphyxia with or without intracranial hemorrhage.' *Journal of Computer Assisted Tomography,* **5,** 663-673.
Francis-Williams, J., Davies, P. A. (1974) 'Very low birthweight and later intelligence.' *Developmental Medicine and Child Neurology,* **16,** 709-728.
Frandsen, A. D. (1960) 'Occurrence of squint.' *Acta Ophthalmologica,* Suppl. 62.
Fraser, G. R. (1964) 'A study of causes of deafness amongst 2,355 children in special schools.' *In:* Fisch, L. (Ed.) *Research in Deafness in Children.* Oxford: Blackwell. pp. 10-13.
—— (1976*a*) 'Preface.' *In: The Causes of Profound Deafness in Childhood: A Study of 3,535 Individuals with Severe Hearing Loss Present at Birth or of Childhood Onset.* London: Balliere Tindall. p. xi.
—— (1976*b*) 'Perinatally acquired deafness.' *In: The Causes of Profound Deafness in Childhood: A Study of 3,535 Individuals with Severe Hearing Loss Present at Birth or of Childhood Onset.* London: Balliere Tindall. pp. 247-267.
Fráter, R., Wohlmuth, G. (1965) 'Electroencephalographic examination of prematurely born school-age children.' *Acta Paediatrica Academiae Scientarum Hungaricae,* **6,** 305-311.
Freeman, L. C. (1965) *Elementary Applied Statistics for Students in Behavioral Sciences.* New York: John Wiley.
Freud, S. (1893) *Zur Kenntniss der Cerebralen Diplegien des Kindesalters. Beiträge zur Kinderheilkunde aus dem Ersten Öffentlichen Kinder-Kranken-Institut in Wien. N.F. III.* Leipzig: Deuticke. pp. 97-101.
Friedman, S. L., Sigman, M. (Eds.) (1981) *Preterm Birth and Psychological Development.* New York: Academic Press.

Fujimura, M., Seryu, J. (1977) 'Velocity of head growth during the perinatal period.' *Archives of Disease in Childhood,* **52,** 105-112.
—— Salisbury, D. M., Robinson, R. O., Howat, P., Emerson, P. M., Keeling, J. W., Tizard, J. P. M. (1979) 'Clinical events leading to intraventricular haemorrhage in the newborn.' *Archives of Disease in Childhood,* **54,** 409-414.
Fuldner, R. V. (1957) 'Labor complications and cerebral palsy.' *American Journal of Obstetrics and Gynecology,* **74,** 159-166.
Fuller, P. W., Guthrie, R. D., Alvord, E. C. (1983) 'A proposed neuropathological basis for learning disabilities in children born prematurely.' *Developmental Medicine and Child Neurology,* **25,** 214-231.
Galaburda, A. M., Kemper, T. L. (1979) 'Cytoarchitectonic abnormalities in developmental dyslexia: a case study.' *Annals of Neurology,* **6,** 94-100.
Gambaro, P. K. (1944) 'Analysis of Vineland Social Maturity Scale.' *American Journal of Mental Deficiency,* **48,** 359-363.
Gans, B. (1959) 'The pupillary membrane in premature infants.' *Archives of Disease in Childhood,* **34,** 292-297.
Gerrard, J. (1952) 'Kernicterus.' *Brain,* **75,** 526-570.
Gesell, A., Amatruda, C. S. (1947) *Developmental Diagnosis, 2nd edn.* New York: Hoeber.
Gillberg, I. C. Gillberg, C. (1983) 'Three-year follow-up at age 10 of children with minor neurodevelopmental disorders. I: Behavioural problems.' *Developmental Medicine and Child Neurology,* **25,** 438-449.
Gleiss, J., Pau, H. (1952) 'Die Entwicklung der Refraktion von der Geburt.' *Klinische Monatsblätte für Augenheilkunde,* **121,** 440-445.
Goetz, E. (1972) 'Auditory growth: development or practice?' *Proceedings of the American Psychopathological Association,* 123-124.
Goldschmidt, E. (1969) 'Refraction in the newborn.' *Acta Ophthalmologica,* **47,** 570-578.
Goldstein, H. (1971) 'Factors influencing the height of seven-year-old children—results from the National Child Development Study.' *Human Biology,* **43,** 92-111.
Goldstein, K. M., Caputo, D. V., Taub, H. B. (1976) 'The effects of prenatal and perinatal complications on development at one year of age.' *Child Development,* **47,** 613-621.
Gomez, M. R. (1967) 'Minimal cerebral dysfunction (maximal neurologic confusion).' *Clinical Pediatrics,* **6,** 589-591.
Graham, F. K., Ernhart, C. B., Thurston, D. B., Craft, M. (1962) 'Development three years after perinatal anoxia and other potentially damaging newborn experiences.' *Psychological Monographs,* No. 522.
Graham, M. V., Gray, O. P. (1963) 'Refraction of premature babies' eyes.' *British Medical Journal,* **1,** 1452-1454.
Graziani, L. J., Dave, R., Desai, H., Branca, P., Waldroup, L., Goldberg, B. (1980) 'Ultrasound studies in preterm infants with hydrocephalus.' *Journal of Pediatrics,* **97,** 624-630.
—— Mason, J. C., Cracco, J. (1981) 'Neurological aspects and early recognition of brain dysfunction in children: diagnostic and prognostic significance of gestational, perinatal and postnatal factors.' *In:* Black, P. (Ed.) *Brain Dysfunction in Children: Etiology, Diagnosis and Management.* New York: Raven Press. pp. 131-169.
Gray, O. P., Ackerman, A., Fraser, A. J. (1968) 'Intracranial haemorrhage and clotting defects in low birthweight infants.' *Lancet,* **1,** 545-548.
Griffiths, R. (1954) *The Abilities of Babies.* London: University of London Press.
Gröpl, H., Derbacher, D. (1971) 'Über das Schicksal von Frühgeborenen.' *Archiv für Kinderheilkunde,* **182,** 16-27.
Gross, G. P., Hathway, W. E., McGaughey, H. R. (1973) 'Hyperviscosity in the neonate.' *Journal of Pediatrics,* **82,** 1004-1012.
Gross, M. D., Wilson, W. C. (1974) *Minimal Brain Dysfunction.* New York: Brunner/Mazel.
Gross, S. J., Kosmetatos, N., Grimes, C. T., Williams, M. L. (1978) 'Newborn head size and neurological status.' *American Journal of Diseases of Children,* **132,** 753-756.
—— Eckerman, C. O. (1983) 'Normative early head growth in very-low-birthweight infants.' *Journal of Pediatrics,* **103,** 946-949.
Gruenwald, P. (1963) 'Chronic fetal distress and placental insufficiency.' *Biologia Neonatorum,* **5,** 215-265.
Gunn, T. R., Aranda, J. V., Little, J. (1978) 'Incidence of retrolental fibroplasia.' *Lancet,* **1,** 216-217.
—— Easdown, J., Outerbridge, E. W., Aranda, J. V. (1980) 'Risk factors in retrolental fibroplasia.' *Pediatrics,* **66,** 1096-1100.

Hack, M., Fanaroff, A., Merkatz, I. R. (1979) 'The low birthweight infant—evolution of a changing outlook.' *New England Journal of Medicine,* **301,** 1162-1165.
Hagberg, B. (1979) 'Epidemiological and preventive aspects of cerebral palsy and severe mental retardation in Sweden.' *European Journal of Pediatrics,* **130,** 71-78.
—— Hagberg, G., Olow, I. (1975*a*) 'The changing panorama of cerebral palsy in Sweden, 1954-1970. I: Analysis of the general changes.' *Acta Paediatrica Scandinavica,* **64,** 187-192.
—— —— —— (1975*b*) 'The changing panorama of cerebral palsy in Sweden, 1954-1970. II: Analysis of the various syndromes.' *Acta Paediatrica Scandinavica,* **64,** 193-200.
—— —— —— (1982) 'Gains and hazards of intensive neonatal care: an analysis from Swedish cerebral palsy epidemiology.' *Developmental Medicine and Child Neurology,* **24,** 13-19.
—— —— —— (1984) 'The changing pattern of cerebral palsy in Sweden. IV: Epidemiological trends, 1959-1978.' *Acta Paediatrica Scandinavica,* **73,** 433-440.
—— Olow, I., Hagberg, G. (1973) 'Decreasing incidence of low birthweight diplegia—an achievement of modern neonatal care?' *Acta Paediatrica Scandinavica,* **62,** 199-200.
Hall, J. G. (1962) 'A histological investigation of the auditory pathways in neonatal asphyxia.' *Acta Laryngologica,* **54,** 369-375.
—— (1963) 'On the neuropathological changes in the central nervous system following neonatal asphyxia with special reference to the auditory system in man.' *Acta Otolaryngologica,* Suppl. 188, 331-338.
—— (1964) 'The cochlea and the cochlear nuclei in neonatal asphyxia.' *Acta Otolaryngologica,* Suppl. 194, 5-93.
Hallahan, D. P., Cruickshank, W. M. (1973) *Psychoeducational Foundations of Learning Disabilities.* Englewood Cliffs, N.J.: Prentice Hall.
Hambleton, G., Wigglesworth, J. S. (1976) 'Origin of intraventricular haemorrhage in the preterm infant.' *Archives of Disease in Childhood,* **51,** 651-659.
Hansen, E. (1960) *Cerebral Palsy in Denmark.* Copenhagen: Munksgaard.
Hanvik, L. J., Nelson, S. E., Hanson, H. B., Anderson, A. S., Dressler, W. H., Zarling, V. R. (1961) 'Diagnosis of cerebral dysfunction in children as made in a child guidance clinic.' *American Journal of Diseases of Children,* **101,** 364-375.
Harper, P. A., Fischer, L. K., Rider, R. V. (1959) 'Neurological and intellectual status of prematures at three to five years of age.' *Journal of Pediatrics,* **55,** 679-690.
—— Wiener, G. (1965) 'Sequelae of low birthweight.' *Annual Review of Medicine,* **16,** 405-420.
Harris, R., Tizard, J. P. M. (1960) 'The electroencephalogram in neonatal convulsions.' *Journal of Pediatrics,* **57,** 501-520.
Harrison, V. C., Heese, H. de V., Klein, M. (1968) 'Intracranial haemorrhage associated with hyaline membrane disease.' *Archives of Disease in Childhood,* **43,** 116-120.
Harvey, D. R., Wallis, S. M. (1979) 'Neurological examination of children who were small-for-dates babies.' *Archives of Disease in Childhood,* **54,** 725-726.
—— Prince, J., Burton, J., Parkinson, C., Campbell, S. (1982) 'Abilities of children who were small-for-gestational-age babies.' *Pediatrics,* 296-300.
Haskins, R., Finkelstein, N. W., Stedman, D. J. (1978) 'Infant-stimulation programs and their effects.' *Pediatric Annals,* **7,** 99-128.
Haworth, J. C., McRae, K. N. (1965) 'The neurological and developmental effects of neonatal hypoglycemia: a follow-up of 22 cases.' *Canadian Medical Association Journal,* **92,** 861-865.
Heath, P. (1950) 'Retrolental fibroplasia as a syndrome.' *Archives of Ophthalmology,* **44,** 245-274.
Heber, R. (1961) *A Manual on Terminology and Classification in Mental Retardation. American Journal of Mental Deficiency, Monograph Supplement,* no. 64.
Hejna, R. (1955) *Developmental Articulation Test.* Madison, Wisconsin: College Printing and Typing Co.
Helper, M. M. (1980) 'Follow-up of children with minimal brain dysfunctions: outcome and predictors.' *In:* Rie, H. E., Rie, E. D. (Eds.) *Handbook of Minimal Brain Dysfunctions.* New York: John Wiley. pp. 75-114.
Herbert, M. (1964) 'The concept and testing of brain damage in children: a review.' *Journal of Child Psychology and Psychiatry,* **5,** 197-217.
Hertzig, M. E. (1981) 'Neurological "soft" signs in low birthweight children.' *Developmental Medicine and Child Neurology,* **23,** 778-791.
—— Bortner, M., Birch, H. G. (1969) 'Neurologic findings in children educationally designated as "brain damaged".' *American Journal of Orthopsychiatry,* **39,** 437-446.
Hervei, S., Bodánsky, H., Miriszlai, E., Csapó, S. (1977) 'Untersuchungen der Gehör- und Vestibular-funktion nach Icterus gravis.' *Monatsschrift für Kinderheilkunde,* **125,** 168-170.

Hess, J. H., Mohr, G. J., Bartelme, P. F. (1934) *The Physical and Mental Growth of Prematurely Born Children.* Chicago: University of Chicago Press.
Hill, A., Perlman, J. M., Volpe, J. J. (1982) 'Relationship of pneumothorax to occurrence of intraventricular hemorrhage in the premature newborn.' *Pediatrics,* **69,** 144-149.
Hinton, G. G., Knights, R. M. (1971) 'Children with learning problems: academic history, academic prediction and adjustment three years after assessment.' *Exceptional Children,* **38,** 513-519.
Hoff-Ginsberg, E., Shatz, M. (1982) 'Linguistic input and the child's acquisition of language.' *Psychological Medicine,* **92,** 3-26.
Hollingshead, A. B. (1957) *Two-factor Index of Social Position. (Mimeographed text available from author.)*
Holm, V. (1982) 'The causes of cerebral palsy.' *Journal of the American Medical Association,* **247,** 1473-1477.
Holmes, G., Rowe, J., Hafford, J., Schmidt, R., Testa, M., Zimmerman, A. (1982) 'Prognostic value of the electroencephalogram in neonatal asphyxia.' *Electroencephalography and Clinical Neurophysiology,* **53,** 60-72.
Hommers, M., Kendall, A. C. (1976) 'The prognosis of the very low-birth-weight infant.' *Developmental Medicine and Child Neurology,* **18,** 745-752.
Honegger, H. (1969) 'Der Augenhintergrund bei Neu- und Frühgeborenen.' *Deutsche ophthalmische Gesellschaft Berichte,* **69,** 156-158.
Horn, R., Grävinghoff, C., Wolf, H. (1969) 'Ergebnisse psychologischer Nachuntersuchungen von ehemals frühgeborenen und ehemals hypotrophen Neugeborenen.' *Monatsschrift für Kinderheilkunde,* **117,** 442-449.
Horwood, S. P., Boyle, M. H., Torrance, G. W., Sinclair, J. C. (1982) 'Mortality and morbidity of 500- to 1499-gram birthweight infants liveborn to residents of a defined geographic region before and after neonatal intensive care.' *Pediatrics,* **69,** 613-620.
Howard, J., Parmelee, A. H., Kopp, C. B., Littman, B. (1976) 'A neurologic comparison of preterm and full-term infants at term conceptional age.' *Journal of Pediatrics,* **88,** 995-1002.
Huessy, H. R., Cohen, A. H. (1976) 'Hyperkinetic behavior and learning disabilities followed over seven years.' *Pediatrics,* **57,** 4-10.
Hunt, J. V. (1978) 'Developmental profile.' *In:* Buros, D. K. (Ed.) *The Eighth Mental Measurements Yearbook.* New Jersey: Gryphon Press. pp. 304-305.
Hurst, J. G. (1962) 'The meaning and use of different scores obtained between performance on Stanford-Binet Intelligence Scale and Vineland Social Maturity Scale.' *Journal of Clinical Psychology,* **18,** 153-160.
Illingworth, R. S., Birch, H. B. (1959) 'The diagnosis of mental retardation in infancy. A follow-up study.' *Archives of Disease in Childhood,* **34,** 269-273.
Ingram, D. (1978) *Phonological Disability.* London: Arnold.
Ingram, T. T. S. (1955) 'The early manifestations and course of diplegia in childhood.' *Archives of Disease in Childhood,* **30,** 244-250.
—— (1964) *Paediatric Aspects of Cerebral Palsy.* Edinburgh: E. & S. Livingstone.
—— Mason, A. W., Blackburn, I. (1970) 'A retrospective study of 82 children with reading disability.' *Developmental Medicine and Child Neurology,* **12,** 271-281.
Ireton, H.,Thwing, E., Gravem, H. (1970) 'Relationships between infant mental development and neurological status, family socio-economic status, and intelligence at age four.' *Child Development,* **41,** 937-945.
James, L. S., Lanman, J. T. (Eds.) (1976) 'History of oxygen therapy and retrolental fibroplasia.' *Pediatrics,* **57,** 591-642.
Janzen, R., Bushart, W., Engel, R. (1968) 'Zur Aussagekraft des EEG beim Neugeborenen.' *Deutsche Zeitschrift für Nervenheilkunde,* **193,** 245-255.
Johnsen, S. (1952) 'Natal causes of perceptive deafness.' *Acta Otolaryngologica,* **42,** 51-63.
Johnston, W. H., Angara, V., Baumal, R., Hawke, W. A., Johnson, R. H., Keet, S., Wood, M. (1967) 'Erythroblastosis fetalis and hyperbilirubinemia.' *Pediatrics,* **31,** 88-92.
Johnstone, F., Inglis, L. (1974) 'Familial trends in low birthweight.' *British Medical Journal,* **3,** 659-661.
Jones, R. A. K., Cummins, M., Davies, P. A. (1979) 'Infants of very low birthweight.' *Lancet,* **1,** 1332-1335.
Kahn, E., Cohen, L. H. (1934) 'Organic drivenness: a brainstem syndrome and an experience.' *New England Journal of Medicine,* **210,** 748-756.
Kalina, R. E., Hudson, W. A., Morgan, B. C. (1972) 'Retrolental fibroplasia in a cyanotic infant.' *Pediatrics,* **50,** 765-768.
Kalverboer, A. F. (1978) 'MBD: discussion of the concept.' *In:* Kalverboer, A. F., van Praag, H. M.,

Mendlewicz, J. (Eds.) *Minimal Brain Dysfunction: Fact or Fiction?* Basel: Karger. pp. 5-17.
—— Touwen, B. C. L., Prechtl, H. F. R. (1973) 'Follow-up of infants at risk for minimal brain dysfunction.' *Annals of the New York Academy of Sciences,* **205,** 173-187.
—— van Praag, H. M., Mendlewicz, J. (Eds.) (1978) *Minimal Brain Dysfunction: Fact or Fiction?* Basel: Karger.
Karch, D., Kästl, E., Sprock, I., Bernuth, H. von (1977) 'Perinatal hypoxia and bioelectric brain maturation of the newborn infant.' *Neuropädiatrie,* **8,** 253-262.
—— Rothe, R., Jurisch, R., Heldt-Hildenbrandt, R,., Lübbesmeier, A., Lemburg, P. (1982) 'Behavioural changes and bioelectric brain maturation of preterm and fullterm newborn infants: a polygraphic study.' *Developmental Medicine and Child Neurology,* **24,** 30-47.
Karlsberg, R. C., Green, W. R., Patz, A. (1973) 'Congenital retrolental fibroplasia.' *Archives of Ophthalmology,* **89,** 122-123.
Kastein, S., Fowler, E. P. (1959) 'Language development among survivors of premature birth.' *Archives of Otolaryngology,* **69,** 131-135.
Katz, C. M., Taylor, P. M. (1967) 'The incidence of low birthweight in children with severe mental retardation.' *American Journal of Diseases of Children,* **114,** 79-87.
Kawi, A. A., Pasamanick, B. (1958) 'Association of factors of pregnancy with reading disorders in childhood.' *Journal of the American Medical Association,* **166,** 1420-1423.
—— —— (1959) 'Prenatal and paranatal factors in the development of childhood reading disorders.' *Monographs of the Society for Research in Child Development,* 24.
Keaster, J., Hyman, C. B. Harris, I. (1969) 'Hearing problems subsequent to neonatal hemolytic disease or hyperbilirubinemia.' *American Journal of Diseases of Children,* **117,** 406-410.
Keleman, G. (1963) 'Hemorrhage: a specific poison to tissue of ampullar cupulae.' *Archives of Otolaryngology,* **77,** 365-375.
Kellaway, P., Crawley, J. (1964) *A Primer of Electroencephalography in the Newborn.* Bethesda: National Institutes of Health.
Kennard, M. (1960) 'Value of equivocal signs in neurological diagnosis.' *Neurology,* **10,** 753-764.
—— Willner, M. D. (1947) 'Significance of paroxysmal patterns in electroencephalograms of children without clinical epilepsy.' *In:* Lennox, W. G., Merritt, H. H., Bamford, T. E. (Eds.) *Epilepsy. Research Publications of the Association for Research in Nervous and Mental Diseases, Vol. 26.* pp. 308-327.
Kenny, T. J., Clemmens, R. L., Hudson, B. W., Lentz, G. A., Cicci, R., Nair, P. (1971) 'Characteristics of children referred because of hyperactivity.' *Journal of Pediatrics,* **79,** 618-622.
Kessel, S. S., Villar, J., Berendes, H. W., Nugent, R. P. (1984) 'The changing pattern of low birthweight in the United States.' *Journal of the American Medical Association,* **251,** 1978-1982.
Kessler, J. W. (1980) 'History of minimal brain dysfunction.' *In:* Rie, H. E., Rie, E. D. (Eds.) *Handbook of Minimal Brain Dynsfunctions.* New York: John Wiley. pp. 18-51.
Kiely, J. L., Paneth, N. (1981) 'Follow-up studies of low birthweight infants: suggestions for design, analysis and reporting.' *Developmental Medicine and Child Neurology,* **23,** 96-100.
—— —— Stein, Z., Susser, M. (1981*a*) 'Cerebral palsy and newborn care. I: Secular trends in cerebral palsy.' *Developmental Medicine and Child Neurology,* **23,** 533-537.
—— —— —— —— (1981*b*) 'Cerebral palsy and newborn care. II: Mortality and neurological impairment in low-birthweight infants.' *Developmental Medicine and Child Neurology,* **23,** 650-659.
Kinsey, V. E. (1956) 'Retrolental fibroplasia: co-operative study of retrolental fibroplasia and the use of oxygen.' *Archives of Ophthalmology,* **56,** 481-543.
—— Arnold, H. J., Kalina, R. E., Stern, L., Stahlman, M., Odell, G., Driscoll, J. M., Elliott, J. H., Payne, J., Patz, A. (1977) 'PaO_2 levels and retrolental fibroplasia: a report of the co-operative study.' *Pediatrics,* **60,** 655-668.
Kitchen, W. H., Richards, A., Ryan, M. M., McDougall, A. B., Billson, F. A., Keir, E. H., Naylor, F. D. (1979) 'A longitudinal study of very low birthweight infants. II: Results of a controlled trial of intensive care and incidence of handicaps.' *Developmental Medicine and Child Neurology,* **21,** 582-589.
—— McDougall, A. B., Naylor, F. D. (1980) 'A longitudinal study of very low birthweight infants. III: Distance growth at eight years of age.' *Developmental Medicine and Child Neurology,* **22,** 163-171.
—— Ford, G., Orgill, A., Rickards, A., Astbury, J., Lissenden, J., Bajuk, B., Yu, V., Drew, J., Campbell, W. (1984) 'Outcome of infants with birthweight 500-999gm: a regional study of 1979 and 1980 births.' *Journal of Pediatrics,* **104,** 921-927.
Klaus, M., Jerauld, R., Kreger, N., McAlpine, W., Steffa, M., Kennell, J. (1972) 'Maternal attachment—importance of the first post-partum days.' *New England Journal of Medicine,* **286,** 460-463.

Knobloch, H., Pasamanick, B. (1959) 'Syndrome of minimal cerebral damage in infancy.' *Journal of the American Medical Association,* **170,** 1384-1387.
—— —— (1960) 'Environmental factors affecting human development before and after birth. *Pediatrics,* **26,** 210-218.
—— Rider, R., Harper, P., Pasamanick, B. (1956) 'Neuropsychiatric sequelae of prematurity.' *Journal of the American Medical Association,* **161,** 581-585.
—— Malone, A., Ellison, P. H., Stevens, F., Zdeb, M. (1982) 'Considerations in evaluating changes in outcome for infants weighing less than 1501 grams.' *Pediatrics,* **69,** 285-295.
Kontras, S. B. (1972) 'Polycythemia and hyperviscosity syndrome in infants and children.' *Pediatric Clinics of North America,* **19,** 919-933.
Korobkin, R. (1975) 'The relationship between head circumference and the development of communicating hydrocephalus in infants following intraventricular hemorrhage.' *Pediatrics,* **56,** 74-77.
Kraushar, M. R., Harper, R. G., Sia, C. C. (1975) 'Retrolental fibroplasia in a full-term infant.' *American Journal of Ophthalmology,* **80,** 106-108.
Krishnamoorthy, K. S., Shannon, D. C., De Long, G. R., Todres, I. D., Davis, K. R. (1979) 'Neurologic sequelae in survivors of neonatal intraventricular hemorrhage.' *Pediatrics,* **64,** 233-237.
Kruuse, E. (1976) 'Reading-retarded pupils' weight at birth.' *Skolepsykolegi,* **13,** 227-231.
Kryter, K. D. (1973) 'Impairment to hearing from exposure to noise.' *Journal of the Acoustical Society of America,* **53,** 1211-1234.
Kudrjavcev, T., Schoenberg, B. S., Kurland, L. T., Groover, R. V. (1983) 'Cerebral palsy—trends in incidence and changes in concurrent neonatal mortality: Rochester, MN, 1950-1976.' *Neurology,* **33,** 1433-1438.
Kumar, S. P., Anday, E. K., Sacks, L. M., Ting, R. Y., Delivoria-Papadopoulos, M. (1980) 'Follow-up studies of very low birthweight infants (1250 grams or less) born and treated within a perinatal center.' *Pediatrics,* **66,** 438-444.
Kurtzberg, D., Vaughan, H. G., Daum, C., Grelling, B. A., Albin, S., Rotkin, L. (1979) 'Neurobehavioural performance of low-birthweight infants at 40 weeks conceptional age: comparison with normal full-term infants.' *Developmental Medicine and Child Neurology,* **21,** 590-607.
Lairy, G. C., Harrison, A. (1968) 'Functional aspects of EEG foci in children.' *In:* Kellaway, P., Petersen, I. (Eds.) *Clinical Electroencephalography of Children.* Stockholm: Almqvist & Wiksell.
Lancet, Leading Article (1980) 'The fate of the baby under 1501g at birth.' *Lancet,* **1,** 461-463.
Lande, L. (1948) 'Clinical signs and development of survivors of kernicterus due to Rh sensitization.' *Journal of Pediatrics,* **32,** 693-705.
Larroche, J. C. (1964) 'Hémorrhagies cérébrales intra ventriculaires chez le prématuré. Partie I (Anatomie et physiopathologie).' *Biologia Neonatorum,* **7,** 26-56.
—— (1972) 'Post-haemorrhagic hydrocephalus in infancy: anatomical study.' *Biology of the Neonate,* **20,** 287-299.
—— Haggai, E. (1967) 'Maturation cérébrale et hypodéveloppement ponderal du nouveau-né.' *Journal of the Neurological Sciences,* **5,** 39-59.
Laubichler, W. (1970) 'Korrelation von Elektroenzephalographie und klinisch-neurologischem Befund bei Säuglingen.' *Archiv für Kinderheilkunde,* **180,** 165-189.
Laufer, M. W. (1962) 'Cerebral dysfunction and behavior disorders in adolescents.' *American Journal of Orthopsychiatry,* **32,** 501-506.
—— (1979) 'Defining the minimal brain dysfunction syndrome.' *In:* Denhoff, E., Stern, L. (Eds.) *Minimal Brain Dysfunction: A Developmental Approach.* New York: Masson. pp. 11-16.
—— Denhoff, E., Solomons, G. (1957) 'Hyperkinetic impulse disorder in children's behavior problems.' *Psychosomatic Medicine,* **19,** 38-49.
Le, C. (1972) *Multiple Classification Analysis: A Computer Program Adapted from ICPR Documentation for the IBM 360/67.* Vancouver: University of British Columbia Computing Centre.
Lee, A. (1977) 'Relationship between birthweight and perceptual motor performance in children.' *Perceptual and Motor Skills,* **45,** 119-122.
Lee, B., Grassi, A. E., Schechner, S., Auld, P. A. (1979) 'Neonatal intraventricular hemorrhage: a serial computed tomography study.' *Journal of Computer Assisted Tomography,* **3,** 483-490.
Lee, K.-S., Tseng, P., Eidelman, A. I., Kandall, S. R., Gartner, L. M. (1976) 'Determinants of neonatal mortality.' *American Journal of Diseases of Children,* **130,** 842-845.
—— Paneth, N., Gartner, L. M., Pearlman, M. A., Gruss, L. (1980) 'Neonatal mortality: an analysis of the recent improvement in the United States.' *American Journal of Public Health,* **70,** 15-21.
Leech, R. W., Kohnen, P. (1974) 'Subependymal and intraventricular hemorrhages in the newborn.'

American Journal of Pathology, **77**, 465-475.
Leiderman, P. H., Seashore, M. J. (1975) 'Mother-infant neonatal separation: some delayed consequences.' *In:* Porter, R., O'Connor, M. (Eds.) *Parent-infant Interaction. Ciba Foundation Symposium, No. 33.* Amsterdam: Elsevier.
Leifer, A. D., Leiderman, P. H., Barnett, C. R., Williams, J. A. (1972) 'Effects of mother-infant separation on maternal attachment behavior.' *Child Development,* **43,** 1203-1205.
Lennox-Buchthal, M. A. (1974) 'Febrile convulsions.' *In:* Vinken, P. J., Bruyn, G. W. (Eds.) *Handbook of Clinical Neurology, Vol. 15: The Epilepsies.* Amsterdam: North Holland.
Levinson, J. D., Gibbs, E. L., Stillerman, M. L., Perlstein, M. A. (1951) 'Electroencephalogram and eye disorders.' *Pediatrics,* **7,** 422-427.
Lindsey, J. D., Frith, G. H. (1981) 'Effects of exceptionality status and art instruction on Goodenough-Harris Standard IQs.' *American Journal of Mental Deficiency,* **85,** 658-660.
Lombroso, C. T. (1975) 'Neurophysiological observations on diseased newborns.' *Biological Psychiatry,* **10,** 527-558.
—— (1981) 'Some aspects of EEG-polygraphy in newborns at risk from neurological disorders.' *In:* Proceedings of the 10th International Congress of Electroencephalography and Clinical Neurophysiology, Kyoto Symposium, No. 2.
—— (1982) 'Neonatal electroencephalography.' *In:* Niedermeyer, E., Da Silva, P. L. (Eds.) *Electroencephalography.* Baltimore: Urban & Schwarzenberg; Part III, Ch. 2.
Lomičkova, H. (1971) 'Health of children of low birthweight at the age of 10 years. VII: Ophthalmological findings.' *(Czech.) Ceskoslovenská Pediatrie,* **26,** 538-539.
—— (1972) 'The development of ocular refraction in children of low birthweight.' *(Czech.) Ceskoslovenská Pediatrie,* **27,** 446-448.
—— Melichar, V. (1968) 'Eye background findings in premature and hypotrophic newborns.' *Biologia Neonatorum,* **12,** 170-174.
London, D. A., Carroll, B. A., Enzman, D. R. (1980) 'Sonography of ventricular size and germinal matrix hemorrhage in premature infants.' *American Journal of Roentgenology,* **135,** 559-564.
Lorber, J., Bhat, U. S. (1974) 'Post-haemorrhagic hydrocephalus: diagnosis, differential diagnosis and long-term results.' *Archives of Disease in Childhood,* **49,** 751-762.
Lou, H. C., Lassen, N. A., Friis-Hansen, B. (1977) 'Low cerebral blood flow in the hypotensive distressed newborn.' *Acta Neurologica Scandinavica,* **64,** 428-429.
—— —— —— (1979) 'Impaired autoregulation of cerebral blood flow in the distressed newborn infant.' *Journal of Pediatrics,* **94,** 118-121.
Low, M. D., Rogers, L. J., Purves, S. J., Dunn, H. G. (1979) 'Spontaneous and evoked cerebral electrical activity and localization of language function in children with minimal cerebral dysfunction.' *In:* Lehmann, D., Callaway, E. (Eds.) *Human Evoked Potentials.* New York: Plenum. pp. 215-234.
Lubchenco, L. O. (1976) *The High Risk Infant.* Philadelphia: W. B. Saunders.
—— Hansman, C., Dressler, M., Boyd, E. (1963*a*) 'Intrauterine growth as estimated from live-born birthweight data at 24 to 42 weeks of gestation.' *Pediatrics,* **32,** 793-800.
—— Horner, L. O., Reed, L. H., Hix, I. E., Metcalf, D., Cohig, R., Elliott, H. C., Bourg, M. (1963*b*) 'Sequelae of premature birth.' *American Journal of Diseases of Children,* **106,** 101-115.
—— Hansman, C., Boyd, E. (1966) 'Intrauterine growth in length and head circumference as estimated from live births at gestational ages from 26 to 42 weeks.' *Pediatrics,* **37,** 403-408.
—— Delivoria-Papadopoulos, M., Butterfield, L. J., French, J. H., Metcalf, D., Hix, I. E., Janick, J., Dodds, J., Downs, M., Freeland, E. (1972*a*) 'Long-term follow-up studies of prematurely born infants. I: Relationship of handicap to nursery routines.' *Journal of Pediatrics,* **80,** 501-508.
—— —— Searls, D. (1972*b*) 'Long-term follow-up studies of prematurely born infants. II: Influence of birthweight and gestational age on sequelae.' *Journal of Pediatrics,* **80,** 509-512.
—— Bard, H., Goldman, A. L., Coyer, W. E., McIntyre, C., Smith, D. M. (1974) 'Newborn intensive care and long-term prognosis.' *Developmental Medicine and Child Neurology,* **16,** 421-431.
Lucas, A., Gore, S. M., Cole, T. J., Bamford, M. F., Dossetor, J. F. B., Barr, I., Dicarlo, I., Cork, S., Lucas, P. J. (1984) 'Multicentre trial in feeding low birthweight infants: effects of diet on early growth.' *Archives of Disease in Childhood,* **59,** 722-730.
Lucas, A. R., Rodin, E. A., Simson, C. B. (1965) 'Neurological assessment of children with early school problems.' *Developmental Medicine and Child Neurology,* **7,** 145-156.
Luria, A. (1959) 'Experimental study of the higher nervous activity of the abnormal child.' *Journal of Mental Deficiency Research,* **3,** 1-22.
Lurie, L. A., Newberger, M., Rosenthal, F. M., Outcalt, L. C. (1941) 'Intelligence quotient and social quotient.' *American Journal of Orthopsychiatry,* **11,** 111-117.

Lütschg, J., Bina, M., Matsumiya, Y., Lombroso, C. T. (1980) 'Brainstem and auditory evoked potentials in asphyxiated and neurologically abnormal newborns.' *Electroencephalography and Clinical Neurophysiology,* **49,** 27.

Lyle, J. G. (1970) 'Certain antenatal, perinatal and developmental variables and reading retardation in middle class boys.' *Child Development,* **41,** 481-491.

Lynch, M. A. (1975) 'Ill health and child abuse.' *Lancet,* **2,** 317-319.

Maccoby, E. E., Jacklin, C. N. (1974) *The Psychology of Sex Differences.* Palo Alto, California: Stanford University Press.

McCormick, A. Q. (1977) 'Retinopathy of prematurity.' *Current Problems in Pediatrics,* **7,** (11).

McDonald, A. D. (1962) 'Neurological and ophthalmic disorders in children of very low birthweight.' *British Medical Journal,* **1,** 895-900.

—— (1964) 'Fits in children of very low birthweight.' *Developmental Medicine and Child Neurology,* **6,** 144-148.

—— (1967) *Children of Very Low Birthweight. M.E.I.U. Monograph No. 1.* London: Spastics Society with Heinemann.

—— (1981) 'Survival and handicap in infants of very low birthweight.' *Lancet,* **2,** 194. *(Letter.)*

McFie, J., Robertson, J. (1973) 'Psychological test results of children with thalidomide deformities.' *Developmental Medicine and Child Neurology,* **15,** 719-727.

McIntosh, E. I., Warren, S. A. (1969) 'Adaptive behavior in the retarded.' *Training School Bulletin,* **66,** 12-22.

Mac Keith, R. (1963) 'Defining the concept of "minimal brain damage".' *In:* Mac Keith, R., Bax, M. (Eds.) *Minimal Cerebral Dysfunction. Clinics in Developmental Medicine, No. 10.* London: Spastics Society with Heinemann.

—— (1974) 'High activity and hyperactivity.' *Developmental Medicine and Child Neurology,* **16,** 543-544.

McLellan, M. S., Strong, J. P., Johnson, Q. R., Dent, J. H. (1962) 'Otitis media in premature infants—a histopathologic study.' *Journal of Pediatrics,* **61,** 53-57.

—— Struck, A. (1965) 'Ear studies in the premature infant: a statistic description of otoscopic landmarks.' *Journal of Pediatrics,* **67,** 122-123.

McMahon, S. A., Greenberg, L. M. (1977) 'Serial neurologic examination of hyperactive children.' *Pediatrics,* **59,** 584-587.

Majima, A., Takahashi, M., Hibino, Y. (1972) 'Clinical studies on retinopathy of prematurity.' *Acta Societatis Ophthalmologiae Japonicae,* **76,** 1030-1036.

Marcus, R. E., Small, H., Emanuel, B. (1963) 'Ototoxic medication in premature children.' *Archives of Otolaryngology,* **77,** 198-204.

Martell, M., Falkner, F., Bertolini, L. B., Diaz, J. L., Nieto, F., Tenzer, F. M., Belitzky, R. (1978) 'Early postnatal growth evaluation in full-term, preterm and small-for-dates infants.' *Early Human Development,* **1,** 313-323.

Mau, G. (1977) 'Entwicklung reifegestörter Neugeborener.' *Medizinische Welt,* **28,** 1423-1426.

May, E. R. (1958) *Ph.D. Thesis, University of Birmingham* (See Crosse and Hill, 1975).

Mehra, K. S., Vaithilingam, E. (1965) 'Refraction in full-term babies.' *British Journal of Ophthalmology,* **49,** 276-277.

Meier, J. H. (1971) 'Prevalence and characteristics of learning disabilities found in second grade children.' *Journal of Learning Disabilities,* **4,** 1-6.

Mendelson, W., Johnson, N., Stewart, M. A. (1971) 'Hyperactive children as teenagers: a follow-up study.' *Journal of Nervous and Mental Diseases,* **153,** 273-279.

Menkes, M. M., Rowe, J. S., Menkes, J. H. (1967) 'A twenty-five year follow-up study on the hyperkinetic child with minimal brain dysfunction.' *Pediatrics,* **39,** 393-399.

Mercer, H. P., Lancaster, P. A. L., Weiner, T., Gupta, J. M. (1978) 'Very low birthweight infants: a follow-up study.' *Medical Journal of Australia,* **2,** 581-584.

Merchant, M. (1974) *Interactive Spline Approximation.* Master's Thesis, University of British Columbia, Department of Computer Sciences.

Merritt, J. C., Sprague, D. H., Merritt, W. E., Ellis, R. A. (1981) 'Retrolental fibroplasia: a multifactorial disease.' *Anesthesia and Analgesia,* **60,** 109-111.

Michaelis, R., Parmelee, A. H., Stern, E., Haber, A. (1972) 'Activity stages in premature and term infants.' *Developmental Psychobiology,* **6,** 209-215.

Millar, J. H. D. (1965) 'Epilepsy and strabismus.' *Epilepsia,* **6,** 43-46.

Miller, F. J. W., Court, S. D. M., Walton, W. S., Knox, E. G. (1960) *Growing Up in Newcastle upon Tyne.* London: Oxford University Press.

Miller, H. C., Hassanein, K. (1971) 'Diagnosis of impaired fetal growth in newborn infants.' *Pediatrics,*

48, 511-522.
——— (1973) 'Fetal malnutrition in white newborn infants: maternal factors.' *Pediatrics,* **52,** 504-512.
Miller, R. G. (1966) *Simultaneous Statistical Inference.* New York: McGraw Hill.
Milligan, D. W. (1980) 'Failure of autoregulation and intraventricular haemorrhages in preterm infants.' *Lancet,* **1,** 896-898.
Milman, D. H. (1979) 'Minimal brain dysfunction in childhood: outcome in late adolescence and early adult years.' *Journal of Clinical Psychiatry,* **40,** 371-380.
Minde, K., Lewin, D., Weiss, G., Lavigueur, H., Douglas, V., Sykes, E. (1971) 'The hyperactive child in elementary school: a 5-year controlled follow-up.' *Exceptional Children,* **38,** 215-221.
Minkowski, A., Amiel-Tison, C., Cukier, F. (1977) 'Long-term follow-up and sequelae of asphyxiated infants.' *In:* Gluck, L. (Ed.) *Intrauterine Asphyxia and the Developing Fetal Brain.* Chicago: Year Book Medical Publishers.
Mohr, G. J., Bartelme, P. F. (1934) 'Physical growth of prematurely born children.' *In:* Hess, J. H., Mohr, G. J., Bartelme, P. F. (Eds.) *The Physical and Mental Growth of Prematurely Born Children.* Chicago: University of Chicago Press.
Monod, N., Dreyfus-Brisac, C. (1962) 'Le tracé paroxystique chez le nouveau-né.' *Revue Neurologique,* **106,** 129-130.
—— Ducas, P. (1968) 'The prognostic value of the electroencephalogram in the first two years of life.' *In:* Kellaway, P., Petersen, I. (Eds.) *Clinical Electroencephalography of Children.* Stockholm: Almqvist & Wiksell. pp. 61-76.
—— Salama, P., Dreyfus-Brisac, C. (1962) 'Le tracé du deuxième trimestre de la vié, sa valeur prognostique, ses relations avec le tracé néonatal.' *Revue Neurologique,* **106,** 131-133.
—— Pajot, N., Guidasci, S. (1972) 'The neonatal EEG: statistical studies and prognostic value in full-term and pre-term babies.' *Electroencephalography and Clinical Neurophysiology,* **32,** 529-544.
Moore, B. C. (1965) 'Relationship between prematurity and intelligence in mental retardation.' *American Journal of Mental Deficiency,* **70,** 448-453.
Morales, N. (1942) 'The social competence of idiots.' *American Journal of Mental Deficiency,* **47,** 209-214.
Morris, N. M., Udry, J. R., Chase, C. L. (1973) 'Reduction of low birthweight rates by the prevention of unwanted pregnancies.' *American Journal of Public Health,* **63,** 935-938.
Mushin, A. S. (1974) 'Retinopathy of prematurity—a disease of increasing incidence.' *Transactions of the Ophthmological Societies of the U.K.,* **94,** 251-257.
Mundo-Vallarta, J. del, Robb, J. P. (1964) 'A follow-up study of newborn infants with perinatal complications.' *Neurology,* **14,** 413-424.
Naeye, R. L., Benirschke, K., Hagstrom, J. W. C., Marcus, C. C. (1966) 'Intrauterine growth of twins as estimated from liveborn birthweight data.' *Pediatrics,* **37,** 409-416.
Neligan, G. A., Robson, E., Watson, J. (1963) 'Hypoglycaemia in the newborn: a sequel of intrauterine malnutrition.' *Lancet,* **1,** 1282-1284.
—— Kolvin, I., Scott, D. McI., Garside, R. F. (1976) *Born too Soon or Born too Small. Clinics in Developmental Medicine, No. 61.* London: S.I.M.P. with Heinemann; Philadelphia: Lippincott.
Nellhaus, G. (1968) 'Head circumference from birth to eighteen years: practical composite international and interracial graphs.' *Pediatrics,* **41,** 106-114.
Nelson, K. B., Deutschberger, J. (1970) 'Head size at one year as a predictor of four-year IQ.' *Developmental Medicine and Child Neurology,* **12,** 487-495.
—— Broman, S. H. (1977) 'Perinatal risk factors in children with serious motor and mental handicaps.' *Annals of Neurology,* **2,** 371-377.
—— Ellenberg, J. H. (1979) 'Neonatal signs as predictors of cerebral palsy.' *Pediatrics,* **64,** 225-232.
——— (1982) 'An epidemiologic approach to the problems of cerebral palsy.' *In:* Fukuyama, Y., Arima, K., Maekawa, K., Yamaguchi, K. (Eds.) *Child Neurology. Excerpta Medica International Congress Series, No. 579.* Amsterdam: Excerpta Medica. pp. 341-350.
Nelson, W. E., Vaughan, V. C., McKay, R. J. (Eds.) (1969) *Textbook of Pediatrics, 9th edn.* Philadelphia: W. B. Saunders. pp. 40-49.
Newby, H. A. (1979) 'Testing the hearing function: Pure tone audiometry; Speech audiometry.' *In: Audiology, 4th edn.* Englewood Cliffs, N.J.: Prentice Hall. Chapters 5 and 6.
Nichols, P., Chen, T. (1981) *Minimal Brain Dysfunction: A Prospective Study.* Hillside, N.J.: Erlbaum.
Nickel, R. E., Bennett, F. C., Lamson, F. N. (1982) 'School performance of children with birthweights of 1000g or less.' *American Journal of Diseases of Children,* **136,** 105-110.
Nihira, K., Foster, R., Shellhaas, M., Leland, H. (1974) *AAMD Adaptive Behavior Scale.* Washington, D.C.: American Association for Mental Deficiency.
Niswander, K. R., Friedman, E. A., Hoover, D. B., Pietrowski, H., Westphal, M. C. (1966) 'Fetal

morbidity following potentially anoxigenic obstetric conditions.' *American Journal of Obstetrics and Gynecology,* **95,** 838-845.
Njiokiktjien, C. J., Kurver, P. (1980) 'Predictive value of neonatal neurological examination for cerebral function in infancy.' *Developmental Medicine and Child Neurology,* **22,** 736-747.
—— Visser, S. L., de Rijke, W. (1977) 'EEG and visual evoked responses in children with learning disorders.' *Neuropädiatrie,* **8,** 134-147.
Nolte, R. J., Schulte, F. J., Michaelis, R., Weisse, U., Gruson, R. (1969) 'Bioelectric brain maturation in small-for-dates infants.' *Developmental Medicine and Child Neurology,* **11,** 83-93.
Norman, M. G. (1978) 'Perinatal brain damage.' *Perspectives in Pediatric Pathology,* **4,** 41-92.
Norman, R. M. (1964) 'Discussion of asphyxia (anoxia) as a cause of congenital deafness.' *In:* Fisch, L. (Ed.) *Research in Deafness in Children.* Oxford: Blackwell. pp. 34-35.
O'Connell, E. J., Feldt, R. H., Stickler, G. B. (1965) 'Head circumference, mental retardation and growth failure.' *Pediatrics,* **36,** 62-66.
O'Connor, M. J. (1980) 'A comparison of preterm and fullterm infants on parameters of habituation at 4 months and performance on the Bayley Scales of Infant Development at eighteen months.' *Child Development,* **51,** 81-88.
Ounsted, M. (1966) 'Unconstrained fetal growth in man.' *Developmental Medicine and Child Neurology,* **8,** 3-8.
—— Ounsted, C. (1968) 'Rate of intrauterine growth.' *Nature,* **220,** 599-600.
Paine, R. S. (1961) 'The early diagnosis of cerebral palsy.' *Rhode Island Medical Journal,* **44,** 522-527.
—— (1962) 'Minimal chronic brain syndromes in children.' *Developmental Medicine and Child Neurology,* **4,** 21-27.
—— Donovan, D. E. (1962) 'The prognostic value of neurological signs in the newborn period.' *Proceedings of the Xth International Congres of Pediatrics, Lisbon.*
—— Brazelton, T. B., Donovan, D. E., Drorbaugh, J. E., Hubbell, J. P., Sears, E. M. (1964) 'Evolution of postural reflexes in normal infants and in the presence of chronic brain syndromes.' *Neurology,* **14,** 1036-1048.
—— Werry, J. S., Quay, H. C. (1968) 'A study of minimal cerebral dysfunction.' *Developmental Medicine and Child Neurology,* **10,** 505-520.
Palmer, P., Dubowitz, L. M. S., Levene, M. I., Dubowitz, V. (1982) 'Developmental and neurologic progress of pre-term infants with intraventricular haemorrhage and ventricular dilatation.' *Archives of Disease in Childhood,* **57,** 748-753.
Paneth, N., Kiely, J. L., Stein, Z., Susser, M. (1981) 'Cerebral palsy and newborn care. III: Estimated prevalence rates of cerebral palsy under differing rates of mortality and impairment of low birthweight infants.' *Developmental Medicine and Child Neurology,* **23,** 801-817.
Papageorgiou, A. N. (1977) 'Recent developments in neonatal-perinatal medicine.' *Canadian Medical Association Journal,* **117,** 109-112.
Pape, K., Wigglesworth, J. S. (1979) *Haemorrhage, Ischaemia and the Perinatal Brain. Clinics in Developmental Medicine, Nos. 69/70.* London: S.I.M.P. with Heinemann; Philadelphia: Lippincott.
—— Buncic, R. J., Ashby, S., Fitzhardinge, P. M. (1978) 'The status at two years of low birthweight infants born in 1974 with birthweights of less than 1001gm.' *Journal of Pediatrics,* **92,** 253-260.
—— Blackwell, R. J., Cusick, G., Sherwood, A., Houang, M. T. W., Thorburn, R., Reynolds, E. O. R. (1979) 'Ultrasound detection of brain damage in preterm infants.' *Lancet,* **1,** 1261-1264.
—— Bennett-Britton, S., Szymonowicz, W., Martin, D., Fitz, C., Becker, L. (1981) 'Incidence and evolution of subependymal and intraventricular haemorrhages: a study of infants with birthweights less than 1500gm.' *Pediatric Research,* **15,** 709. *(Abstract.)*
Papile, L. A., Burstein, J., Burstein, R., Koffler, H. (1978) 'Incidence and evolution of subependymal and intraventricular hemorrhage: a study of infants with birth weights of less than 1500gm.' *Journal of Pediatrics,* **92,** 539-544.
Parkinson, C. E., Wallis, S., Harvey, D. (1981) 'School achievement and behaviour of children who were small-for-dates at birth.' *Developmental Medicine and Child Neurology,* **23,** 41-50.
Parks, M. M. (1975) *Ocular Motility and Strabismus.* Hagerstown, Maryland: Harper & Row. pp. 70 & 83.
Parmelee, A. H. (1981) 'Auditory function and maturation in preterm infants.' *In:* Friedman, S. L., Sigman, M. (Eds.) *Preterm Birth and Psychological Development.* New York: Academic Press. pp. 127-150.
—— Haber, A. (1973) 'Who is the "risk infant"?' *Clinical Obstetrics and Gynecology,* **16,** 376-387.
—— Schulte, F. J., Akiyama, Y., Wenner, W. H., Schultz, M. A., Stern, E. (1968) 'Maturation of EEG activity during sleep in premature infants.' *Electoencephalography and Clinical Neurophysiology,*

24, 319-329.
—— Minkowski, A., Saint Anne-Dargassies, S., Dreyfus-Brisac, C., Lézine, I., Bergès, J., Chervin, G., Stern, E. (1970) 'Neurological evaluation of the preterm infant.' *Biology of the Neonate,* **15,** 65-78.
—— Kopp, C. B., Sigman, M. (1976) 'Selection of developmental assessment techniques for infants at risk.' *Merrill-Palmer Quarterly,* **22,** 177-199.
Pasamanick, B., Knobloch, H. (1960) 'Brain damage and reproductive casualty.' *American Journal of Orthopsychiatry,* **30,** 298-305.
—— Lilienfeld, A. M. (1955) 'Association of maternal and fetal factors with the development of mental deficiency. I: Abnormalities in the prenatal and paranatal periods.' *Journal of the American Medical Association,* **159,** 155-160.
Patz, A. (1957) 'The role of oxygen in retrolental fibroplasia.' *Pediatrics,* **19,** 504-524.
—— (1968) 'The ophthalmologist in the premature nursery.' *American Journal of Ophthalmology,* **66,** 970-972.
Paykel, E. S. (1971) 'Classification of depressed patients: a cluster analysis derived grouping.' *British Journal of Psychiatry,* **118,** 275-288.
Perlman, J. M., Fainmesser, P., Sohmer, H. (1983) 'Auditory nerve-brainstem responses in hyperbilirubinemic neonates.' *Pediatrics,* **72,** 658-664.
Perlstein, M. A. (1952) 'Infantile cerebral palsy—classification and clinical correlations.' *Journal of the American Medical Association,* **149,** 30-34.
—— (1960) 'The late clinical syndrome of posticteric encephalopathy.' *Pediatric Clinics of North America,* **7,** 665-687.
Peters, J. E., Romine, J. S., Dykman, R. A. (1975) 'A special neurological examination of children with learning disabilities.' *Developmental Medicine and Child Neurology,* **17,** 63-78.
Petersen, I., Eeg-Olofsson, O., Sellden, U. (1968) 'Paroxysmal activity in EEG of normal children.' *In:* Kellaway, P., Petersen, I. (Eds.) *Clinical Electroencephalography of Children.* Stockholm: Almqvist & Wiksell. pp. 167-187.
Pharoah, P. O. D., Alberman, E. D. (1981) 'Mortality of low birthweight infants in England and Wales, 1953 to 1979.' *Archives of Disease in Childhood,* **56,** 86-89.
Phelps, D. L. (1981) 'Retinopathy of prematurity: an estimate of vision loss in the United States—1979.' *Pediatrics,* **67,** 924-926.
—— (1982) 'Vitamin E and retrolental fibroplasia in 1982.' *Pediatrics,* **70,** 420-425.
Pincus, J. H., Glaser, G. H. (1966) 'The syndrome of "minimal brain damage" in childhood.' *New England Journal of Medicine,* **275,** 27-35.
Pomerance, J. J., Breger, B., Brown, S. (1982) 'Incidence of retrolental fibroplasia.' *Clinical Research,* **30,** 122A. *(Abstract.)*
Pond, D. A. (1961) 'Psychiatric aspects of epileptic and brain-damaged children.' *British Medical Journal,* **2,** 1377-1382; 1454-1459.
Prader, A., Tanner, J. M., von Harnack, G. A. (1963) 'Catch-up growth following illness or starvation. An example of developmental canalization in man.' *Journal of Pediatrics,* **62,** 646-659.
Prechtl, H. F. R. (1965) 'Prognostic value of neurological signs in the newborn infant.' *Proceedings of the Royal Society of Medicine,* **58,** 3-4.
—— (1967) 'Neurological sequelae of prenatal and perinatal complications.' *British Medical Journal,* **4,** 763-767.
—— (1968) 'Neurological findings in newborn infants after pre- and paranatal complications.' *In* Jonxis, J. H. P., Visser, H. K. A., Troelstra, J. A. (Eds) *Aspects of Praematurity and Dysmaturity.* Springfield, Ill: C. C. Thomas.
—— (1974) 'The behavioral states of the newborn (a review).' *Brain Research,* **76,** 185-212.
—— Dijkstra, J. (1960) 'Neurological diagnosis of cerebral injury in the newborn.' *In: Prenatal Care.* Groningen: Noordhoff. pp. 222-231.
—— Theorell, K., Blair, A. W. (1973) 'Behavioural state cycles in abnormal infants.' *Developmental Medicine and Child Neurology,* **15,** 606-615.
Preston, M. S., Guthrie, J. T., Childs, B. (1974) 'Visual evoked responses in normal and disabled readers.' *Psychophysiology,* **11,** 452-457.
Pringle, M. L. K. (1966) *Social Learning and its Measurement.* London: Longman Green.
Procianoy, R. S., Garcia-Prats, J. A., Hittner, H. M., Adams, J. M., Rudolph, A. J. (1981) 'An association between retinopathy of prematurity and intraventricular hemorrhage in very low birthweight infants.' *Acta Paediatrica Scandinavica,* **70,** 473-477.
Rabinovitch, M. S., Bibace, R., Caplan, H. (1961) 'Sequelae of prematurity: Psychological test findings.' *Canadian Medical Association Journal,* **84,** 822-824.

Rapin, I. (1982) 'Disorders of oral and written language.' *In: Children with Brain Dysfunction.* New York: Raven Press. Ch. 10, pp. 131-156.
Rapoport, J. L., Ferguson, H. B. (1981) 'Biological validation of the hyperkinetic syndrome.' *Developmental Medicine and Child Neurology,* **23,** 667-682.
Rawlings, G., Reynolds, E. O. R., Stewart, A., Strang, L. B. (1971) 'Changing prognosis for infants of very low birthweight.' *Lancet,* **1,** 516-519.
Rawson, M. B. (1968) *Developmental Language Disability: Adult Accomplishments of Dyslexic Boys.* Baltimore: Johns Hopkins University Press.
Reese, A. B. (1955) 'An epitaph for retrolental fibroplasia.' *American Journal of Ophthalmology,* **40,** 267-269.
Riddle, K. D., Rapoport, J. L. (1976) 'A 2-year follow-up of 72 hyperactive boys.' *Journal of Nervous and Mental Diseases,* **162,** 126-134.
Rider, R. V., Taback, M., Knobloch, H. (1955) 'Associations between premature births and socio-economic status.' *American Journal of Public Health,* **45,** 1022-1028.
Rie, H. E. (1975) 'Hyperactivity in children.' *American Journal of Diseases of Children,* **129,** 783-789.
—— (1980) 'Definitional problems.' *In:* Rie, H. E., Rie, E. D. (Eds.) *Handbook of Minimal Brain Dysfunctions.* New York: John Wiley. pp. 3-17.
—— Rie, E. D. (Eds.) (1980) *Handbook of Minimal Brain Dysfunctions.* New York: John Wiley.
Roberton, N. R. C. (1979) 'Intensive care and the very-low-birthweight infant.' *Lancet,* **2,** 362.
—— Tizard, J. P. M. (1975) 'Prognosis for infants with idiopathic respiratory distress syndrome.' *British Medical Journal,* **2,** 271-274.
Robertson, A. M., Crichton, J. U. (1969) 'Neurological sequelae in children with neonatal respiratory distress.' *American Journal of Diseases of Children,* **117,** 271-275.
Robinson, G. C., Anderson, D. O., Moghadam, H. K., Cambon, K. G., Murray, A. B. (1967) 'A survey of hearing loss in Vancouver school children.' *Canadian Medical Association Journal,* **97,** 1199-1207.
Robinson, N. M., Robinson, H. B. (1965) 'A follow-up study of children of low birthweight and control children at school age.' *Pediatrics,* **35,** 425-433.
Robinson, R. O. (1971) 'The preterm baby.' *British Medical Journal,* **4,** 416-419.
—— (1979) 'Pathogenesis of intraventricular haemorrhage in the low birthweight infant.' *Developmental Medicine and Child Neurology,* **21,** 815-819.
Rocissano, L., Yatchmink, Y. (1983) 'Language skill and interactive patterns in prematurely born toddlers.' *Child Development,* **54,** 1229-1241.
Rodin, E., Lucas, A., Simpson, C. (1964) 'A study of behavior disorders in children by means of general purpose computers.' *In:* Enslein, K. (Ed.) *Data Acquisiton and Processing in Biology and Medicine, Vol. 3.* Oxford: Pergamon. pp. 115-124.
Rogers, L. J., McBurney, A. K., Dunn, H. G., Crichton, J. U., Low, M. D. (1980) 'Multivariate analysis indicating relations between cerebral lateralization (as measured by EEG, EP and CNV) and IQ scores, for normal and MCD children.' *In:* Lechner, H., Aranibar, A. (Eds.) *Proceedings of the 2nd European Congress of EEG and Clinical Neurophysiology, Salzburg, Austria, September 1979. Excerpta Medica International Congress Series, No. 526.* Amsterdam: Elsevier. pp. 329-337.
Rose, A. L., Lombroso, C. T. (1970) 'Neonatal seizure states: a study of clinical, pathological and electroencephalographic features in 137 full-term babies with a long-term follow-up.' *Pediatrics,* **45,** 404-425.
Rosegger, H., Haidvogl, M., Stern, E. (1980) 'Frühernährung mit Frauenmilch: Erfahrungen bei Frühgeborenen und Neugeborenen mit niedrigem Geburtsgewicht. I: Schädel- und Körperwachstum im ersten Lebensmonat.' *Monatsschrift für Kinderheilkunde,* **128,** 186-190.
Rosen, M. (1978) 'Cain-Levine Social Competency Scale.' *In:* Buros, D. (Ed.) *The Eighth Mental Measurements Yearbook.* New Jersey: Gryphon Press. pp. 718-720.
Rosenblith, J. F. (1964) 'Prognostic value of behavioural assessment of neonates'. *Biologia Neonatorum,* **6,** 76-103.
—— (1966) 'Prognostic value of neonatal assessment.' *Child Development,* **37,** 623-631.
Rosenfeld, G. B., Bradley, C. (1948) 'Childhood behavior sequelae of asphyxia in infancy with special reference to pertussis and asphyxia neonatorum.' *Pediatrics,* **2,** 74-84.
Ross, D. M., Ross, S. A. (1982) *Hyperactivity: Current Issues, Research and Theory, 2nd edn.* New York: John Wiley.
Ross, E. M., Peckham, C. S., West, P. B., Butler, N. R. (1980) 'Epilepsy in childhood: findings from the National Child Development Study.' *British Medical Journal,* **1,** 207-210.
Ross, G. S. (1980) 'Parental responses to infants in intensive care: the separation issue revisited.' *Clinics in Perinatology,* **7,** 47-60.

Rossier, A. (1962) 'The future of the premature infant.' *Developmental Medicine and Child Neurology,* **4,** 483-487.

Rothberg, A. D., Maisels, M. J., Bagnato, S., Murphy, J., Gifford, K., McKinley, L., Palmer, E. A., Vannucci, R. C. (1981) 'Outcome for survivors of mechanical ventilation weighing less than 1250 gm at birth.' *Journal of Pediatrics,* **98,** 106-111.

Rourke, B. P., Orr, R. R. (1977) 'Prediction of the reading and spelling performances of normal and retarded readers: a four-year follow-up.' *Journal of Abnormal Child Psychology,* **5,** 9-20.

—— Dietrich, D. M., Young, G. C. (1973) 'The significance of WISC verbal-performance discrepancies for younger children with learning disabilities.' *Perceptual and Motor Skills,* **36,** 275-282.

Rubin, R. A., Rosenblatt, C., Balow, B. (1973) 'Psychological and educational sequelae of prematurity.' *Pediatrics,* **52,** 352-363.

Ruiz, M. P. D., LeFever, J. A., Hakanson, D. O., Clark, D. A., Williams, M. L. (1981) 'Early development of infants of birthweight less than 1000 grams with reference to mechanical ventilation in newborn period.' *Pediatrics,* **68,** 330-335.

Russell, E. M. (1960) 'Correlation between birthweight and clinical findings in diplegia.' *Archives of Disease in Childhood,* **35,** 548-551.

Rutter, M. (1977) 'Brain damage syndromes in childhood: concepts and findings.' *Journal of Child Psychology and Psychiatry,* **18,** 1-21.

—— Martin, J. A. M. (Eds.) (1972) *The Child with Delayed Speech. Clinics in Developmental Medicine, No. 43.* London: S.I.M.P. with Heinemann.

—— Yule, W. (1975) 'The concept of specific reading retardation.' *Journal of Child Psychology and Psychiatry,* **16,** 181-197.

—— Lebovici, S., Eisenberg, L., Sneznevskij, A. V., Sadoun, R., Brooke, E., Lin, T. Y. (1969) 'A tri-axial classification of mental disorders in childhood.' *Journal of Child Psychology and Psychiatry,* **10,** 41-61.

—— Tizard, J., Whitmore, K. (1970) *Education, Health and Behaviour.* London: Longman.

—— Cox, A., Tupling, C., Berger, M., Yule, W. (1975) 'Attainment and adjustment in two geographical areas. I: The prevalence of psychiatric disorder.' *British Journal of Psychiatry,* **126,** 493-509.

—— Chadwick, D., Schacher, R. (1980) 'Hyperactivity and minimal brain dysfunction: epidemiological perspectives on questions of cause and classification.' Mary Elaine Meyer O'Neal Award Lecture. Omaha: University of Nebraska Medical Center.

Sacks, L. M., Schaffer, D. B., Anday, E. K., Peckham, C. J., Delivoria-Papadopoulos, M. (1981) 'Retrolental fibroplasia and blood transfusion in very low birthweight infants.' *Pediatrics,* **68,** 770-774.

Saint-Anne Dargassies, S. (1962) 'Le nouveau-né à terme: aspect neurologique.' *Biologia Neonatorum,* **4,** 174-200.

—— (1977) 'Long-term neurological follow-up study of 286 truly premature infants. I: Neurological sequelae.' *Developmental Medicine and Child Neurology,* **19,** 462-478.

Sameroff, A. J., Chandler, M. J. (1975) 'Perinatal risk and the continuum of caretaking casualty.' *In:* Horowitz, F., Hetherington, M., Scarr-Salapatek, S., Siegel, C. (Eds.) *Review of Child Development Research, Vol. 4.* Chicago: University of Chicago Press.

Sandberg, S. T., Rutter, M., Taylor, E. (1978) 'Hyperkinetic disorders in psychiatric clinic attenders.' *Developmental Medicine and Child Neurology,* **20,** 279-299.

Sanders, D. Y., Eliot, D. S., Cramblett, H. G. (1967) 'Retrospective study for possible kanamycin ototoxicity among neonatal infants.' *Journal of Pediatrics,* **70,** 960-962.

Satran, R., Rosen, M. (1967) 'Serial EEG observations on the premature infant.' *Electroencephalography and Clinical Neurophysiology,* **23,** 97.

Satz, P., Radin, D., Ross, J. (1971) 'An evaluation of a theory of specific developmental dyslexia.' *Child Development,* **42,** 2009-2021.

Satterfield, J. (1973) 'EEG issues in children with minimal brain dysfunction.' *Seminars in Psychiatry,* **5,** 35-46.

—— Lesser, L. I., Saul, R. E., Cantwell, D. P. (1973) 'EEG aspects in the diagnosis and treatment of minimal brain dysfunction.' *Annals of the New York Academy of Sciences,* **205,** 274-282.

Scarr, S., Williams, M. (1971) 'The assessment of neonatal and later status in low-birthweights infants.' *Paper presented to the Society for Research in Child Development, Minneapolis.*

Scarr-Salapatek, S., Williams, M. L. (1973) 'The effects of early stimulation on low birthweight infants.' *Child Development,* **44,** 94-101.

Scharf, J., Zonis, S., Zeltzer, M. (1978) 'Refraction in premature babies: a prospective study.' *Journal of Pediatric Ophthalmology and Strabismus,* **15,** 48-50.

Scher, M. S., Tharp, B. R., Sylvestri, L. O. (1982) 'Significance of focal abnormalities in neonatal electro-encephalograms: radiological correlation and outcome.' *Annals of Neurology,* **12,** 217A.
Scherzer, A. L., Miké, V. (1974) 'Cerebral palsy and the low birthweight child.' *American Journal of Diseases of Children,* **128,** 199-203.
Schleifer, M., Weiss, G., Cohen, N., Elman, M., Cvejic, H., Kruger, E. (1975) 'Hyperactivity in preschoolers and the effect of methylphenidate.' *American Journal of Orthopsychiatry,* **45,** 38-50.
Schneeweiss, B., Klehn, P. E., Matz, J. (1970) 'Clinical follow-up studies in late prognosis.' *Pädiatrie und Grenzgebiete,* **9,** 208-211.
Schulman, J. L., Reisman, J. M. (1959) 'An objective measure of hyperactivity.' *American Journal of Mental Deficiency,* **64,** 455-456.
—— Kasper, J. C., Throne, F. M. (1965) *Brain Damage in Children.* Springfield, Ill.: C. C. Thomas.
Schulman-Galambos, C., Galambos, R. (1975) 'Brain stem auditory evoked responses in premature infants.' *Journal of Speech and Hearing Research,* **18,** 456-465.
Schulte, F. J. (1966) 'Neonatal convulsions and their relation to epilepsy in early childhood.' *Developmental Medicine and Child Neurology,* **8,** 381-392.
—— Hermann, B. (1965) 'Elektroencephalographie beim Neugeborenen. Zuordung zu anatomischen Befunden und prognostische Bedeutung.' *Monatsschrift für Kinderheilkunde,* **113,** 457-465.
—— Stennert, E. (1978) 'Hearing defects in preterm infants.' *Archives of Disease in Childhood,* **53,** 269-270.
—— Hinze, G., Schrempff, G. (1971) 'Maternal toxemia, fetal malnutrition and bioelectric brain activity of the newborn.' *Neuropädiatrie,* **2,** 439-446.
—— Stennert, E., Wulbrand, H., Eichhorn, W., Lenard, H. G. (1977) 'The ontogeny of sensory perception in preterm infants.' *European Journal of Pediatrics,* **126,** 211-224.
Scobee, R. G. (1951) 'Esotropia: incidence, etiology and results of therapy.' *American Journal of Ophthalmology,* **34,** 817-833.
Scott, K. E., Usher, R. (1966) 'Fetal malnutrition: its incidence, causes and effects.' *American Journal of Obstetrics and Gynecology,* **94,** 951-963.
Scott, W. R., New, P. F. J., Davis, K. R., Schnurr, J. A. (1974) 'Computerized axial tomography and intraventricular hemorrhage.' *Radiology,* **112,** 73-80.
Seleny, F. L., Streczyn, M. (1969) 'Noise characteristics in the baby compartments of incubators.' *American Journal of Diseases of Children,* **117,** 445-450.
Setzer, E. S., Webb, I. B., Wassenaar, J. W., Reeder, J., Mehta, P. S., Gitzman, D. V. (1982) 'Platelet dysfunction and coagulopathy in intraventricular hemorrhage in the premature infant.' *Journal of Pediatrics,* **100,** 599-605.
Shaffer, D. (1978) 'Longitudinal research and the minimal brain damage syndrome.' *In:* Kalverboer, A. F., van Praag, H. M., Mendlewicz, J. (Eds.) *Minimal Brain Dysfunction: Fact or Fiction?* Basel: Karger. pp. 18-34.
—— McNamara, N., Pincus, J. H. (1974) 'Controlled observations on patterns of activity, attention and impulsivity in brain-damaged and psychiatrically disturbed boys.' *Psychological Medicine,* **4,** 4-18.
Shambaugh, G. E., Derlacki, E. L., Harrison, W. H., House, H., House, W., Hildyard, V., Schuknecht, H., Shea, J. J. (1959) 'Dihydrostreptomycin deafness.' *Journal of the American Medical Association,* **170,** 1657-1660.
Shaywitz, S. E., Cohen, D. J., Shaywitz, B. A. (1978) 'The biochemical basis of minimal brain dysfunction.' *Journal of Pediatrics,* **92,** 179-187.
—— Hunt, S. E., Jatlow, P., Cohen, D. J., Young, J. G., Pierce, R. N., Anderson, G. M., Shaywitz, B. A. (1982) 'Psychopharmacology of attention deficit disorder.' *Pediatrics,* **69,** 688-694.
Sheehan, P., Barry, P. J. C., O'Brien, N. G. (1977) 'Resuscitation at birth and subsequent development to six years.' *Irish Medical Journal,* **70,** 107-111.
Sheridan, M. (1972) 'Reported incidence of hearing loss in children of seven years.' *Developmental Medicine and Child Neurology,* **14,** 296-303.
Shirley, M. (1939) 'A behavior syndrome characterizing prematurely born children.' *Child Development,* **10,** 115-128.
Shohat, M., Reisner, S. H., Krikler, R., Nissenkorn, I., Yassur, Y., Ben-Sira, I. (1983) 'Retinopathy of prematurity: incidence and risk factors.' *Pediatrics,* **72,** 159-163.
Siegel, L. S. (1983) 'Correction for prematurity and its consequences for the assessment of the very low birthweight infant.' *Child Development,* **54,** 1176-1188.
—— Saigal, S., Rosenbaum, P., Morton, R. A., Young, A., Berenbaum, S., Stoskopf, B. (1982) 'Predictors of development in preterm and full-term infants: a model for detecting the at risk child.' *Journal of Pediatric Psychology,* **7,** 135-148.
Silver, A. A., Hagin, R. A. (1964) 'Specific reading disability: follow-up studies.' *American Journal of*

Orthopsychiatry, **34,** 95-102.
Silverman, W. A. (1981) 'Outcome for infants of very low birthweight.' *Lancet,* **1,** 1319.
Sinclair, J. C., Coldiron, J. S. (1969) 'Low birthweight and postnatal physical development.' *Developmental Medicine and Child Neurology,* **11,** 314-329.
Sloan, W. (1955) 'The Lincoln-Oseretsky motor development scale.' *Genetic Psychology Monographs,* **51,** 183-251.
Small, L. (1982) *The Minimal Brain Dysfunction Syndrome.* New York: Free Press.
Smith, A. C., Flick, G. L., Ferriss, G. S., Sellmann, A. H. (1972) 'Prediction of developmental outcome at seven years from prenatal, perinatal and postnatal events.' *Child Development,* **43,** 495-507.
Smith, V. H. (1963) 'A survey of strabismus in cerebral palsy.' *In:* Smith, V. H. (Ed.) *Visual Disorders in Cerebral Palsy. Little Club Clinics in Developmental Medicine, No. 9.* London: National Spastics Society with Heinemann.
Sneath, P. H. A., Sokal, R. R. (1973) *Numerical Taxonomy.* San Francisco: Freeman.
Song, A. Y., Jones, S. E. (1982) 'Vineland Social Maturity Scale norm examined—the Wisconsin experience with 0- to 3-year-old children.' *American Journal of Mental Deficiency,* **86,** 428-431.
Sorsby, A., Benjamin, B., Sheridan, M. (1961) 'Refraction and its components during the growth of the eye from the age of three.' *Medical Research Council Special Report Series, No. 301.* London: H.M.S.O.
Spector, G. J., Pettit, W. J., Davis, G., Strauss, M., Rauchbach, E. (1978) 'Fetal respiratory distress causing CNS and inner ear hemorrhage.' *Laryngoscope,* **88,** 764-784.
Speer, M. E., Blifeld, C., Rudolph, A. J., Chadda, P., Holbein, M. E. B., Hittner, H. M. (1984) 'Intraventricular hemorrhage and vitamin E in the very low-birth-weight infant: evidence for efficacy of early intramuscular vitamin E administration.' *Pediatrics,* **75,** 1107-1112.
Stanley, F. J. (1981) 'Spastic cerebral palsy: changes in birthweight and gestational age.' *Early Human Development,* **5,** 167-178.
—— (1982) 'Using cerebral palsy data in the evaluation of neonatal intensive care: a warning.' *Developmental Medicine and Child Neurology,* **24,** 93-94.
Statistics Canada, Health and Welfare Divison (1972) *Vital Statistics. Preliminary Annual Report, 1970.* Ottawa: Statistics Canada.
Stave, U., Ruvalo, C. (1980) 'Neurological development in very low birthweight infants. Application of a standardized examination and Prechtl's optimality concept in routine evaluations.' *Early Human Development,* **4,** 229-241.
Stennert, E., Schulte, F. J., Vollrath, M. (1977) 'Incubator noise and hearing loss.' *Early Human Development,* **1,** 113-115.
Stephenson, P. S. (1975) 'The hyperkinetic child: some misleading assumptions.' *Canadian Medical Association Journal,* **113,** 764-769.
Stern, L., Denton, R. L. (1965) 'Kernicterus in small premature infants.' *Pediatrics,* **35,** 483-485.
Stevens, D. A., Boydstun, J. A., Dykman, R. A., Peters, J. E., Sinton, D. W. (1967) 'Presumed minimal brain dysfunction in children.' *Archives of General Psychiatry,* **16,** 281-285.
Stevens, J. R., Sachdev, K., Milstein, V. (1968) 'Behavior disorders of childhood and the electroencephalogram.' *Archives of Neurology,* **18,** 160-177.
—— Milstein, V. (1970) 'Severe psychiatric disorders of childhood: electroencephalographic and clinical correlates.' *American Journal of Diseases of Children,* **120,** 182-192.
Stewart, A., Abramovich, S. (1979) 'Hearing conservation in premature infants.' *Journal of the Royal Society of Medicine,* **72,** 298.
Stewart, A. L., Reynolds, E. O. R. (1974) 'Improved prognosis for infants of very low birthweight.' *Pediatrics,* **54,** 724-735.
—— Turcan, D. M., Rawlings, G., Reynolds, E. O. R. (1977) 'Prognosis for infants weighing 1000g or less at birth.' *Archives of Disease in Childhood,* **52,** 97-104.
—— —— Lipscomb, A. P. (1981) 'Outcome for infants of very low birthweight: survey of world literature.' *Lancet,* **1,** 1038-1041.
Stewart, M. A., Mendelson, W. B., Johnson, N. E. (1973) 'Hyperactive children as adolescents: how they describe themselves.' *Child Psychiatry and Human Development,* **4,** 3-11.
Stillerman, M. L., Gibbs, E. L., Perlstein, M. A. (1952) 'Electroencephalographic changes in strabismus.' *American Journal of Ophthalmology,* **35,** 54-63.
Strauss, A. A., Werner, H. (1942) 'Disorders of conceptual thinking in the brain-injured child.' *Journal of Nervous and Mental Diseases,* **96,** 153-172.
—— Kephart, N. C. (1955) *Psychopathology and Education of the Brain-injured Child Vol. II.* New York: Grune & Stratton.

—— Lehtinen, L. E. (1947) *Psychopathology and Education of the Brain-injured Child.* New York: Grune & Stratton.
Strauss, J. S., Bartko, J. J., Carpenter, W. T. (1973) 'The use of clustering techniques for the classification of psychiatric patients.' *British Journal of Psychiatry,* **122,** 531-540.
Strother, C. R. (1973) 'Minimal cerebral dysfunction: an historical overview.' *Annals of the New York Academy of Sciences,* **205,** 6-17.
Svedbergh, B. (1975) 'Retrolental fibroplasia or congenital encephalo-ophthalmic dysplasia.' *Acta Paediatrica Scandinavica,* **64,** 891-894.
Symann-Louett, N., Gascon, G. G., Matsumiya, Y., Lombroso, C. T. (1977) 'Wave form differences in visual evoked responses between normal and reading disabled children.' *Neurology,* **27,** 156-159.
Taub, H. B., Goldstein, K. M., Caputo, D. V. (1977) 'Indices of neonatal prematurity as discriminators of development in middle childhood.' *Child Development,* **48,** 797-805.
Teberg, A., Hodgman, J. E. Wu, P. Y. K., Spears, R. L. (1977) 'Recent improvements in outcome for the small premature infant.' *Clinical Pediatrics,* **16,** 307-313.
—— Wu, P. Y. K., Hodgman, J. E., Mitch, C., Garfinkle, S., Azen, S., Wingert, W. A. (1982) 'Infants with birthweight under 1500g: physical, neurological and developmental outcome.' *Critical Care Medicine,* **10,** 10-14.
Tharp, B. R., Cukier, F., Monod, N. (1981) 'The prognostic value of the electroencephalogram in premature infants.' *Electroencephalography and Clinical Neurophysiology,* **51,** 219-236.
Thom, D. A. (1942) 'Convulsions of early life and their relations to the chronic disorders and mental defect.' *American Journal of Psychiatry,* **98,** 574-580.
Thompson, T., Reynolds, J. (1977) 'The results of intensive care therapy for neonates.' *Journal of Perinatal Medicine,* **5,** 59-75.
Thorburn, R. J., Lipscomb, A. P., Stewart, A. L., Reynolds, E. O. R., Hope, P. L., Pape, K. (1981) 'Prediction of death and major handicap in very preterm infants by brain ultrasound.' *Lancet,* **1,** 1119-1121.
Tibbles, J. A. R., Prichard, J. S. (1965) 'The prognostic value of the electroencephalogram in neonatal convulsions.' *Pediatrics,* **35,** 778-786.
Torres, F., Blaw, M. E. (1968) 'Longitudinal EEG-clinical correlations in children from birth to 4 years of age.' *Pediatrics,* **41,** 945-954.
Touwen, B. C. L. (1979) *Examination of the Child with Minor Neurological Dysfunction, 2nd edn. Clinics in Developmental Medicine no. 71.* London: S.I.M.P. with Heinemann Medical; Philadelphia: Lippincott.
Towbin, A. (1971) 'Organic causes of minimal brain dysfunction.' *Journal of the American Medical Association,* **217,** 1207-1214.
Tsiantos, A., Victorin, L., Relier, J. P., Dyer, N., Sundell, H., Brill, A. B., Stahlman, M. (1974) 'Intracranial hemorrhage in the prematurely born infant.' *Journal of Pediatrics,* **85,** 854-859.
Twitchell, T. E. (1963) 'The neurological examination in infantile cerebral palsy.' *Developmental Medicine and Child Neurology,* **5,** 271-278.
Uddenberg, G. (1955) 'Diagnostic studies of prematures.' *Acta Psychiatrica Scandinavica,* Suppl. 104.
Ungerer, J. A., Sigman, M. (1983) 'Developmental lags in preterm infants from one to three years of age.' *Child Development,* **54,** 1217-1228.
Usher, R. H. (1970) 'Clinical and therapeutic aspects of fetal malnutrition.' *Pediatric Clinics of North America,* **17,** 169 183.
—— McLean, F. (1969) 'Intrauterine growth of live-born Caucasian infants at sea level: standard obtained from measurements of infants born at between 25 and 44 weeks of gestation.' *Journal of Pediatrics,* **74,** 901-910.
Vancouver General Hospital, Medical Records Department (1973) *Personal communication.*
van den Berg, B. J., Yerushalmy, J. (1969) 'Studies on convulsive disorders in young children. I: Incidence of febrile and non-febrile convulsions by age and other factors.' *Pediatric Research,* **3,** 298-304.
Vernon, M. (1967) 'Prematurity and deafness: the magnitude of the problem among deaf children.' *Exceptional Children,* **33,** 289-298.
Visser, S. L., Njiokiktjien, C. J., de Rijke, W. (1982) 'Neurological condition at birth in relation to the electroencephalogram (EEG) and visual evoked potential (VEP) at the age of 5.' *Electroencephalography and Clinical Neurophysiology,* **54,** 458-464.
Vohr, B. R., Oh, W. (1983) 'Growth and development in preterm infants small for gestational age.' *Journal of Pediatrics,* **103,** 941-945.
—— —— Rosenfield, A. G., Cowett, R. M. (1979) 'The preterm small-for-gestational age infant: a two-year follow-up study.' *American Journal of Obstetrics and Gynecology,* **133,** 425-431.

Volpe, J. J. (1976) 'Perinatal hypoxic-ischemic brain injury.' *Pediatric Clinics of North America,* **23,** 383-397.
—— (1977) 'Neonatal intracranial hemorrhage: pathophysiology, neuropathology and clinical features.' *Clinical Perinatology,* **4,** 77-102.
—— Pasternak, J. F., Allan, W. C. (1977) 'Ventricular dilation preceding rapid head growth following neonatal intracranial hemorrhage.' *American Journal of Diseases of Children,* **131,** 1212-1215.
Voss, O. (1923) 'Geburtstrauma und Gehörorgan.' *Zeitschrift für Hals-, Nasen- und Ohrenheilkunde,* **6,** 182-219.
Walzer, S., Wolff, P. H. (Eds.) (1973) *Minimal Cerebral Dysfunction in Children.* New York: Grune & Stratton.
Warkany, J., Monroe, B. C., Sutherland, B. S. (1961) 'Intrauterine growth retardation.' *American Journal of Diseases of Children,* **102,** 249-279.
Watanabe, K., Iwase, K. (1972) 'Spindle-like fast rhythms in the EEGs of low birthweight infants.' *Developmental Medicine and Child Neurology,* **14,** 373-381.
—— Miyazaki, S., Hara, K., Hakamada, S. (1980) 'Behavioral state cycles, background EEGs and prognosis of newborns with perinatal hypoxia.' *Electroencephalography and Clinical Neurophysiology,* **49,** 618-625.
Weber, H., Ströder, J. (1973) 'Bleibende Schaden nach Rh-Erythroblastose, ABO-Erythroblastose und Hyperbilirubinämie in der Neugeborenenperiode.' *Klinische Pädiatrie,* **185,** 383-399.
Weiss, G., Minde, K. K., Douglas, V. I., Werry, J. S., Nemeth, E. (1971) 'Studies on the hyperactive child. VIII: Five-year follow-up.' *Archives of General Psychiatry,* **24,** 409-414.
—— Kruger, E., Danielson, U., Elman, M. (1975) 'Effect of long-term treatment of hyperactive children with methylphenidate.' *Canadian Medical Association Journal,* **112,** 159-160.
Wender, P. H. (1971) *Minimal Brain Dysfunction in Children.* New York: John Wiley.
—— (1976) 'Hypothesis for a possible biochemical basis of minimal brain dysfunction.' *In:* Knights, R.M., Bakker, D. J. (Eds.) *The Neuropsychology of Learning Disorders.* Baltimore: University Park Press. pp. 111-122.
Wepman, J. M. (1958) *Auditory Discrimination Test.* Chicago: Wepman.
Werner, E. (1957) 'Milieu differences in social competence.' *Journal of General Psychology,* **91,** 239-249.
—— Simonian, K. (1966) 'The social maturity of preschool children in Hawaii.' *Journal of Social Psychology,* **69,** 197-207.
—— Honzik, M. P., Smith, R. S. (1968) 'Prediction of intelligence and achievement at ten years from twenty months pediatric and psychologic examinations.' *Child Development,* **39,** 1063-1075.
—— Bierman, J. M., French, F. E. (1971) *The Children of Kauai: A Longitudinal Study from the Prenatal Period to Age Ten.* Honolulu: University of Hawaii Press.
Werner, S. S., Stockard, J. E., Bickford, R. G. (1977) 'Ontogenesis of the electroencephalogram in prematures.' *In: Atlas of Neonatal Electroencephalography.* New York: Raven Press.
Werry, J. S. (1968) 'Studies on the hyperactive child. IV: An empirical analysis of the minimal brain dysfunction syndrome.' *Archives of General Psychiatry,* **19,** 9-16.
Wiener, G. (1962) 'Psychologic correlates of premature birth: a review.' *Journal of Nervous and Mental Diseases,* **134,** 129-144.
—— (1968) 'Scholastic achievement at age 12-13 of prematurely born infants.' *Journal of Special Education,* **2,** 237-250.
—— (1970) 'The relationship of birthweight and length of gestation to intellectual development at ages 8 to 10 years.' *Journal of Pediatrics,* **76,** 694-699.
—— Rider, R. V., Oppel, W. C., Fischer, L. K., Harper, P. A. (1965) 'Correlates of low-birth-weight: psychological status at six to seven years of age.' *Pediatrics,* **35,** 434-444.
—— —— —— Harper, P. A. (1968) 'Correlates of low birthweight. Psychological status at eight to ten years of age.' *Pediatric Research,* **2,** 110-118.
Wigglesworth, J. S., Keith, I. H., Girling, D. J., Slade, S. A. (1976) 'Hyaline membrane disease, alkali and intraventricular haemorrhage.' *Archives of Disease in Childhood,* **51,** 755-762.
Wikler, A., Dixon, J. F., Parker, J. B. (1970) 'Brain function in problem children and controls: psychometric, neurological and electroencephalographic comparisons.' *American Journal of Psychiatry,* **127,** 634-645.
Willerman, L., Broman, S. H., Fiedler, M. (1970) 'Infant development, pre-school IQ and social class.' *Child Development,* **41,** 69-77.
Windle, W. F. (1961) 'Anoxia and asphyxia: experiments in fetal and neonatal monkeys.' *In:* Fields, W. S., Desmond, M. M. (Eds.) *Disorders of the Developing Nervous System.* Springfield, Ill.: C. C. Thomas. Ch. 7.
Winick, M. (1968) 'Changes in nucleic acid and protein content of the human brain during growth.'

Pediatric Research, **2,** 352-355.
—— Rosso, P. (1969) 'Head circumference and cellular growth of the brain in normal and marasmic children.' *Journal of Pediatrics,* **74,** 774-778.
Winkel, S., Bonding, P., Larsen, N. K., Roosen, J. (1978) 'Possible effects of kanamycin and incubation in newborn children with low birthweight.' *Acta Paediatrica Scandinavica,* **67,** 709-715.
Wise, B. L., Ballard, R. (1976) 'Hydrocephalus secondary to intracranial hemorrhage in premature infants.' *Child's Brain,* **2,** 234-241.
Wolff, P. H., Hurwitz, J. (1973) 'Functional implications of the minimally brain damaged syndrome.' *Seminars in Psychiatry,* **5,** 105-115.
Woods, D. L., Malan, A. F., Heese, H. de V. (1979) 'Patterns of retarded fetal growth.' *Early Human Development,* **3,** 257-262.
Woods, G. E. (1957) *Cerebral Palsy in Childhood.* Bristol: John Wright.
World Health Organization (1948-49) *Manual of the International Statistical Classification of Diseases, Injuries and Causes of Death.* Geneva: W.H.O.
—— (1954) *The Mentally Subnormal Child. Technical Report Series, No. 75.* Geneva: W.H.O.
—— (1961) *Public Health Aspects of Low Birthweight, 3rd Report, Expert Committee on Maternal and Child Health. Technical Report Series, No. 217.* Geneva: W.H.O.
—— (1977) 'Recommended definitions, terminology and format for statistical tables related to the perinatal period and use of a certificate for cause of perinatal deaths.' *Acta Obstetrica et Gynecologica Scandinavica,* **56,** 247-253.
Wright, F. H., Blough, R. R., Chamberlin, A., Ernest, T., Halstead, W. C., Meier, P., Moore, R. Y., Naunton, R. F., Newell, F. W. (1972) 'A controlled follow-up study of small prematures born from 1952 through 1956.' *American Journal of Diseases of Children,* **124,** 506-512.
Yannet, H., Lieberman, R. (1946) 'Central nervous system complications associated with kernicterus.' *Journal of the American Medical Association,* **130,** 335-340.
Yerushalmy, J., van den Berg, B. J., Erhardt, C. L., Jacobziner, H. (1965) 'Birthweight and gestation as indices of "immaturity".' *American Journal of Diseases of Children,* **109,** 43-57.
Ylöppö, A. (1919) 'Das Wachstum der Frühgeborenen von der Geburt bis zum Schulalter.' *Zeitschrift für Kinderheilkunde,* **24,** 111-178.
Yow, M. D., Tengg, N. E. (1961) 'The use of kanamycin sulfate as a therapeutic agent for infants and children.' *Journal of Pediatrics,* **58,** 538-547.
Yu, V. Y. H., Hollingsworth, E. (1980) 'Improving prognosis for infants weighing 1000g or less at birth.' *Archives of Disease in Childhood,* **55,** 422-426.
Yule, W. (1978) 'Diagnosis: developmental psychological assessment.' *In:* Kalverboer, A. F., van Praag, H. M., Mendlewicz, J. (Eds.) *Minimal Brain Dysfunction: Fact or Fiction?'* Basel: Karger, pp. 35-54.
Ziegler, A. L., Calame, A., Marchand, C., Passera, M., Reymond-Goni, L. S., Prod'hom, L. S. (1976) 'Cerebral distress in full-term newborns and its prognostic value: a follow-up study of 90 infants.' *Helvetica Paediatrica Acta,* **31,** 299-317.
Zivin, L., Marsan, C. A. (1968) 'Incidence and prognostic significance of "epileptiform" activity in the EEG of non-epileptic subjects.' *Brain,* **91,** 751-778.

Index

Abbreviations
See p. vi

A
AAMD Adaptive Behaviour Scale 217
Abruptio placentae 238
Absence seizure 91
Alpern and Boll Scale 217
Antibiotics, hearing loss due to 151, 152, 161
Apgar score 21, 239
Apnoea 238
Asymmetries 87, 88
Attention deficit 19
Attention deficit disorder (organic behaviour syndrome) 19, 100, 106-7, 118-119, 252, 268
  EEG abnormalities 107
  evolution 6½-13 years 260-1
Audiometric tests 152-5
Autism 69 (table)
Autoregulation failure 6

B
Balthazar Scales of Adaptive Behaviour 217
Behaviour syndrome 15-17, 268
Birthweights ≤2500g as % of live births 10 (table), 24
Blink response to light 238
Blood pressure fluctuation 6
Brain, immature, pathological features 5-8
Brain-damaged children/syndromes 15, 97
  see also Minimal brain dysfunctions
Brainstem auditory evoked responses 151
British Columbia study 23 34
  births and deaths of LBW infants, British Columbia/Vancouver General Hospital 26 (table)
  births and infant deaths by weight groups (1958, 1966) 24 (tables)
  cohort 25-30
  findings 29-30
  flow-chart of children 33 (fig.)
  follow-up 30-4
    completeness 33-4, 91-3
    developmental testing 31
    educational achievement 31-2
    EEG 31
    eye examination 31
    home visit 31
    intelligence testing 31
    nursery assessment 30-1
    speech/hearing evaluation 31
  racial origin 28-9
  singletons 27 (table), 28 (table)
  social class 32-3
  statistics 24-5
  twins 28 (table)
British surveys 3, 23

C
Caine-Levine Social Competency Scale 217
Cat, deaf white 151
Cataracts, congenital bilateral 145
Catch-up growth 49
  SGA infants 35-6
Cerebral anoxia
  hearing loss due to 151, 159
  prevention 11
  psychological findings at 3 years 20-1
Cerebral palsy 13-14, 69 (table), 82-9
  age of ascertainment/assessment 14
  antecedents 85
  ataxia 69 (table)
  ataxic diplegia 13
  choreo-athetoid 7
  evolution 85-8
  incidence 82
    in Sweden 14, 82
  intellectual outcome 88
  neurological findings at 1 year 88
  perinatal characteristics 85, 239
  singletons 84
  social class 84-5
  spastic, increase in W. Australia 13
  spastic crural monoplegia 69 (table), 87-8
  spastic diplegia 7, 13, 69 (table), 82, 83-4
    evolution 85-6
    intelligence 88-9
  spastic hemiplegia 69, 84, 87
  spastic paraplegia 7
  spastic quadriplegia 69 (table), 86-7
  strabismus 133, 138
  twins 84
Child guidance clinic, proportion of children with brain damage 18
Clusters with respect of MBD
  analysis 115
  mean WISC Full-scale IQ 122 (table)
  percentage male 122 (table)
  percentage SGA 122 (table)
  qualitative features 120 (table)
  quantitative features 119 (table)
Coagulation mechanism defects 6
Cochlea
  deaf white cats 151
  perinatal anoxia damage 151
Cochlear nucleus, damage due to:
  anoxia 151
  jaundice 150
Collis test 86
  asymmetric 87
Communication skills 168-78
  discussion 176-7

method 169-71
analysis of data 171
assessment 169
procedure 170-1
speech/language at 4 years 169-70
results 171-6
boys' vs. girls' language scores 173-4
comparison of language scores 171-2
EEGs related to language scores 176
neurological status related to language scores 174, 175 (table)
Competence scales 217-18; *see also* Vineland Social Maturity Scale
Conceptional age 36
Congenital malformations, incidence 1, 7
Continuum of reproductive casualty 3-4, 14
Convulsions, febrile 89, 91

D

Deafness *see* Hearing loss
Developmental canalization 49
Developmental test scores 54-67
method 55
results 55-64
birthweight and test performance 56-9
discussion 64-7
LBW children *vs.* FBW controls 55-6
light/heavy babies in LBW group 59 (table)
longitudinal findings 63-4
psychometric tests, LBW children *vs.* FBW controls 57 (table)
sex differences 56
SGA preterm *vs.* SGA term infants 59
SGA *vs.* preterm AGA children 58, 60
socio-economic status 59-63
study sample 55
Dihydrostreptomycin 151, 161
Duane's retraction syndrome 91, 137
Dyslexia 114, 194-7, 200, 251
Dysphasia 69 (table), 171-6

E

Educational achievement 179-204, 263-6
discussion 200-3
method/material 180-2
information from teachers 181-2
school placement 182
socio-economic status 181
standardized achievement testing 181
results 182-203
birthweight categories 188-9, 190 (figs.)
classroom behaviour 197-200
comparisons within LBW sample 186
educational progress 182-6
neurological status 194, 195 (table), 196 (table), 199-200
reading disability 194-7
sex differences 187-8, 189 (figs.), 192-3
SGA *vs.* AGA preterm within social class 193-4
socio-economic status 190-3
Electroencephalograms 219-37
abnormal 219-26
discussion 232-6
material/method 221-3
minimal brain dysfunctions 101, 230-2, 236, 250
evolution 6¾-15 years 261-3, 269-70
neonates 219-21
results 222 (tables), 223-32
at about 1 year 224, 225 (table)
at about 6¾ years 224-6
correlation neonatal EEG/neurological status and IQ at 6¾ years 227
correlation neonatal EEG/subsequent EEG 226-7
correlation 1 year 228-9
correlation 1/6¾ years 228-9
correlation 1 year/neurological status and IQ 6¾ years 229-30
correlation 6¾ years/neurological status and IQ 230
'late neonatal' 222 (table), 224, 232
neonatal records 222 (table), 223-4
sensorineural hearing defect 232
SGA children 9
social class 232, 233 (table), 236
strabismus 134, 136 (table), 232, 233 (table), 236
Emmetropia, premature infants 139
Encephalopathy, anoxic-ischaemic, pathological features 5-6
Epilepsy 69 (table), 89-91
absence seizures (true petit mal) 91
febrile/non-febrile convulsions 89-90
idiopathic febrile convulsions 90-1
Erythroblastosis, hearing loss due to 150
Esotropia
accommodative 137
intermittent 137
variable, with hypertropia 137
Exotropia 135-7

F

Factor analysis 115

G

Growth 35-33; *see also* Physical growth

H

Haemolytic disease of newborn, hearing loss due to 150
Haggerty-Olson-Wickman behaviour ratings 208
Hand-preference 87
Head circumference 43-9, 51-2, 78-9
norms 42 (table)
small 79-80
Hearing loss 147-67
classification 153
conductive 153, 161-2

incidence 154 (table), 155
material/method 152-3
minimal high-frequency 162
results 152-7
sensorineural 7, 14, 69 (table), 147-8, 150 (fig.), 153
anoxia induced 151, 159
clinical conditions associated 155
discussion 157-9
due to: anoxia 151, 159
birth injury 152
haemorrhage into inner ear 149
jaundice 150, 152
ototoxic drugs 151-2
prematurity 152
EEGs 232
gamma correlation coefficients 155
hyperbilirubinaemia induced 150, 159
incidence 157
incubator time 159-61
neurological states 157, 161
prediction from selected variables 156
pure-tone air condition thresholds 154 (table)
High-risk newborns, transient neurological abnormalities 17
Hyaline membrane disease 6
Hydrocephalus, post-haemorrhagic 5, 7, 14, 78-9
Hyperactivity 16, 99-100, 110, 123
adult men 251
children at 12 years 267
function of psychiatric disturbance 19
situational/true 19
Hyperbilirubinaemia 7
hearing loss due to 150, 159
Hyperkinetic syndrome, doubtful existence 18
Hypermetropia
at birth 138
older children 139
Hyperviscosity syndrome 7
Hypotension 6
Hypothermia 6
Hypoxia 6

I
Incubator time/noise 159-61, 177
Infancy, predictor variables, neurological status at 6½ years 242, 243 (table)
Infant mortality (British Columbia), by birthweight 11 (table)
Inferior colliculi nuclei damage due to anoxia 150
Intelligence quotient, prediction at 6½ years 19-21, 247
Intensive care nurseries 11
Intracranial haemorrhage 5-6
CT scan 6
ultrasound 7
VLBW infant 7
Intra-uterine growth curves 5
Intra-uterine growth retardation 14
Intravenous fluid overload 6
Intraventricular haemorrhage 5
amount/severity of neurological impairment 21

J
Jaundice, deafness due to 150, 152, 155-9

K
Kanamycin 152, 161
Kernicterus 7
deafness due to 150
Knots 38

L
Labour, complications of 2
Leukomalacia 5, 84, 85
Light-for-dates child, compared with infant of short gestation 9
Low birthweight (LBW) infants
categories 4-9
correlation of developmental/intelligence test scores, various ages 64-5 (table)
diminished frequency 10
follow-up studies 2-4
hazards 6 (table)
high risk group 21
improved outlook for survivors 12
incidence 1
mental development 14, 54-67
morbidity 1, 11-13
mortality 1, 9-11
prediction and infant 'at risk' 19-22, 238-48
proportions with abnormalities at 6½ years (FBW controls) 118 (table)
risk of neurological/intellectual sequelae 20
school performance 19, 179-204
scoring systems 22

M
Maternal efficiency 66
Mental retardation 69 (table), 80-2, 94 (table)
lower social classes incidence 81
Minimal brain dysfunctions 15-18, 97, 126, 249-72
abnormal behavioural findings 100, 101
abnormal neurological signs 99-100
abnormal psychological findings 100, 110-11
adolescence 250, 269
adult life 269
aetiology of behavioural symptoms 18
age at diagnosis 68, 72, 249
antecedents 108
attention deficit disorder *see* Attention deficit disorder
behaviour syndrome 268
Bender Visual-Motor Gestalt Test 101, 103, 104 (table), 110

borderline low-normal intelligence children 111
brothers as controls 249
cerebral dysfunction, more than minimal 108-9, 111
characteristics 114
congenital stigmata 109
criteria 98-109
definition 16
depressive tendencies 250
discussion 109-11
EEG 101, 230-2, 236, 250, 261-3, 269
emotional relationships 268
evolution to 12-15 years 249-72
discussion 266-71
educational achievement 263-6, 270
EEGs 261-3
emotional relationships 257-60
material/method 251-3
motor proficiency testing 254-6
neurological abnormalities 253-4
psychological assessment 257
results 253-6
social relationships 257-61
Goodenough-Harris Draw-a-person Test 100, 103-5, 110, 252
history 97-8
hyperkinesis 18, 19
interaction of variables related to IQ 105
LBW infants 17-18, 108 (table), 271
long-term follow-up 269
medication 259, 268
neurological signs 267
neuropsychological examination 267
parents 250, 259
prognosis 251
psychiatric disorder 259, 268
psychological performances 267-8
psychotherapy 251
remedial education 251
school performance 19, 249-50
SGA infants, 9, 17
social relationships 257-61, 268
socio-economic status 101, 110
speech 100
statistical analysis 114-26
cluster analysis of LBW subgroups 116-22
comparison of LBW and control groups 115-16
description/coding of variables 125-6
discussion 122-3
subsyndromes 17, 120-3
teenage behaviour 250
teenage re-assessment 251
WISC Verbal-Performance IQ Scores 102-3
Monofixation syndrome 137
Moro response 74-6, 86, 238, 241, 244-6
Mother-child relationship, disturbance 2
Myopia of prematurity 131
Myopia
at birth 138-9
older children 139
premature infants 139

N
Neonatal mortality rates 10
Neurological correlations/predictions 238-48
discussion 245-7
material/method 239-40, 241 (tables), 243 (table)
results 240-4
boys' predictive variables 244-5
girls' predictive variables 242-4
Neurological sequelae 68-96
adverse prognostic indicators 239
autism 69 (table)
borderline low normal intelligence 69 (table)
cerebral palsy *see* Cerebral palsy
dysphasia 69 (table)
epilepsy *see* Epilepsy
infants at risk 239
mental retardation 69 (table), 80-2
minimal brain dysfunctions 69 (table); *see also* Minimal brain dysfunctions
postural response 73-8
asymmetrical tonic neck reflex 78
Moro response 74-6
parachute response 76-7
plantar response 77-8
sensorineural hearing defect 69 (table)
strabismus 88
survivors lost from study 91-2, 93 (table)
visual defects 69 (table)

O
Obstetric risk score 238
Ophthalmic disorders 127-46
corrected visual acuity at 6½-7 years 141 (table)
material/method 127-9
mean refractive values 141 (tables)
results 128-9
retinal vessel tortuosity 131
see also Refraction; Retinopathy of prematurity; Strabismus
Organic behaviour syndrome 15-16, 109
behavioural abnormalities akin to 17
see also Attention deficit disorder
Ototoxic drugs 151-2
Overactivity *see* Hyperactivity
Overperfusion, cerebral 6
Oxygen administration, monitoring 11

P
Palmar grasp 238
Parachute response 76-7
asymmetric 87
Photic response latencies, neonatal 238
Physical growth 35-53
catch-up-growth 49

developmental canalization 49
head circumference 43-4, 51-2
relationship to neurological/psychological outcome 45-9
length/height 41-2, 50-1
material/method of study 37-9
smaller ('runt') twin 35
weight 39-41, 49-50
Plantar responses 77-8, 86, 238
Pneumothorax 6
Polynomial curves 38
Postural responses 73-8
Prediction
neurological 238-47
IQ 247
school achievement 247-8
Prematurity, definition 1
Preterm AGA child 5
audiometric testing 152
Griffiths Scale results 8
growth 39-45
hearing loss 155
intelligence testing 9
learning difficulties 9
management 10-11
reading tests 9
Psychological test scores 54-67
discussion 64-7
method 55
results 55-64
birthweight and test performance 56-9
LBW children *vs.* FBW controls 55-6
light/heavy babies in LBW group 59 (table)
longitudinal findings 63-4
psychometric tests, LBW children *vs.* FBW controls 57 (table)
sex differences 56
SGA preterm *vs.* SGA term infants 59
SGA *vs.* preterm AGA children 58, 60
socio-economic status 59-63
study sample 55

Q
Quinine 152

R
Refraction 138-42
results 140-2
Respiratory distress syndrome 176-7
Retinal vessel tortuosity 131
Retinopathy of prematurity (retrolental fibroplasia) 5, 14, 129-32
discussion 142-3
frequency of minor forms 143-4
pathogenesis 130-1
prevention 144
results 131
Retrolental fibroplasia *see* Retinopathy of prematurity

S
School, maladjustment at 15, 258-9
School achievement prediction from measures in infancy/early childhood 248
Sensorineural hearing loss *see under* Hearing loss
Single parent 1
Sleep states, polygraphic recordings 238
Small for gestational age (SGA) infant 5, 35-53
at term 5
boys/girls 8
brain 7-8
catch-up growth 35-6
head circumference 8, 35, 42 (table), 43-5, 51-2
relationship to neurological/psychological outcome 45-9
intelligence tests results 8
length/height 41-3, 50-1
mental retardation 8
neurological sequelae 9
pathological conditions 7
school performance 8-9
seizures 8
skull growth *in utero* 36
stature 8, 35
weight 39-41, 49-50
Social class
EEG abnormalities 232, 233 (table), 236
GQ and IQ 62-3
mental retardation 81
Social growth 205-18
clinical abnormalities 213-14
EEG abnormalities 213
family group factors 211-12
intellectual characteristics 213
maternal factors 212-13
nursery history 213
physical characteristics 213
see also Vineland Social Maturity Scale; Vineland Social Quotient
Socio-economic status 1, 32, 181, 190-3
Sonogram 22
Strabismus 132-8
associated features 137-8
brain dysfunction associated 133-4
cerebral palsy associated 133
convergent 132
Crawford Dexterity Test 138
discussion 144
EEGs 134, 136 (table), 232, 233 (table), 236
FBW controls 137
incidence 132
LBW children 132-3
learning and 138
matched pairs, neurologically normal children 136 (table)
neurological status *vs.* visual acuity 136 (table)
results 134-5
school placement 137-8

types 135-7
vision 137
Streptomycin 151, 152, 161
Subependymal haemorrhage 6-7
Sucking reflex 238

T

Term, definition 5
Tonic neck reflex, asymmetrical 78

V

Ventriculomegaly 79
Very low birth weight (VLBW) infant
acidaemia, severe neonatal 21
Apgar score, prediction of cerebral palsy 21
blindness incidence 130
cerebral palsy incidence 14
hypothermia 21
improved outlook for survivors 12-13
intracranial haemorrhage 7
mental retardation 80
retinopathy of prematurity 14
Vestibular function 163-7
discussion 166-7
material/method 165
normal findings, audiological/vestibular tests 164 (table)
results 165-6
audiology 165-6
vestibular function 166
Vineland Social Maturity Scale 205-7
revision 218
Vineland Social Quotient 206-7
at 2½, 4 years 207
discussion 215-18
relation to IQ 208
sex differences at 2½, 4 years 208
SQ-IQ differences 210 (table)
SQ-IQ scores
at 2½, 4 years 210-11, 214 (fig.), 215 (fig.)
predictors of responses at 6½ years 214-15
singletons/twins 212
see also Social growth
Vitamin E 144